OXFORD MEDICAL PUBLICATIONS

Cancer incidence and mortality in England and Wales:
trends and risk factors

This book is to be returned on or be
the ⌐st⌐ ⌐ ⌐ ⌐ ⌐ ⌐ ⌐ow

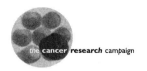

Cancer incidence and mortality in England and Wales: trends and risk factors

ANTHONY SWERDLOW, ISABEL DOS SANTOS SILVA, and RICHARD DOLL

Section of Epidemiology, Institute of Cancer Research,
Department of Epidemiology and Population Health,
London School of Hygiene and Tropical Medicine,
and Epidemiological Studies Unit, University of Oxford

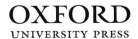

OXFORD
UNIVERSITY PRESS

Great Clarendon Street, Oxford OX2 6DP

Oxford New York

Oxford University Press is a department of the University of Oxford.
It futhers the University's objective of excellence in research, scholarship,
and education by publishing worldwide in
Oxford New York

Athens Auckland Bangkok Bogota Buenos Aires Calcutta
Cape Town Chennai Dar es Salaam Delhi Florence Hong Kong Istanbul
Karachi Kuala Lumpur Madrid Melbourne Mexico City Mumbai
Nairobi Paris São Paulo Singapore Taipei Tokyo Toronto Warsaw
and associated companies in
Berlin Ibadan

Oxford is a registered trade mark of Oxford University Press
in the UK and in certain other countries

Published in the United States
by Oxford University Press Inc., New York

A catalogue record for this title is available from the British Library
(Data available)

Library of Congress Cataloging in Publication Data

1 3 5 7 9 10 8 6 4 2

ISBN 0 19 262748 1

Typeset by
EXPO Holdings, Malaysia

Printed in Great Britain on acid free paper by
The Bath Press, Avon

Contents

Preface

The twentieth century saw improvements in health at least as great as those that had occurred in the previous century from the discovery of pathogenic micro-organisms and the provision of pure water supplies. The expectation of life at birth increased from 50 to 77 years and, most notably, from 11 to 17 years at 65 years of age, at which period of life it had previously changed very little. Pulmonary tuberculosis as a cause of death was reduced by 98%; chronic obstructive lung disease, which had been nicknamed 'the British disease', became uncommon under 50 years of age, and in recent decades even myocardial infarction and stroke began to become less common and, in the case of the former, less fatal. Cancer, however, has seemed to be an exception. There have recently been some remarkable discoveries about the changes in cells that cause cancer, but it will be some years before they can be expected to lead to practical methods for the control of the disease. Meanwhile the importance of cancer as a cause of death progressively increased until it became responsible for a quarter of all deaths in 1997 against less than ten percent at the start of the century, and for over half of all deaths in women between 45 and 55 years of age. The prevalence of people who have had the disease has also increased, as treatment has led to longer survival, and seems to have increased much more than it actually has, because it is talked about more openly and knowledge of its occurrence is no longer suppressed. It is not surprisingly, therefore, that many people believe that the risk of developing cancer has increased and are unable to understand how the claims for improved treatment can be justified.

The impression of rising risks is long-standing. A century ago, when the Registrar General (RG) analysed the data then available on cancer trends in England and Wales (RG, 1890), he concluded that 'in face of the constant and great growth of mortality under this heading [cancer], and the expressed belief of medical practitioners specially engaged in dealing with this class of diseases that they are really becoming more and more common, ... it must be admitted, as at any rate highly probable, that a real increase is taking place in the frequency of these malignant affections'.

The true trends, however, need careful consideration. There have in fact been major improvements in treatment in recent decades that have reduced the fatality of many types of cancer. The impression, despite this, of increasing frequency of cancer, has been due to several factors. Everyone dies sooner or later, and the large reductions in deaths from many major diseases, especially infections, have had the inevitable consequence that the proportion of overall deaths due to other diseases that have not decreased so much, such as cancer, has risen. This is accentuated for cancer, the risk of which increases rapidly with age, by the increased proportion of people living into old age. Also, for certain cancers, improved medical diagnostic techniques have led to better detection of cancer as a cause of death.

As for the recorded incidence of cancer, here too there have been apparent large changes over time, and again the actual trends are not always as they seem. Interpretation has been confused by improved medical services and new diagnostic methods that have allowed many cases to be diagnosed that would previously have not been recognised, while the screening of apparently healthy people has compounded the problem by detecting cases that, seen under the microscope have to be described as cancer, but which might never have caused symptoms and led to clinical diagnosis before the individual had died of some other cause. These changes alone must have accounted for much, if not all, of the recorded increases in incidence of several types of cancer. In addition there have been real changes in occurrence rates as the extent of exposure to factors that cause or prevent cancer has altered, most notably for lung cancer, which became very much more common in the first seven decades as a result of increased consumption of cigarettes, before beginning to decline.

In England and Wales, data about mortality from cancer have been collected nationally for over a century and there has been a national cancer registration scheme for several decades. In addition, data have been collected, in some instances for a hundred years or more, but in others only recently, on trends nationally in a wide range of risk factors for cancer. Many of these data, however, are not easy to find, or are not fully published. We have, therefore, brought together and analysed in this book information about trends in cancer in England and Wales and trends in factors that have been suspected of causing, or in some cases been shown to cause, one or more types of cancer, to enable readers to draw conclusions about the changes that have been occurring in rates of cancer incidence and mortality, and the reasons for these changes.

It is our hope that the publication of these data in a compact form will help the understanding of the changes in cancer rates, the progress that has been made in control, and of what now constitute the most urgent problems for research.

Acknowledgements

Preparation of this book would not have been possible without the patient and careful collection of cancer mortality data by the staff of the General Register Office and its successors for over 100 years, and of cancer incidence data over recent decades by the regional cancer registries of England and Wales, as well as the collation of these regional data by OPCS/ONS. We are grateful to the Cancer Research Campaign (CRC), who funded work on the book, to Professor J. G. McVie, Dr A. Galpine, and Ms J. Toms at the CRC for their encouragement, and to the Medical Research Council who funded the Epidemiological Monitoring Unit, within which the work was mainly undertaken.

We are most grateful to Dr T. Davies, Mrs M. Page, and Ms D. Stockton of the East Anglia Cancer Registry for their generous provision of unpublished cancer survival data. We also thank the following for data displayed in the book: Dr M. Catchpole for data on trends in sexually transmitted diseases; Dr C. Driscoll for data on solar ultraviolet radiation measurements by the National Radiological Protection Board; Dr B. Evans for data on trends in AIDS and cancer in AIDS patients; Dr J. Hodgson for data on trends in asbestos imports; Dr J. Stather for data on radioactive fallout; Dr C. Stiller for Childhood Cancer Research Group data on survival from childhood cancer; and the UK Transplant Support Service Authority for data on trends in organ transplantation. At ONS we thank in particular Dr P. Babb, Ms J. Jones, and Dr M. Quinn for providing cancer registration data and Mr C. Chantler for mortality data.

We are grateful for their advice to Professor E. Alberman, Sir A. Alment, Sir I. Chalmers, Professor D. Crawford, Dr T. Kenny, Professor D. C. Linch, Mrs K. Neel, Professor J. Pemberton, Professor J. M. Tanner, Dr A. Thomas, and Dr A. Webb.

We thank for permission to publish Figures reproduced in this book: Cambridge University Press, Central Statistics Office, *Journal of Infectious Diseases*, *Journal of Radiological Protection*, Kluwer Publishers, Medical Research Council, MRC Environmental Epidemiology Unit, ONS, and *The Lancet*.

The computing to produce the statistics in the Tables and to draw the Figures was conducted by Andrew Reid and Zongkai Qiao, and the many drafts of the text were typed by Evelyn Middleton. We thank them not only for their careful and dedicated work, but also for their patience with the numerous revisions we foisted upon them. We are grateful to Oxford University Press for their help in preparing the publication, and for their tolerance.

Abbreviations

AIDS	Acquired immunodeficiency syndrome
ALL	Acute lymphocytic leukaemia
BBR	Birmingham Births Register
CCRG	Childhood Cancer Research Group
CDSC	Communicable Disease Surveillance Centre
CI	Confidence interval
CLL	Chronic lymphoid leukaemia
CML	Chronic myeloid leukaemia
CT	Computed tomography
DZ	Dizygotic
EBV	Epstein-Barr virus
EMF	Electromagnetic (radiation) field
GB	Great Britain
GDP	Gross domestic product
GNP	Gross national product
HIV	Human immunodeficiency virus
HMSO	His/Her Majesty's Stationery Office
HPV	Human papilloma virus
HRT	Hormone replacement therapy (postmenopausal)
HSE	Health and Safety Executive
ICD (1, 2 etc.)	International Classification of Diseases (First, Second, etc. revisions)
MAFF	Ministry of Agriculture, Fisheries, and Food
MRI	Magnetic resonance imaging
NCDS	National Child Development Study
NFS	National Food Survey
NHL	Non-Hodgkin's lymphoma
NK	Not known
NOS	Not otherwise specified
NRPB	National Radiological Protection Board
NSAIDs	Non-steroidal anti-inflammatory drugs
NSHD	National Survey of Health and Development
OC	Oral contraceptive
ONS	Office for National Statistics
OPCS	Office of Population Censuses and Surveys
OSCC	Oxford Survey of Childhood Cancers
RG	Registrar General
SCIR	Standardized cohort incidence ratio
SCMR	Standardized cohort mortality ratio
T	Tesla
TURP	Transurethral resection of the prostate

UK	United Kingdom
UKTSSA	United Kingdom Transplant Support Service Authority
UVR	Ultraviolet radiation
WHO	World Health Organization

1 | *Introduction*

Science has nothing to offer more inviting in speculation than the laws of vitality, the variations of those laws in the two sexes at different ages, and the influence of civilization, occupation, locality, seasons, and other physical agencies, either in generating diseases and inducing death, or in improving the public health.

William Farr, Letter to the Registrar-General, 6th May 1839

Approximately 250 000 cancers occur each year in England and Wales, and cancer accounts for about 140 000 deaths. As the impact of other diseases, especially infections, has decreased over time, so cancer has come to constitute an increasing proportion of mortality. In 1911–15, neoplasms accounted for 8% of deaths in England and Wales; now they account for 25% (Figure 1.1).

In order to enable a balanced assessment of cancer trends over time, and the reasons for these trends, this book presents new analyses of trends in cancer incidence and mortality in England and Wales, concentrating particularly on the last few decades, but also for certain cancers extending as far back as data allow (to 1868 at the earliest). Also, in order to consider possible reasons for these trends, information is provided on trends in survival from cancer, artefactual influences on recorded rates, and trends in factors that may cause or prevent cancer.

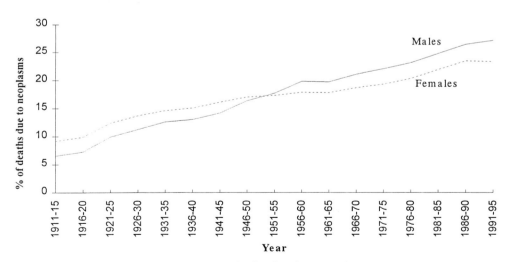

Figure 1.1   Percentage of all deaths due to neoplasms, England and Wales, 1911–95.

2 | *History*

Mortality statistics

The collection and publication of statistics on cause of death in England and Wales has a long history. Notification of deaths can be traced back to the London Bills of Mortality of 1532, which each week recorded burials in parishes of London and the probable causes of the deaths. Similar records were kept at the time in all the parishes of the Kingdom, although they were not always complete. The compilation and publication of information was an object-lesson in timeliness: 'When anyone dies, then, either by tolling or ringing of a bell, or by bespeaking of a grave of the sexton, the same is known to the searchers, corresponding with the said sexton. The searchers hereupon (who are ancient matrons sworn to their office) repair to the place where the dead corpse lies, and...examine by what disease or casualty the corpse died. Hereupon they make their report to the parish clerk, and he, every Tuesday night, carries in an accompt of all the burials...and on Thursday published and dispersed to the several families who will pay four shillings per annum for it' (Graunt 1662). Now, several hundred years later, we have high-powered computers, the data collection is not by ancient matrons, and of course the information is not published with such alacrity.

National statutory death registration in England and Wales was initiated on 1 July 1837, and since then the Registrar General has collected and published national mortality data. Initially these data included cancer only as an overall category with no subdivision by site, and they are not, therefore, of much value for epidemiology. The first site-specific cancer data were published for 1868 (Registrar General 1890) and 1888 (Registrar General 1890), with regular annual data starting from 1897 (Registrar General 1899) and age-specific data from 1901 (Registrar General 1903). The validity of diagnosis and certification in these early years, however, is uncertain.

Until 1958, mortality data for England and Wales were processed entirely clerically, without the use of computers. No materials now exist (other than the original death certificates) to enable analyses from those years disaggregated beyond the information contained in the published tables; these, for instance, only present numbers of cases by 5-year age group, and do not give data on mortality by year of birth. The individual death records for 1959 onwards, however, are held on computer, and therefore can be analysed in greater detail. For the present book we therefore concentrated primarily on data since 1960, for which we could conduct new analyses, although for certain cancers we also analysed trends in earlier years, recalculating rates from published data.

Cancer registration statistics

Cancer registration in England and Wales began under the aegis of the Radium Commission in the 1920s. A national system was started in 1945 (Stocks 1950), and since 1947 the data collected by local cancer registries have been collated by the General Register Office (subsequently incorporated into the Office of Population Censuses and Surveys (OPCS), and then the Office for National Statistics (ONS))[1]. The system is based on

---

[1] To avoid complex mentions of these three different institutions for different calendar periods, we have sometimes referred to them collectively, without discrimination of calendar period, as the 'Registrar General['s Office]'.

central collation of data collected by local cancer registries—in the 1950s there were 75 of these around the country, but with amalgamations the numbers have been reduced to 10. The scheme attained full national geographical coverage in 1962 and was reorganized in 1971 in a way that probably improved its completeness. Since 1971 there have been considerable artefactual changes in some regions and we have, therefore, not analysed incidence trends by region. The impact on the national data overall has, however, been small (Swerdlow *et al.* 1993), and since completeness is particularly important when examining trends we have therefore limited cancer registration analyses in this book to national data for the period from 1971 onwards.

Publications on trends

Traditionally, mortality data for England and Wales have been published by the Registrar General in single-year 'Annual Review Volumes'. These volumes consisted mainly of standard tables for the year under review, but there was also, in the volumes before 1968, a large 'Commentary', in which trend analyses were sometimes included. In addition, there have been *ad hoc* publications, both from the Registrar General's Office and from academic sources.

In the early twentieth century, consideration of cancer trends focused on whether the apparent large increases in mortality rates seen at that time were real or an artefact of better diagnosis and certification (Newsholme 1923). It was a point in favour of artefact in some analyses (Newsholme 1923; Greenwood 1935), but not others (Registrar General 1919), that the increases were far larger for cancers of inaccessible than of accessible sites. In the middle of the twentieth century, concern centred particularly on the rising mortality from lung cancer, the extent to which this rise was real or artefactual, and the possible reasons for its occurrence if real (Stocks 1953*a*). There was also, during this period, development of methods for analysis of cancer trends in relation to birth cohort (i.e. grouped year of birth), using information on death

rates by quinquennium of death and 5-year age group at death to estimate year of birth (Stocks 1953*a,b*; Case 1956*a*). Tables were compiled (Case 1956*b*; McKenzie *et al.* 1957) and analyses conducted (Case 1956*b*) of trends in cancer mortality for numerous sites since early in the twentieth century. These tables were subsequently updated (OPCS 1975*a*), and then data were presented with the range of cancer sites slightly increased for mortality from 1951–80 (Osmond *et al.* 1983).

Trends in cancer incidence in adults have not been considered systematically for England and Wales. Data have been published in single-year Annual Review Volumes, which contain a single table giving a limited comparison with data from the few years before the year of the volume.

Cancer trends in children have been analysed in a series of publications from the Childhood Cancer Research Group (Toms *et al.* 1981; Draper *et al.* 1982, 1994; Stiller *et al.* 1991; Draper 1995), mainly presenting mortality (1953–90) and incidence (1953–91) data for Great Britain overall, but with mortality data for leukaemia and all other neoplasms combined (1971–90) examined only for England and Wales (Draper 1995).

Certain publications on international trends in cancer have included data for England and Wales, although inevitably with relatively little detail—these have charted mortality to 1985 (Kurihara *et al.* 1989) or 1989 (La Vecchia *et al.* 1992; Levi *et al.* 1992; Coleman *et al.* 1993) and incidence to 1987 (Coleman *et al.* 1993). None of the above publications have considered trends in risk factors for cancer alongside the cancer trends themselves. Useful general consideration of trends internationally and explanations of these trends, but without systematic presentation of international or of British data, can be found in the volumes edited by Magnus (1982), Davis and Hoel (1990), and Doll *et al.* (1994).

There has been no such examination of geographical variation in cancer trends within England and Wales, except once by Stocks (1970) who examined mortality trends by region for breast and uterine cancers.

3 | *Materials and methods*

Mortality 1960–97

Data were extracted from national mortality files on all deaths in residents of England and Wales occurring in 1960–97 that were coded to a malignant neoplasm as the underlying cause of death[1]. In addition, we extracted data on deaths from brain and nervous system tumours that were coded as benign or of unspecified or uncertain behaviour. Cause of death data in the national files were coded to three different revisions of the International Classification of Diseases (ICD) over the study period, as shown in Table 3.1. To provide a uniform classification for analysis, we re-grouped ('bridge coded') the ICD Seventh Revision (ICD7), ICD8, and ICD9 data to give, as far as possible, constant diagnostic categories (WHO 1978) as detailed in Figures 6.1 to 6.35. Because the analyses were conducted from the original individual records, we were able to categorize deaths by year of death rather than by year of registration of death; the latter has been used in previously published statistics, for administrative convenience, but is not in principle the measure of interest. The difference between the two methods is small, but it is the reason why our results differ slightly from those in official volumes.

Table 3.1 Data years for which each ICD revision has been used by the Registrar General for cause coding of England and Wales mortality statistics.

ICD revision	Years of use	Reference for double coding of data to this revision and the previous one	Reference for equivalence between coding categories in this revision and the previous one
–[a]	1901–10		
2	1911–20		
3	1921–30		Registrar General 1923
4	1931–39		Registrar General 1932
5	1940–49	Registrar General 1944*a,b*; McKenzie *et al.* 1957	Registrar General 1944*b*
6	1950–57	Registrar General 1953	Registrar General 1953
7[b]	1958–67	Registrar General 1959	Registrar General 1959
8	1968–78	Registrar General 1971	Nectoux 1976
9	1979–present[c]	OPCS 1983*a*	OPCS 1983*a*; Percy 1987

[a] Un-numbered Registrar General's classification similar to ICD1.
[b] Plus fourth-digit codes devised by the Registrar General for cancer sites within certain three-digit ICD categories (upper aerodigestive tract, respiratory, and unknown primary cancers).
[c] Coding of mortality data to ICD9 will continue until 2000; coding to ICD10 is planned to begin in 2001. (For cancer registrations, coding to ICD 10 started in 1995).

---

[1] All of the mortality analyses presented in this book relate to the underlying cause rather than other mentioned causes of death; the latter have only been coded occasionally by the Registrar General's Office, and we have drawn on a published analysis of them (see p. 12) when commenting on potential reasons for certain trends.

We calculated age-standardized mortality rates for 1960–4, 1995–7, and the intermediate five-year periods, standardizing directly by single year of age to the census population of England and Wales in 1981. Rates were calculated for the age-bands 0–14, 15–34, 35–49, 50–69, and 70–84 as well as 0–84 and 15–84. We omitted data for ages 85 and above partly because information on cause of death at these ages may be seriously unreliable and partly because the rate at ages 85 years and above is substantially affected by demographic changes in the proportion living to extreme old age. For each age-band we calculated the rate in each time period as a percentage of the rate in 1960–4. These percentages rather than the actual rates are presented in most of the Figures because they facilitate the display of trends at different ages within the same graph. Age-bands with small numbers of cases and hence instability of rates have been omitted from the Figures, but the data can be found in the Tables in Appendix C.

As well as assessing rates over calendar time ('secular trends') we also analysed mortality rates during 1960–97 in relation to year of birth ('birth cohort trends'). For this analysis we used the data on year of birth of each case contained in the computer records of the individual deaths, and estimated populations at risk by year of birth and age[2], to calculate age-specific and birth year-specific death rates. From these death rates we calculated directly age-standardized cohort mortality ratios (SCMRs) by 5-year period of birth, plus, where of interest, by single year of birth. Standardization was by single year of age to the population of England and Wales in 1981. Exact 95% confidence intervals for the SCMRs were calculated, based on the Poisson distribution (Bailar and Ederer 1964). The SCMRs summarize the risk in each birth cohort, at the ages they had reached in the study period, relative to mortality at the same ages in the study population overall, with allowance for differences in population age structure between different cohorts. The use of actual year of birth to demarcate the birth cohorts avoids the imprecision in the traditional birth cohort analyses where quinquennium of birth is estimated from 5-year age-group and 5-year calendar period (Case 1956*a*).

The calculation of SCMRs enables a summary measure to be obtained across age groups, with the advantage over age-specific rates that larger numbers give more stable risk estimates. In principle, if a cohort interpretation of risk pertains, risks at different ages can be combined because each represents a different segment of the same generation-based risk. This will apply, however, only across the age range for which aetiology is homogeneous. Because the aetiology of cancer in children may differ from that in adults, we have not included childhood ages with adult ones in the cohort analyses. For similar reasons, we have generally not included young adult ages (under 35 years) in analyses for adults overall, although we have done so where there is reason to believe that aetiology in young adults is similar to that at older ages, for instance for cervical cancer. Thus for most cancers we have analysed SCMRs for ages 35–84, but for certain sites we decided on different age divisions to accord with epidemiological knowledge on likely age ranges within which there is aetiological homogeneity—for instance, dividing testicular cancer in adults into cases at ages 15–49 and 50–84 years, and Hodgkin's disease into cases in childhood (0–14), young adulthood (15–44), and older adult ages (45–84). The age ranges analysed for each cancer site are indicated when presenting data for that site.

In similar fashion to the secular analyses, for which we did not display in the Figures those age groups at which there were few cases and hence instability of rates, for the cohort analyses we did not display in the Figures birth cohorts in which there were few cases. Because the numbers of cases varied between the sexes, there is therefore sometimes a different range of cohorts displayed in the Figures for men and women, but fuller data can be found in the Tables in Appendix C.

We did not calculate SCMRs for cancer overall because there is great heterogeneity by age in the individual cancer sites that are most common, and hence a cohort analysis combining data across a broad age range would effectively be a comparison that emphasized different malignancies in different birth cohorts. For leukaemia, we did not analyse data by cohort except in children, because in adults there are several aetiological entities whose age distributions overlap considerably.

Unlike the analyses presented by secular period, for which the same age range of data was available for each period analysed, the cohort analyses had to contend with the difficulty that the data available for different cohorts were for different age intervals, because information for the entire life-span was not

---

[2] See 'Denominators', p. 7 for method of estimation.

available. Thus for early cohorts, cancers at young ages occurred before the time period for which we had data, and conversely recent cohorts had not yet reached older ages and hence data were only available for them when young. The method used to calculate SCMRs provides a statistically appropriate method to overcome this problem (Breslow and Day 1987). Interpretation must take into account, however, the fact that the SCMRs are calculated to a baseline (i.e. SCMR = 100) that applies only to the age range of the particular SCMR calculation, and hence is not precisely equivalent for different cohorts because the age range available for analysis differs between them. For practical purposes, the method should provide a good comparison between the risk in a particular cohort and that in cohorts born in nearby years, but a less satisfactory one when comparing cohorts born several decades apart. It should also be noted that the SCMRs will tend to be slightly conservative, because of the (inevitable) use of the overall data set, including data for the cohort under analysis, to provide the expected values[3].

As well as analysing cancer mortality trends for England and Wales overall, we also used the individual records to assess secular trends by region of residence. For this, we calculated directly age-standardized mortality rates[4] for ages under 85 years in each health board region in 1960–4 and 1990–4 (the data after 1994 are not coded to the same regions), and then calculated the percentage change from the former to the latter period. The geographical locations of the regions are mapped in Swerdlow and dos Santos Silva (1993). There were boundary changes to certain of the regions in 1974, shown in the map just cited, but these were not large and were unlikely to have affected trends appreciably. (The rates calculated for each period were based on contemporary regional numerators and denominators.)

Mortality 1911–60

For selected cancer sites we extended the secular analyses back to 1911 by use of published material. Data for

these years were only available in the degree of detail for which aggregated statistics have been published (for instance in 5-year age groups), not as individual records. We therefore age-standardized the rates by 5-year age group to the England and Wales population of 1981, and examined these data for 5-year periods from 1911 to 1960[5] alongside the newly calculated data from the computer files for 1961 onwards. The 'bridge coding' used for different ICD revisions is shown in Figures 6.1 to 6.35.

Mortality 1868–1910

Data on deaths from certain cancers at ages 35 years and above in 1868 and 1888 were published by the Registrar General in 1890. The rates published were crude, not age-standardized, and no age-specific data were given. Age-specific cancer mortality rates for the period 1901–10 (but not for all of the individual calendar years within this) were published by the Registrar General (1912). To analyse trends in mortality since 1868 for selected cancers, allowing for changes in age distribution as far as possible, we used the crude rates for 1868 and 1888, and we age-standardized the rates in 1901–97 at ages 35 years and above to the age distribution of the population of England and Wales in 1871. The cause coding categories used for the data before 1911 are shown in the appropriate Figures in Chapter 6.

Incidence 1971–92

We obtained from the national cancer registration files at the Office for National Statistics, data on cancers incident[6] in 1971–92 in residents of England and Wales. We included for analysis all malignant neoplasms except non-melanoma skin cancers, for which the data are seriously incomplete (Lloyd Roberts 1990; Ko *et al.* 1994). In addition, we extracted data on nervous system tumours coded as benign or of unspecified or uncertain behaviour. Cancer sites were coded in the files to the ICD, with the same dates of use of consecutive revisions as in the mortality data (Table 3.1). We conducted bridge coding between ICD revisions as for the mortality analyses (see Figures 6.1 to 6.35). Age-standardized incidence rates were calculated for 1971–4, 1990–2, and the 5-year periods in between. Rates in each period were then calculated as a percentage of the 1971–4 rate, and standardized cohort incidence ratios (SCIRs) calculated, again following the methods for the mortality analyses. For certain sites where the age distribution of incidence is of particular interest, we also produced Figures of rates by 5-year age group or single year of age.

Although cancer registration data for England and Wales are available before (and after) the period 1971–92, we restricted the analyses to these years because of the need for comparability of completeness of registration if trends are to be examined. National registration data are available since 1962, but a re-organization of data collection in 1971 appreciably improved completeness, and therefore we did not analyse data from years before this. Similarly, data have continued to be collected after 1992, but substantial numbers of registrations for these more recent years had yet to reach the national registration files when we undertook the analyses, so these years were also omitted.

Cancer in people with AIDS

There is no national registration system that records and identifies as such all cancers occurring in AIDS patients, but data are collected by the Communicable Disease Surveillance Centre (CDSC) on initial AIDS-defining illnesses. Because Kaposi's sarcoma tends to occur early in the course of AIDS, the data on this tumour as an AIDS-defining illness give a reasonable proxy for all AIDS-associated cases. Incidence data by sex and 5-year age group from the CDSC were used to calculate incidence rates for this tumour. The main other malignancy associated with AIDS is lymphoma, which tends to occur late in the course of the disease.

Data from the CDSC on lymphoma cases as the initial AIDS-defining illness are presented, but need cautious interpretation as a proxy for all cases because they omit lymphomas occurring later.

Since 1993, ONS have allocated a separate cause code to deaths for which the underlying cause was coded to HIV and in which a cancer was also mentioned on the death certificate. The coding employed does not enable the cancer site to be identified, however, and as only one-third of AIDS deaths are categorized as such by ONS, the data for AIDS-related cancer deaths are likely to be substantial under-estimates. We have therefore not presented trend data using this coding.

Cancer in people who have received organ transplants

The UK Transplant Support Service Authority receives notification from all transplant centres in the UK on cancers causing death in transplant patients. The data are believed to be virtually complete since 1984, and therefore data for 1984 onwards were analysed.

Denominators

The denominators used to calculate national and regional cancer rates by calendar year in this book come from decennial censuses and inter-censal population estimates prepared by the Registrar General's Office, except that because population estimates for 1997 were not yet available, we used the 1996 estimates for that year.

Population data are not available by year of birth, so to gain denominators for calculation of cancer rates by birth cohort, we estimated these from population estimates by single calendar year and single year of age. For each age versus calendar year combination, two adjacent years of birth were possible, and we partitioned the population between these two years in proportion to the numbers of births in the years.

4 | *Issues to consider in interpretation of trends*

Numerous factors complicate the interpretation of apparently straightforward trends in the recorded cancer rates described in this volume. These factors are described in general terms here, but their impact differs greatly between different cancer sites and they are therefore also highlighted as appropriate when discussing particular cancers.

Mortality data

Use of medical care, medical diagnostic ability, and diagnostic labelling

The extent to which cancers, when they occur, are detected and diagnosed, can be altered by changes in the propensity of patients to present for diagnosis, the availability and competence of medical services, the ability of doctors to make diagnoses (including their diagnostic effort and aptitude, and the impact of technological advances), and the extent of screening. Improved diagnosis may either increase the number of cancers identified, or decrease them by correcting previously erroneous diagnoses of cancer. Errors in diagnosis that may be diminished by better diagnostic methods can also be made between cancers of different sites, for instance of the lung and pleura. Metastases to sites such as the lung, liver, bone, and brain may be mistaken for primary cancers of these sites, and improved diagnosis may identify the primary site of these cancers or of cancers that would previously have been diagnosed as 'primary site unknown'. Thus a specific cancer may appear to become more common over time because it has become more readily diagnosed, or conversely the frequency of a non-specific

diagnostic category such as 'cancer, primary site not known' may diminish if better diagnosis removes cancers to more-specific categories.

Changes in the diagnostic labels given to different diseases (for instance, in the categorization of lesions on the borderline between benign and malignant neoplasia), can also affect apparent trends in cancer.

These issues affect different cancer sites in different ways. For instance, diagnostic artefacts are less likely to be pertinent to trends in easily diagnosed sites such as the testis, breast, or oesophagus than to trends of cancers of deep internal organs such as the pancreas, or cancers whose diagnosis needs complex diagnostic technology, such as myeloma and brain cancer. Changes in categorization or diagnosis of borderline lesions will particularly have affected trends in tumours of sites where borderline lesions are common and/or often undiagnosed, such as the prostate and bladder. These potential artefacts are therefore discussed as relevant when considering specific cancers in this book.

For most of the diagnostic factors discussed above, data to judge the extent of change over time are not available, but for one relevant source of diagnostic information, autopsy, the Registrar General has long published statistics. Autopsy can substantially increase the number of cancers diagnosed at certain sites, such as the lung, ovary, and kidney (Heasman and Lipworth 1966), while diminishing the numbers of cancers of unknown primary site. Figure 4.1 shows time trends in the proportion of deaths in England and Wales certified after autopsy since 1928, when such data were first compiled. The overall prevalence of post-mortems increased until the early 1980s and then decreased a little. Within this overall trend, however, there were differing trends for two types of post-mortem[1] that

---

[1] For the shorter period for which data by type of post-mortem are available.

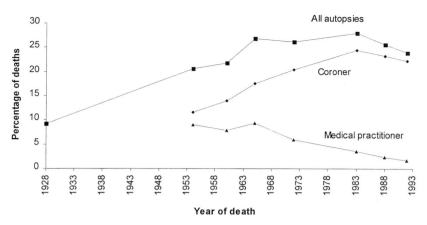

Figure 4.1 Percentage of deaths in England and Wales for which autopsy stated on death certificate, 1928–92, by type of certifier (data by type of certifier not available for 1928).

have different consequences for cancer statistics. Coroners' post-mortems, which are undertaken when the cause of death might have been criminal or otherwise of public interest, have increased considerably, but cancer is infrequently the final diagnosis of these examinations (in about 5% of instances). Post-mortems for medical reasons, which much more often reveal cancer (in about a quarter of cases), have declined greatly.

Efficacy of treatment, and survival

Trends in cancer mortality depend not just on trends in the incidence and diagnosis of new cases, but also on the efficacy of treatment, the risk of intercurrent disease (such as myocardial infarction) if survival is prolonged, and if the cancer is fatal on whether the certifier enters the cancer as the underlying cause of death. For many of the common cancers, these factors do not seriously affect interpretation of trends because survival has been poor. In these circumstances the artefacts in cancer registration data, described later, are likely to be greater than those in mortality data, and therefore the latter are likely to give a better indication of trends in underlying incidence. For certain cancers where treatment and consequently survival has greatly improved, such as Hodgkin's disease and testicular cancer, greater emphasis needs to be given to registra-

tion data when assessing trends in incidence, and indeed the mortality data have ceased to be of value for this purpose, and have become of more use as a way to describe at a population level the consequences of the success of treatment.

In order to help the consideration of comparative trends in incidence and mortality, Figures A1–A26 show trends in 5-year survival for patients with cancers incident from 1971 to 1992. Because reliable national survival data are not available throughout this period[2], the data presented are for East Anglia, the only region in the country for which the cancer registry has continued active follow-up of cancer patients until the present. It should be noted, however, that the survival data, like those for incidence and mortality, may be subject to artefact. In particular, one of the main artefacts in registration data applies to survival too: if changes in detection or categorization of neoplasms lead to the registration of more lesions of low malignancy, then apparent survival will improve for this reason alone. Also, if cancers are diagnosed earlier in their natural history, for instance because of improved diagnostic procedures or screening, this will cause 5-year survival to appear better, artefactually, because the date from which survival is measured has been moved earlier. Therefore increases in recorded survival cannot in themselves necessarily be taken to indicate

---

[2] Except for children, see below.

that a divergence between recorded incidence and mortality trends is real and a consequence of more successful treatment.

National cancer survival data for England and Wales have been subject to considerable inaccuracy, primarily because of incomplete follow-up (which since 1971 has been conducted passively by linkage to records of the National Health Service Central Register). A particular recent effort has been made, however, to improve the quality of data for survival of cases incident in 1981 and 1989 (ONS 1998a). These data are presented[3] in the Figures alongside those for East Anglia. It should be noted, however, that the data are still of appreciably lower quality than those for East Anglia. For instance, 8.7% of national registrations in 1981 and 9.7% in 1989 had to be excluded from analysis because the date of death was equal to the recorded date of incidence[4], compared with 3.1% in East Anglia. The national data also excluded patients not traceable at the National Health Service Central Register (about 3.5% in 1981 and almost 3% in 1989)[5], as well as the 10% or so of incident cancers not registered in the National Cancer Registry (see p. 13), compared with perhaps 4% or less incompleteness for East Anglia (Swerdlow et al, 1993). Thus in total, it appears that about 22% of incident cancers were omitted from the national analysis compared with about 7% from the East Anglia analysis. The extent of loss to follow-up in the national data set is not published, but again is likely to be above the low figure of 0.6% in East Anglia. Furthermore, site-specific survival analyses must exclude cancers of unknown primary site, and because these tend to have much worse survival than cancers of known site overall, apparent survival at known sites will be artefactually improved by this exclusion; again this will have had a greater effect for the England and Wales data, in which by 1985–9 6%[6] of cases were of unspecified primary site, than in East Anglia, where the corresponding percentage over the study period was 0.4 to 0.5%[7]. The East Anglia data, however, only derive from a small proportion of the country, so that one cannot be certain that they are entirely representative of the whole (although the direction of trends is likely to be), and for less common sites the confidence intervals around the survival rates are wide.

Although the above data are the most reliable that we could obtain for survival of cancer patients overall in England and Wales, for childhood cancer highly complete incidence and survival data have been collected by the Childhood Cancer Research Group (Draper et al. 1982; Stiller and Bunch 1990; Stiller 1994). We used published CCRG results and unpublished data kindly supplied by the CCRG to graph 5-year survival for cases incident in Great Britain 1962–91. The results are presented in Figures B1–B8.

Death certification and enquiries to improve precision of certification

Death certification data for England and Wales are believed to be virtually complete for the fact of death, at least since 1927 when an Act of Parliament came into force making it unlawful to dispose of the body of a dead person before a registrar's certificate or coroner's order had been issued. Completeness of registration does not of itself ensure that the cause of death is always competently certified, although the proportion of deaths not certified by a qualified person has been low and falling. In the late nineteenth and early twentieth centuries, a few per cent of deaths were registered without certification by a medical practitioner or coroner (2.7% in 1891 (Registrar General 1892), 1.8% in 1901 (Registrar General 1903)), but by 1928 this had decreased to under 1% (Registrar General 1930).

The certifier enters information about the death onto a death certificate, the format of which follows WHO requirements. Thus cancer trends will be affected by the extent to which diagnosed fatal cancers are entered correctly onto death certificates. The form of the death certificate was changed in July 1927, but probably with no substantial effect on cancer statistics (Stocks 1953a). It was changed again for neonates in 1986, such that no underlying cause of death could any longer be classified for this age-group; the effect on cancer statistics will have been negligible, how-

---

[3] Survival rates, but not confidence intervals, which were not published.
[4] Presumptively these cases were registered solely from death certificates and hence their actual date of incidence was not known.
[5] There were no such cases for East Anglia, where follow-up did not depend on the NHS Central Register.
[6] Percentage of cancers other than non-melanoma skin cancer, at ages 0–84.
[7] Percentage of cancers other than non-melanoma skin cancer, at ages 0–84.

ever, since very few cancers occur at such a young age. Completed death certificates are sent to the Registrar General's Office, where coding is undertaken.

When the information about cause of death entered on the death certificate is insufficiently precise, the Registrar General may send a 'medical enquiry' to the certifier requesting clarification. These enquiries, which started in the nineteenth century and continued until the end of 1992, have tended to increase the number of deaths coded to cancer overall, and within this to increase apparent mortality from certain well-specified cancer categories (notably in the present analyses, cancers of the pleura, corpus uteri, eye, and brain) and to decrease it for less well specified categories (especially cancer of the uterus of unspecified subsite, and cancer of unspecified primary site). As a consequence, changes over time in the age groups or diagnostic categories for which enquiries have been made can artefactually affect apparent mortality trends. Notably this occurred when enquiries were temporarily discontinued in 1967 and 1981–2, and for certain cancers in 1974, and when they ceased permanently for ages 75 and above in 1984, and for all other ages in 1993. Further details on these enquiries and other similar enquiries by the Registrar General after post-mortems, and on

their effects, can be found in Swerdlow (1989); important site-specific effects are discussed under the relevant cancer sites, below, and shown in Table 4.1.

A general indication of the degree of precision of specification of cause of death in mortality statistics can be gained from examination of the proportion of deaths coded to vague categories such as 'debility' or 'old age'. The percentage coded to symptoms, signs, and ill-defined conditions decreased from 2.0% in 1950 to 0.4% in 1980, but then increased to 0.9% in 1990 and 1.9% in 1996. Although these figures are small in themselves, they may be representative of trends in imprecision affecting far more deaths certified to poorly specified categories, which overall could substantially affect apparent cancer mortality, at least at older ages (Grulich *et al.* 1995).

Coding of cause of death and selection of underlying cause

Since 1911, mortality data for England and Wales have been coded to the International Classification of Diseases (ICD), and hence mortality statistics have been affected each time a new revision of the ICD has been adopted. Table 3.1 shows the dates of use of each

Table 4.1 Percentage effects of certain artefacts on secular trends in recorded cancer mortality in England and Wales, selected cancer sites.

Cancer site	Year and nature of artefact		
	1940. Introduction of ICD5[a]	1984. Altered interpretation of ICD coding rule 3[a]	1993. Reversion to pre-1984 interpretation of rule 3, plus cessation of medical enquiries[b]
Stomach	−1.9	+2.3	−3.1
Colon and rectum	—	+3.7	−6.6
Lung[c]	−1.5	+1.0	−2.3
Pleura	—	0	−23.3
Melanoma of skin[d]	−10.4	+1.7	+3.9
Breast, female	−6.0	+3.9	−4.2
Prostate	−3.8	+6.3	−6.4
Eye	—	+1.3	−23.6
Brain	—	+2.3	−8.7
Non-Hodgkin's lymphoma	—	+3.9	—
Myeloma	—	+6.0	—
Leukaemia	−3.0	+4.0	−4.0
Site unspecified	—	+2.7	+7.5
All neoplasms[e]	−2.9	+2.8	−2.9

[a] From data double-coded to successive coding systems (Registrar General 1944*b*; OPCS 1985).
[b] Implied from effects of medical enquiries, 1992 (OPCS 1995) plus effect of rule 3 change in 1984 (OPCS 1985).
[c] Lung plus pleura in 1940.
[d] All skin in 1940.
[e] All malignancies in 1940.
— Data not available.

ICD revision in England and Wales. The effect of changes in ICD revision on the numbers of deaths in England and Wales coded to particular cancer sites are indicated by the results of exercises in which the Registrar General has double-coded single years of data to successive revisions, for the changes from ICD4 to 5 onwards; references are given in Table 3.1. References are also given there to publications detailing the equivalence between codes for specific cancers in successive ICD revisions.

From the viewpoint of cancer statistics, the change from ICD4 to 5 in 1940 was particularly important because the method of ascription of underlying cause of death when more than one cause was mentioned on the death certificate was changed. Previously, arbitrary rules of precedence were applied; each type of disease was given a ranking, and the highest ranking disease on the certificate was selected as the underlying cause, ignoring the order in which the certifier had entered the causes on the certificate. Cancer was given a high precedence among diseases in this system. From ICD5 onwards, the certifier's preference, as expressed in the order of causes on the certificate, was taken into account. The effects of this change are shown in Table 4.1.

Certain other changes have been made to mortality coding for England and Wales independent of the adoption of new ICD revisions. Of particular consequence was a change in 1984 in the OPCS application of ICD coding rule 3, which governs the circumstances in which a cause that is stated by the certifier as only contributory to death should nevertheless be selected as the underlying cause of death for mortality statistics. From that year, when certain vague conditions such as bronchopneumonia were specified as an apparently underlying cause on a death certificate, they were discounted by OPCS mortality coders in favour of more likely underlying causes such as cancer, when these were specified on the same certificate, even if this required disregarding the order in which the causes had been specified by the certifier. Bridge coding for this change is given in OPCS (1985), and further discussion is given in Grulich *et al.* (1995). The effects for major cancer sites are shown in Table 4.1. Also of importance was that in 1993 coding of causes of death and selection of underlying cause of death were altered from a clerical to a computerized operation. The computerized coding, based on software developed by the US National Center for Health Statistics, reversed the 1984 change in interpretation of ICD rule 3 referred to above, reverting to the previous selection procedure. With the introduction of computerized coding, OPCS also ceased to send 'medical enquiries' to certifiers when the original information on a death certificate was unclear or was not final (see above). No double-coding exercise was undertaken to ascertain the effects of these two changes in 1993, but it can be implied that they were approximately the opposite of those described above for the introduction of the rule 3 change in 1984 and the effect of medical enquiries in 1992 (Table 4.1).

Order of causes on the death certificate

Changes by certifying doctors in the ordering of the causes stated on death certificates can affect apparent mortality rates because selection of the underlying cause of death has, since 1940, taken account of the order in which the certifier has entered onto the death certificate the conditions he/she believes to be causally related to the death. Comparison of data for 1976 and 1986 suggests that changes in the position of recording of cancer on death certificates have tended to raise apparent cancer rates by a few per cent in recent years, with greater effects at older than younger ages, and with substantial effects for breast cancer, prostatic cancer, and leukaemia at older ages (Grulich *et al.* 1995).

Cancer registration data

The diagnostic and coding artefacts discussed above with regard to mortality data apply also to cancer registrations, although sometimes with different force. In particular, changes in diagnostic completeness will have much more impact on incidence data than on mortality data and changes in the categorization of borderline malignant tumours will have affected only incidence data as such tumours are very unlikely to cause death. This is one of the reasons why, if effectiveness of treatment has not altered substantially, mortality trends may be easier to interpret than registration trends. A particular source of identification of borderline lesions that might not otherwise have been detected can be the introduction of a screening programme.

In addition to these artefacts, there are others specific to cancer registrations, which will be discussed in this section. The England and Wales cancer registration scheme is based on national aggregation of data collected by independent regional cancer registries. Cancer registration is voluntary. The number of registries, their data sources, and their individual geographical coverages have altered over the years. Data quality has varied between the registries as well as within the registries over time, but there is limited information from which to assess quality in the national system. An outline is given below. Further discussion of the registries, their data sources, and quality can be found in Swerdlow (1986) and OPCS (1990*a*). Information on individual registries can be found in their own reports and occasional publications on data quality (West 1976; Nwene and Smith, 1982; Benn *et al.* 1982; Gulliford *et al.* 1993; Lancaster *et al.* 1994; Seddon and Williams 1997) and, for most, in their entries in *Cancer Incidence in Five Continents* (Parkin *et al.* 1997).

Completeness and accuracy

The possibility that trends in recorded incidence may reflect changed completeness of registration rather than true changes in occurrence is the main disadvantage of cancer registration compared with mortality data. Although the completeness of cancer registration data for England and Wales has not been examined comprehensively, available indications suggest that it may have been about 90% or better[8] through the period 1971–84 (Villard-Mackintosh *et al.* 1988; Hawkins and Swerdlow 1992; Swerdlow *et al.* 1993) and did not change greatly during those years (Swerdlow *et al.* 1993). A change in 1985 that may have had an appreciable impact on national trends was the amalgamation of the North East and North West Thames registries with the registry for South Thames. The North Thames registries had long been substantially incomplete, and the amalgamation probably increased completeness appreciably for cancers in their 7 million catchment population.

There are no data on trends in accuracy of cancer registration data for England and Wales, although it

Table 4.2　Data quality of cancer registrations: percentage of registrations with histological verification, selected regional registries in England and Wales, around 1970, 1980, and 1990[a]

Registry		% histologically verified All cancers[b]			Testicular cancer		
		1970	1980	1990	1970	1980	1990
Birmingham and	Male	62	68	—	97	97	—
West Midlands	Female	74	76	—			
Mersey	Male	47	43	70	78	66	96
	Female	57	49	71			
North Western	Male	—	60	64	—	94	95
	Female	—	68	67			
Oxford	Male	69	76	74	98	99	98
	Female	78	80	77			
South Thames	Male	67	80	63	97	98	86
	Female	74	83	64			
South Western	Male	65	68	75	95	93	95
	Female	75	71	74			
Trent	Male	55	62	—	95	88	—
	Female	67	67	—			

[a] Periods of data reported in *Cancer Incidence in Five Continents* vols III (Waterhouse *et al.* 1976), V (Muir *et al.* 1987), and VII (Parkin *et al.* 1997): generally 1968–72, 1978–82 and 1988–92, but with slight variations.
[b] All malignancies except non-melanoma skin cancer.
— Data not available.

[8] Completeness when 5 years had elapsed after the year of incidence. It takes this long for all data to be collected and reach the national register—see 'Late registrations', below.

may to some extent have parallelled the completeness of the recording system. The proportion of tumours for which histological verification is available gives some indication of likely diagnostic accuracy. Such information is not available nationally, but is available for certain regional registries, and is shown in Table 4.2. The Table presents data for cancer overall, and also for a tumour site, the testis, for which one would expect histological verification to be obtained in almost all cases. It can be seen that there has been considerable variation between registries in the degree of completeness of histological verification, and also surprisingly large variations within certain registries over time, but there is no overall indication that the national data set is likely to have become appreciably more, or less, complete over the years analysed in this book.

Duplication, and registration of multiple primary cancers

Cancer registration data, unlike those for mortality, can be substantially erroneous through duplicate registrations of a cancer—for instance, because it is reported to a regional registry from more than one clinical source, or it is reported to the national registry from more than one regional registry. In 1978, in order to reduce unintended duplication of registrations (although it is not known to what extent it was successful in this), the system changed from registration based on region of treatment (or diagnosis) to registration by region of residence[9]. There are no data on the extent of duplication in the national register for England and Wales. A recent systematic exercise has been undertaken by the national registry to identify potential duplicates since 1971 and return them to regional registries for checking. This exercise should not have erased registrations of genuine bilateral cancers or multiple primary cancers, but is believed to have reduced duplicate registrations in the data used in this book to well under 1% of the total (M. Quinn, personal communication).

Apparent cancer incidence rates from registration data can also vary over time because of changes in rules or methods for registration of multiple primary cancers occurring in the same person; again a problem not encountered for mortality data. The data in the England and Wales files analysed in this book are based on registrations of incident cancers, without differentiation of first and subsequent cancers occurring in the same person. Thus if more than one primary cancer is found to have occurred in a person, each is counted as a separate registration. Ambiguity and scope for artefact in registration trends can occur if the rules and methods for distinguishing between duplicate registrations and multiple primary cancers alter over time; this can occur particularly for tumours of different histology occurring at the same anatomical site, and for tumours occurring in opposite paired organs (e.g. breasts, testes, ovaries). According to OPCS (1983*b*) a change in 1978 to OPCS rules for decision between duplicates and multiple primary cancers led to a 13% decrease in registrations for Wales and a 1% decrease for England and Wales overall. A further change to the rules occurred for registrations processed from mid-March 1982 onwards (Swerdlow 1986), whereby contralateral primaries in paired organs such as the breast, testis, and ovary were to be counted as one registration rather than two, as previously. If this change was fully implemented, it would presumably have appreciably reduced apparent rates for breast and testicular cancers, at least—about 5% of breast cancers and of testicular cancers are bilateral. Examination of rates of these tumours in the single calendar years around 1982 (not shown), however, leaves it uncertain whether there was an artefactual decrease: there were lower rates in 1982 and 1983 (but not 1984–5) than in 1981 for testicular cancer, for which year to year fluctuations in rates are anyway appreciable, but there was no clear decrease in 1982–3 for breast cancer.

Late registrations

It takes several years for all registrations relating to a particular year of incidence of cancers to be collected by the regional cancer registries and transmitted to the national register. Almost all (about 99%) of the eventual registrations have reached the national register by 5 years after the incidence year (Hawkins and Swerdlow 1992), so the trends presented here should not be materially incomplete through late registrations—indeed this was the reason why 1992 is the last year of incidence to

---

[9] This may also have altered completeness for patients crossing regional boundaries for treatment.

have been included in this book. It is a consequence, however, that the numbers of cases presented often differ from the numbers in published annual data from OPCS/ONS, which omit late registrations (and late cancellations and alterations) to the data files after the publication.

Comparison of mortality and incidence trends

As well as the issues discussed above, it should be noted when comparing the mortality and incidence trends in the Figures that as the mortality data are presented for a longer period than those for incidence, if rates of change in each are equal, the total percentage change over the period studied will be larger for mortality than incidence. Also, because the deaths will generally be of persons in whom cancer was incident several years earlier (the mean duration varying by cancer site), the mortality trends comparable with those for incidence will be some years later.

Consideration of trends at young and older ages

In general, cancer trend data are easier to interpret at young than at older ages. Diagnostic artefacts are particularly likely to affect cancer trends at older ages, both because there have probably been changes over time in the extent to which intensive diagnostic investigation is pursued for ill elderly people, and because multiple pathology is more common in the elderly. Trends at younger ages, say under 65, are therefore more likely to be reliable, especially for cancer sites that are difficult to diagnose or need complex technologies for their diagnosis.

Trends at young adult ages are also of importance for a second reason: they represent the likely future. For most common cancers, all-age rates are dominated by cancers at older ages, so that current rates depend mainly on cancers in persons born 60 or 70 years ago, and likewise rates in 20 or 30 years' time will mainly reflect cancers incident in the generations who are now young and middle-aged adults. The future rates of cancer in these recent generations are, for most cancer sites, likely to be well-predicted by their current rates as young adults, because incidence of these cancers relates to exposures decades earlier and/or to patterns of behaviour (e.g.

smoking) established at young ages. On the other hand, current rates of cancer at older ages are important too, although for a different reason—because of their current public health and health care implications.

Age and sex composition of the population

Cancer rates vary greatly by age and between the sexes. Comparison of cancer rates at different times, when the age and sex distributions of the population have differed, will therefore be influenced by these demographic changes, unless allowance is made for them. This potential artefact is overcome in the present analyses by considering all rates separately for each sex and adjusted for age. Age adjustment, however, provides a summary measure across different ages at the potential expense of missing differences in effect between them. Therefore the secular data have mainly been considered for broad age groups (age-adjusted within these age groups), with less emphasis generally given to the results for all ages combined. The cohort analyses, too, were conducted for broad age groups (age-adjusted within these groups) chosen on aetiological grounds as described on p. 5.

Accuracy of denominators

Inaccuracies in denominators are likely to have been of negligible importance to analyses of national cancer rates in recent decades, because both censal and intercensal population estimates have been highly accurate. For instance, it is estimated that the 1981 census undercounted the population overall by 0.5%, with the greatest age-specific error for children under 5 years of age, for whom there is estimated to have been a 1.2% undercount (OPCS 1984). For intercensal estimates too, accuracy has been high: the estimate of the 1981 population based on the 1971 census was only 0.2% less than the actual count from the 1981 census (OPCS 1982), with the greatest age-specific difference an underestimate of 1.2% at ages 45–64 years. Similarly, differences in definitions between the census and cancer data—for instance with regard to inclusion of overseas visitors and Britons temporarily abroad—have only been of slight importance for national rates (Swerdlow 1986).

It should be noted that unlike in several previous publications, the numerator and denominator data for both sexes during 1915–20, and for males from 3 September 1939 to 31 December 1949 and females from 1 June 1941 to 31 December 1949, analysed in this book, refer to mortality in the civilian plus military population rather than the civilian population alone. Considerable perturbations occurred to all-cause civilian mortality rates in young adults, especially men, in these periods (Swerdlow 1987) because the civilian population was heavily weighted with persons who were unfit for military service or had been discharged from service because of medical incapacity (Campbell 1965). If civilian data alone are analysed, cancer mortality rates in young adults in these years are overestimated because incidence of cancer would have led to military discharge.

Artefacts detectable in data on incidence and mortality by single calendar year

One method to try to detect artefacts in cancer trend data is to examine rates by single calendar year, to see whether sudden increases or decreases have occurred that are too large to be plausibly real and which might reflect changes in coding, data collection, diagnostic fashion, or other artefacts. Figure 4.2 shows mortality rates for all-cancers and cancer of unspecified primary site by single year since 1960. An artefactual increase can be seen in the all-cancer data for females and less clearly for males in 1984, due to the change in OPCS interpretation of ICD coding rule 3 discussed above, and a decrease can be seen in each sex in 1993 when this coding change was reversed. For cancer of unspecified primary site, there was a decrease in each sex in 1968, when ICD8 was introduced, and a large increase in 1979 plus the three years subsequently, after the introduction of ICD9 and industrial action by Registrars; there was in each sex an oscillation in rates in the years leading to the 1984 change in interpretation of ICD coding rule 3, and a substantial increase in 1993, when medical enquiries (see p. 11) ceased (and the rule 3 change was reversed and cause coding automated).

Figure 4.3 shows incidence by single calendar year for the same categories of neoplasm. For all-cancers, there was a sudden increase in each sex in 1985 when the Thames Cancer Registry was formed, presumably because of better registration in the North Thames regions, but surprisingly the increase was not sustained in the years immediately following. There was also a peak in females, and perhaps males, in 1974, the

reason for which is unclear. Although 1974 was the first year in which cases registered solely from death certificates were included in the published national data, these cancers had been included in the computer files for 1971–3 (OPCS 1979), so that the rates we calculated from data in these files should not have been deficient.

For cancer of unspecified primary site, a peak of incidence can be seen in 1974, perhaps for the same (but unknown) reason as the all-cancer increase in that year. There was also, as in mortality data, an oscillation in 1982–4, for reasons unclear. A peak in 1985, when the Thames Cancer Registry was formed, is apparent in females but not males. Finally, there was a large peak in 1987, which on examination by region (not shown) was the consequence of increases in the Thames and West Midlands regions, for reasons which are not apparent.

Overall, there has been a substantial rise over the period analysed in the rates of cancer of unspecified primary site, especially for mortality, which implies that the true trends in cancers of specified primary sites, particularly those that are difficult to diagnose, have been somewhat more upward than they appear from the recorded rates.

Chance

All data on disease occurrence contain an element of random variation, and hence chance is a possible explanation of trends, although not in general a likely one for the trends discussed in this book because of the large numbers of cases on which they are based. We have not presented any uniform testing of statistical significance of trends, since the appropriate test will depend on the question the reader wishes to address, and in general the trends to which attention is drawn are based on numbers which are far too large for chance to be a plausible explanation.

Aetiology

As well as the various potential artefactual reasons for trends in cancer rates discussed above, and changes in survival, trends can also, of course, reflect real changes in incidence consequent on changes in factors causing, or preventing, cancer. Trends in these factors are discussed in the next chapter.

(a) All malignant neoplasms

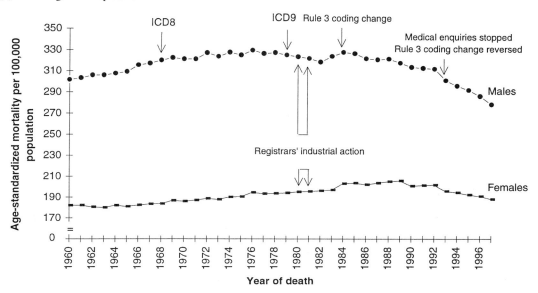

(b) Cancer of unspecified primary site

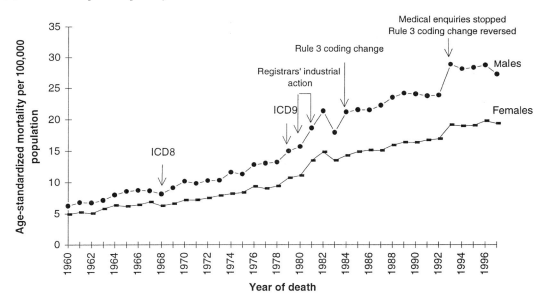

Figure 4.2 Age-standardized mortality from (a) all malignant neoplasms (ICD7 140–207, 292.3, 294; ICD8 140–209; ICD9 140–208, 238.4, 289.8), (b) cancer of unspecified primary site (ICD7 156, 165, 198, 199; ICD8 195–199; ICD9 155.2, 195–199), ages 0–84, 1960–97.

(a) All malignant neoplasms except non-melanoma skin cancer

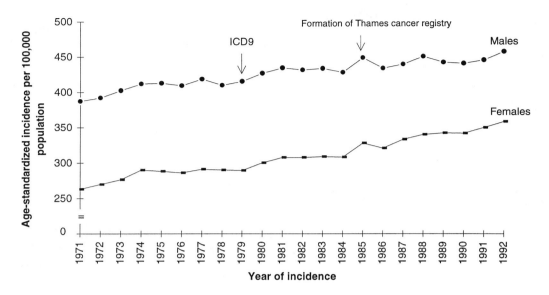

(b) Cancer of unspecified primary site

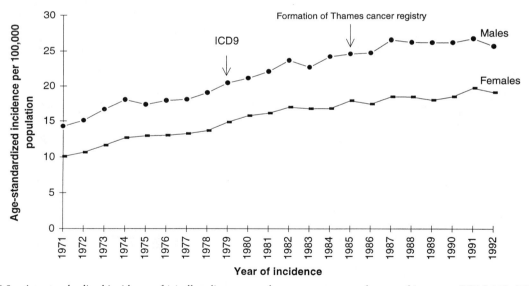

Figure 4.3   Age-standardized incidence of (a) all malignant neoplasms except non-melanoma skin cancer (ICD8 140–172, 173.5, 174–209; ICD9 140–172, 174–208, 238.4, 289.8), (b) cancer of unspecified primary site (ICD8 195–199; ICD9 155.2, 195–199), ages 0–84, 1971–92.

5 | Trends in factors that may cause or prevent cancer

One of the main reasons for interest in cancer trend data is to compare them with trends in putative risk factors in the same population. Although such 'ecological' comparisons, examining exposure and disease rates in populations rather than in individuals, generally give weak evidence on aetiology, they can be useful in suggesting which factors are plausible as major risk factors and which are not. This can help to identify factors needing closer investigation as potentially aetiological, and to decide whether new epidemics of cancer are explicable by known causes or indicate the need to search for 'new' factors. Thus, for instance, in the 1940s when it was noted that lung cancer rates were rising, potential reasons for this epidemic were sought by considering which respirable factors were increasing. It is illustrative, however, of the fallibility of ecological comparisons to identify a cause, as opposed to constraining the plausibility of hypothesized causes, that the factors deemed most likely at the time were coal smoke and motor car fumes, rather than smoking (Doll 1967).

The exposure data available at a population level are limited in several respects. Direct information about population exposure to many known or suspected risk factors for cancer has not been collected, and thus for some variables no data are presented and for others only proxies for the exposure can be shown. The calendar years for which exposure data have been collected are often not ideal—for many variables, the data are not available for as long ago as would be desirable. The geographical area for which data can be obtained varies. When available, we have presented exposure data for England and Wales, but for certain variables information is only available for Britain or the United Kingdom overall. As the population of England and Wales constitutes 91% of the population of Britain and 88% of that of the United Kingdom, this should make no material difference.

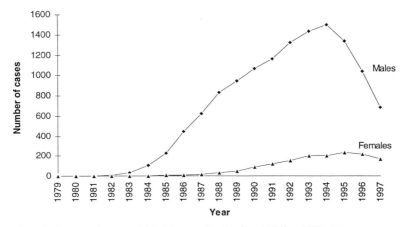

Figure 5.1   Number of newly diagnosed cases of AIDS by sex, England and Wales, 1979–97.

We have included exposure data to the most recent date available, although this is sometimes beyond the period relevant to current cancer rates, because the exposure trends are of intrinsic interest and also because they are of relevance to future cancer trends. The factors are presented in alphabetical order.

Acquired immune deficiency syndrome (AIDS)

Figure 5.1 uses data from the Communicable Disease Surveillance Centre to show the progress of the AIDS epidemic in England and Wales, which reached a peak in males in 1994 and in females in 1995.

Air pollution

Information on concentrations of various outdoor air pollutants are available from national surveys (Department of the Environment 1978). Daily measurements have been made by local authorities since 1960, and in some towns since earlier years. Measurements made on a regular basis are available from about 700–800 sites, mainly urban, throughout the country.

Data were extracted from http:\www.environment. detr.gov.uk\airq\aqinfo.htm for 1970 onwards. For earlier years, data were extracted from Central Statistical Office (1974) and were only available for black smoke and sulphur dioxide. The results are shown in Figure 5.2. Smoke emissions have decreased greatly since the early 1950s, whereas sulphur dioxide emissions have declined since 1970. Emissions of carbon monoxide decreased slightly in the early 1970s and more markedly since the late 1980s. Emissions of methane, nitrogen oxides, and volatile organic compounds increased from the early 1970s into the 1980s, but have since declined. Emissions of particulate matter decreased markedly from 1970 to 1996.

Monitoring of ozone levels in the United Kingdom began only in 1986/7 and was initially restricted to a small number of rural sites. Measurements in urban areas began only in 1992/3. Given the paucity of data it is not possible to examine national trends in ozone levels.

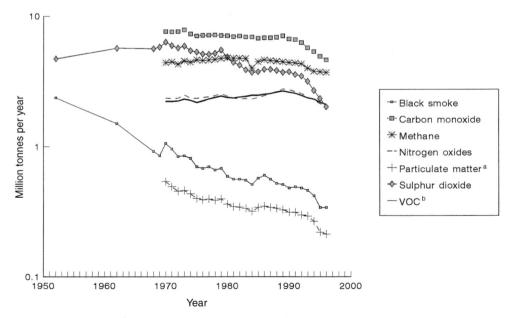

a Less than 10 µg.
b VOC=Volatile organic compounds excluding methane.

Figure 5.2   Air pollution in the United Kingdom, 1952–96: trends in emissions of certain pollutants (logarithmic scale).

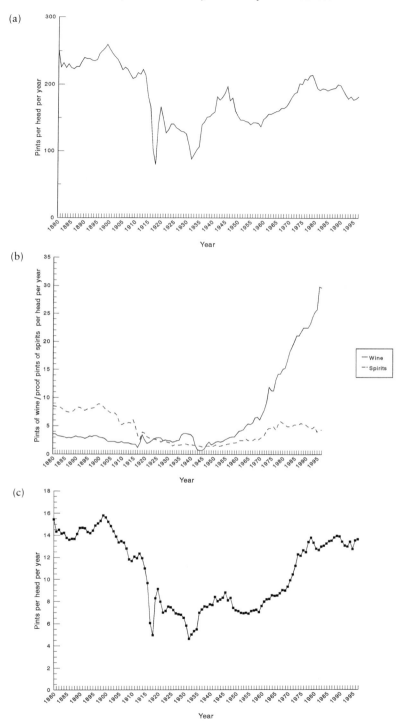

Figure 5.3 Trends in alcohol consumption in both sexes combined, United Kingdom, 1880–1997: (a) beer, (b) wine and spirits, (c) total alcohol (as equivalent in absolute alcohol). (One pint = 0.568 litres).

Alcohol consumption

Data on wine, beer, and spirits consumption in the United Kingdom, as estimated from supplies, were extracted from Wilson (1940) and Spring and Buss (1977) for the years 1880–1922 and from the Brewers and Licensed Retailers Association (1993, 1998) for 1923 onwards. Total absolute alcohol consumption was estimated by assuming that spirits contained 40% ethyl alcohol, wine 12%, and beer 4%. Beer consumption was high before the First World War, low in the inter-war years, reached a peak in 1946, and then increased from 1959 until 1980 but not subsequently (Figure 5.3a). Consumption of spirits (Figure 5.3b), and of alcohol in total (Figure 5.3c), followed a similar trend except that the peak in the 1940s was less marked for alcohol overall and absent for spirits. Wine consumption was low until the 1960s but has since increased greatly (Figure 5.3b).

Data on self-reported alcohol consumption by sex have been collected since 1978 by the General House-

Table 5.1 Trends in self-reported alcohol consumption by sex. Persons aged 18 years and over, Great Britain, 1978–96. (Data for 1978–84 from OPCS (1986) and for 1984–96 from ONS (1998*b*))

Year	Men		Women	
	% moderate drinkers[a]	% heavy drinkers[b]	% moderate drinkers[a]	% heavy drinkers[b]
1978	15	25	4	4
1980	14	23	4	2
1982	14	21	4	1
1984	14	20	4	2
	% moderate drinkers (11–21 units per week)	% heavy drinkers (>21 units per week)	% moderate drinkers (8–14 units per week)	% heavy drinkers (>14 units per week)
1984	21	25	14	9
1986	22	27	14	10
1988	22	27	14	10
1990	22	28	14	11
1992	22	27	15	11
1994	22	27	15	13
1996	23	27	16	14

[a] Defined as five to six units of alcohol at least once a week or more than six units once or twice a month (1 unit = 9 grams of alcohol).
[b] Defined as seven or more units at least once a week.

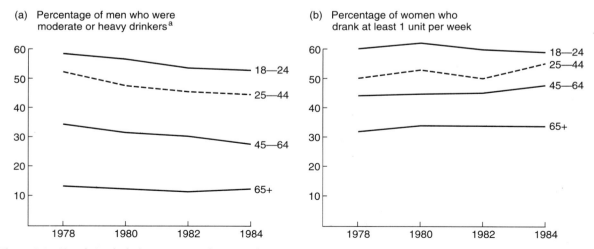

(a) Percentage of men who were moderate or heavy drinkers[a]

(b) Percentage of women who drank at least 1 unit per week

Figure 5.4 Trends in alcohol consumption by sex and age, Great Britain, 1978–84. (Reproduced from OPCS 1986 with permission from the Office for National Statistics; Crown Copyright 2000.) [a] Definitions as in Table 5.1.

hold Survey (OPCS 1986; ONS 1998*b*), although there is a discontinuity in the data because they were collected on a different basis up to 1984 and from then onwards. The levels of consumption were higher in men than in women throughout, but in each sex there was no clear trend except for a modest decrease in men from 1978–84 and an increase in women in the most recent years (Table 5.1).

Trends in self-reported alcohol consumption by age are shown in Figure 5.4 and Table 5.2, on the different bases for which data are available at different dates. The proportion of men who were moderate or heavy drinkers declined during 1978–84 in all age groups under 65 years (Figure 5.4a), but there were only small changes in consumption during 1992–6 (Table 5.2). The proportion of women who drank at least one unit

of alcohol per week increased during 1978–84 in all age groups except 18–24 years (Figure 5.4b), and at all ages consumption by women increased during 1992–6 (Table 5.2).

The proportion of heavy smokers who were also heavy drinkers declined slightly from 1988 to 1996 in each sex (Table 5.3), although the proportion of light smokers who were heavy drinkers increased.

In order to obtain an indirect indication of sex-specific trends in alcohol consumption over a longer period than available from the General Household Survey, we extracted data on mortality from cirrhosis of the liver from various sources (Wilson 1940; Registrar General 1925, 1934, 1944*b*, 1952, 1962; OPCS 1972*a*; OPCS, ONS 1977–98). The results are shown in Figure 5.5. In each sex the trends are fairly

Table 5.2 Mean weekly self-reported alcohol consumption in units, by sex and age. Persons aged 16 years and over, Great Britain, 1992–6. (Data from ONS (1998*b*))

Age (years)	Men			Women		
	1992	1994	1996	1992	1994	1996
16–24	19.1	17.4	20.3	7.3	7.7	9.5
25–44	18.1	17.5	17.6	6.3	6.2	7.2
45–64	15.6	15.5	15.6	5.3	5.3	5.9
65+	9.7	10.0	11.0	2.7	3.2	3.5

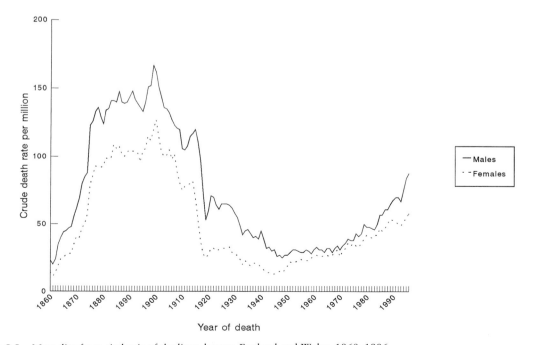

Figure 5.5 Mortality from cirrhosis of the liver, by sex, England and Wales, 1860–1996.

Table 5.3   Proportion of men and women in each smoking category who were heavy drinkers[a]. Persons aged 16 years and over, Great Britain, 1988–96. (Data from OPCS (1990*b*, 1996) and ONS (1998*b*))

Year	Current cigarette smokers		Current non-smokers of cigarettes	
	Heavy (20+ per day)	Light (<20 per day)	Ex-regular smokers	Never/only occasionally
Men				
1988	43	30	24	20
1994	43	33	25	20
1996	40	34	26	21
Women				
1988	24	13	11	6
1994	23	19	15	9
1996	21	21	15	10

[a] Defined as more than 21 units per week for men and more than 14 units per week for women.

similar to those for alcohol consumption in Figure 5.3, with a rapid decrease from 1900 to 1920, a lesser decrease to a minimum in 1950, and subsequently an increase, mainly since 1970.

Anthropometric characteristics

Body mass index

National data on weight are available from the 1980 Survey of Heights and Weights in Great Britain (Knight 1984), the 1987 Dietary and Nutritional Survey in Great Britain (Gregory *et al.* 1990), and the Health Surveys of England conducted in 1991–95 (White *et al.* 1993; Bennett *et al.* 1995; Colhoun *et al.* 1996; Bost *et al.* 1997).

The body mass index (BMI) is a measure of obesity standardized for height, which is calculated as weight (in kg)/height (in m)^2. The mean BMI increased from 24.3 in 1980 to 26.1 in 1995 for men and from 23.9 to 25.9 for women. The proportions of men and women with a BMI over 30 (obese) also increased during this

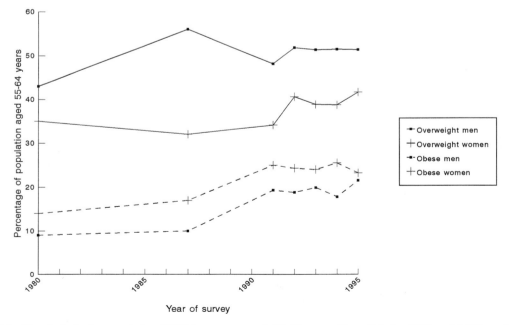

Figure 5.6   Trends in body mass index (BMI) in persons aged 55–64 years, Great Britain, 1980 and 1987, and England, 1991–5. Overweight defined as a BMI greater than 25 but not greater than 30; obesity defined as a BMI greater than 30.

period, as did the proportion overweight (BMI greater than 25 but not greater than 30). The increases in the proportion overweight or obese have been greatest in those aged 35 years and over, and in particular in those aged 55–64 years (Figure 5.6), but at younger adult age-groups there were also substantial increases (not shown).

Height

Long-term trends in height of men from the middle of the eighteenth to the beginning of the twentieth century are available from Floud *et al.* (1990). These estimates are based on a sample of about 170 000 recruits to the Army, the Royal Marines, the Royal Military Academy at Sandhurst, and the Marine Society of London. Recruitment into the armed services was voluntary until 1916, but published statistics show that recruits were drawn widely from the working class throughout Britain. Therefore, it is possible to base estimates of the height of that population on the evidence of the heights of the recruits. Military recruiters, however, were concerned to select men who were healthy and fit enough to cope with military life, and therefore minimum height limits were imposed. Floud *et al.* used special statistical methods to correct for this bias and thus to estimate the average height of the whole population. For more recent years, Floud *et al.* obtained data on height from various national surveys. There was a long-term increase in height up to men born in the 1830s, then a fall in those born in the next 30 years, and then a rising trend (Figure 5.7).

Data on mean adult male and female height for successive 5-year cohorts of men and women born from 1900 to 1940 and for the cohorts born in 1946 and 1958 were extracted from Kuh *et al.* (1991). These estimates were based on 50 000 measurements taken from members and their parents in two British birth cohort studies: the Medical Research Council's National Survey of Health and Development (NSHD) and the National Child Development Study (NCDS) (Kuh *et al.* 1991). The NSHD is a longitudinal study of a sample of 5362 children born in one week in 1946, and collected data on mother's and father's height when the child was aged 6 years. The NCDS included practically all children born in Britain in one week in 1958, and collected data on mother's height at antenatal examination and father's height when the child was aged 11 years. Mean adult height increased for successive generations of men and women born from 1900 to 1958, except for a small interruption for cohorts born during 1936–40 (based on 854 men and 3079 women) (Figure 5.8).

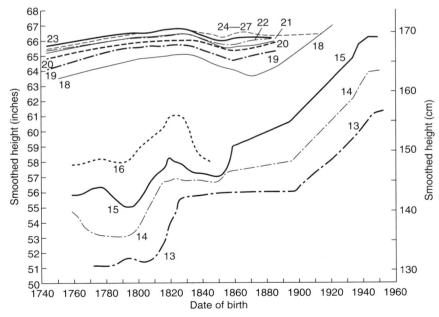

Figure 5.7 Long-term age-specific trends in the heights of male adolescents and adults in Britain, by year of birth. (Reproduced with permission from Floud *et al.* 1990.)

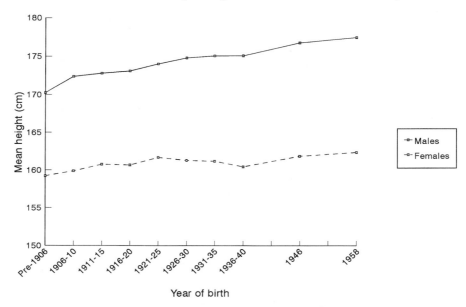

Figure 5.8   Mean adult height for generations of men and women born in Britain from 1900 to 1958.

Asbestos

Figure 5.9 shows asbestos imports to the UK, by type of asbestos, since 1900. The data for 1900–77 are from reports and evidence submitted to the Advisory Committee on Asbestos, those for 1978–83 and 1990–5 from the Asbestos Information Council, and those for 1984–9 from Eurostat. During the Second World War much of the asbestos was used in shipbuilding, and for women there was substantial exposure in gas-mask manufacture and manufacture of other asbestos goods. In the 1960s and 1970s, however, most asbestos was used in the construction industry (Peto *et al.* 1995), and therefore substantial exposures have continued to occur many years after initial use, during renovation, maintenance, and demolition of buildings.

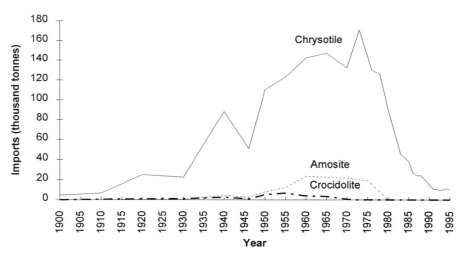

Figure 5.9   Trends in asbestos imports to the United Kingdom, 1900–95.

Birth order

Data on number of previous liveborn children to the mother are available for legitimate livebirths in England and Wales since 1938 (OPCS 1987; OPCS, ONS 1985–97). We used these data to calculate mean birth order and the percentage of children who were firstborn. Before 1978, illegitimate births were under 10% of all births, so the omission of birth order for them should have had little effect. The proportion illegitimate has since risen, however, exceeding 20% in 1986, so that recent data may be less representative of all births.

Mean birth order decreased unevenly from 1938–78, but has since changed little (Figure 5.10). The percentage of children who were firstborn decreased unevenly from 1938 to 1964, and has since increased slightly (Figure 5.11).

Birthweight

Data on birthweights of liveborn children in England and Wales have been collected systematically on a national basis since 1975. Initially, data collection was very incomplete, and results of it have been published only since 1977 (OPCS 1980–8; OPCS, ONS 1990–8). Before 1975, data on birthweight are available from two national sample studies, of all births in one week in March 1958 and one week in April 1970 (Alberman 1977), and from notifications to the Department of Health from 1953–72 of all babies weighing under

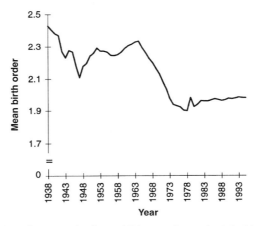

Figure 5.10 Mean birth order (number of previous liveborn children to the mother), legitimate livebirths, England and Wales, 1938–95.

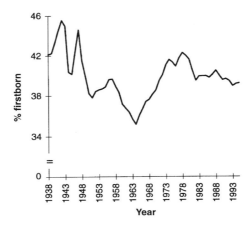

Figure 5.11 Percentage of legitimate livebirths for which the mother had delivered no previous liveborn child, England and Wales, 1938–95.

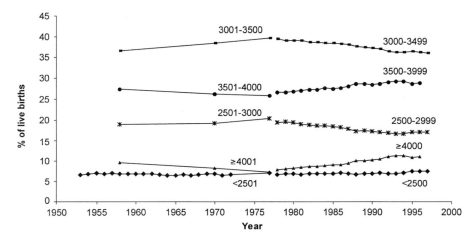

Figure 5.12   Birthweight of livebirths, England and Wales, 1953–97.

2501 g (but not heavier) (Alberman 1974). Figure 5.12 therefore shows the percentage of liveborn babies of low birthweight since 1953, using the Department of Health data for the period 1953–72, and the complete birthweight distribution of livebirths in 1958, 1970, and 1977–97[1], from the national sample surveys and the subsequent routine data collection system. Data for 1977–82 from the national routine system should be considered cautiously because birthweight was then recorded for under 90% of births (compared with more than 95% thereafter).

There is a discontinuity in Figure 5.12 in 1978, because birthweight was categorized slightly differently before then (<2501 g, 2501–3000, etc.) and from then onwards (<2500 g, 2500–2999, etc.); this change reduced the percentages in each of the two lowest birthweight categories in the Figure by about 0.4–1.2%, and increased the percentage in each of the two highest categories by about 0.3–0.6% (OPCS 1980–8).

The percentage of low-birthweight livebirths remained unchanged from 1953–72, but has since increased a little, from 6.6% under 2500 g in 1978 to

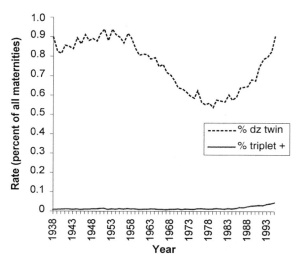

Figure 5.13   Rates of dizygotic (DZ) twin maternities and of triplet or higher-order maternities, England and Wales, 1938–95.

---

[1] Except that data are not available dividing 3500–3999 from ≥4000 g in 1997.

7.4% in 1997. The proportion of livebirths in the greatest birthweight category appeared to decrease in the early years (although based on one week sample data), but has subsequently increased from 7.9% in 1978 to 10.9% in 1996.

Dizygotic twins

Rates of dizygotic twin birth were estimated by the Weinberg method (Hrubec and Robinette 1984) from counts of all twin births and of same-sex twin births in England and Wales, which are available for 1938 onwards (except 1981) (OPCS 1987; OPCS, ONS 1985–97). The data presented in Figure 5.13 are for counts of maternities (pregnancies resulting in still or livebirths) rather than of offspring, and include maternities from which one or more of the offspring were stillborn as well as those from which they were liveborn. The number of higher-order births has also been shown because these give a marker of the extent of multiple births due to hormonal treatment of infertility, which would have affected dizygotic twinning rates. From 1938–58 dizygotic twinning rates showed no consistent trend, but then there was a marked decline in the rate until 1979, and then a steep increase from the mid-1980s to 1995. This latter increase, however, was accompanied by a huge rise in the triplet and higher-order birth rate, indicating that much or all of the increase in dizygotic twinning may have been due to infertility treatment rather than endogenous changes in women.

Ethnic minority populations

Ethnic minority groups (i.e. non-whites) represent 6% of the total population of England and Wales according to the 1991 census (Peach 1996), the first one to collect information on ethnicity (Table 5.4).

Table 5.4 Population of England and Wales by self-defined ethnicity, 1991. (Data from Peach (1996))

Ethnic group	Population size	Percentage
White	46 937 861	94.0
Black-Caribbean	499 030	1.0
Black-African	209 589	0.4
Black-Other[a]	175 755	0.4
Indian	830 205	1.7
Pakistani	455 363	0.9
Bangladeshi	161 701	0.3
Chinese	146 462	0.3
Other Asian[b]	192 930	0.4
Other[c]	281 381	0.6
Total population	49 908 593	100

[a] Mainly second-generation Afro-Caribbeans.
[b] Includes people with origin in Sri Lanka, Japan, the Phillipines, Mauritius, Malaysia, and Vietnam.
[c] Residual category. The largest single group is of Arab or Middle Eastern descent.

Indirect estimates of changes over time in the sizes of the various ethnic minority groups have been made from data on country of birth collected at various censuses in conjunction, since 1981, with data from the Labour Force Survey (Table 5.5). The latter is an annual sample survey of approximately 150 000 residents in private households, which includes questions on both country of birth and self-reported ethnicity (OPCS 1992).

Food and nutrient consumption

Data on food and nutrient consumption per person for the years 1940 to 1997 were obtained from the National Food Survey (MAFF 1991*a,b*, 1992, 1993–8). The National Food Survey (NFS) started in 1940 as a survey covering mainly working-class households, but since 1950 it has been based on a representative national sample of households. The NFS asks the housewife to keep a record of her purchases of food for

Table 5.5 Caribbean, Indian, Pakistani, and Bangladeshi ethnic populations in Great Britain, 1951–91: estimated population sizes by calendar year. (Modified from Peach (1996))

Year	West Indian or Caribbean	Indian	Pakistani	Bangladeshi
1951	28 000	31 000	10 000	2 000
1961	210 000	81 000	25 000	6 000
1966	402 000	223 000	64 000	11 000
1971	548 000	375 000	119 000	22 000
1981	545 000	676 000	296 000	65 000
1991	500 000	840 000	477 000	163 000

one week and from this the average quantity of food eaten per person is calculated. Nutrient intakes are calculated from these consumption figures, by reference to published tables of food composition. To provide information on food intake for the period before the start of the NFS and the years when its sample was not representative of the entire population of the country, data on total food supplies to the United Kingdom and their nutritional value for the years 1909–50 were extracted from Greaves and Hollingsworth (1966). These estimates are not directly comparable to those derived from the NFS because food supplies do not take into account food wasted at the production level or used for purposes other than human consumption. They provide, nevertheless, a reasonable picture of the national trends in food intake in the first half of the twentieth century.

Measurements of individual fat consumption in males and females for the years 1930–85 were available from a compilation of results from all studies conducted in the United Kingdom in which individual dietary assessment was carried out and fat intake reported (Stephen and Sieber 1994). Estimates of total dietary fibre intake were extracted from Southgate *et al.* (1978), Bingham *et al.* (1979), Bingham and Cummings (1980), and MAFF (1991*b*, 1995, 1998).

Fat, protein, and carbohydrates

Total per caput fat intake increased in the UK from the early part of the century until the 1930s (Table 5.6),

but reduced to some extent during the Second World War and the immediate post-war period. Thereafter, it rose to 120 g per person per day in 1969 (Figure 5.14), after which a decline began, continuing into the 1990s. Despite the recent fall in fat consumption, the proportion of total energy derived from fat, which had increased in the immediately post-war decades, has since changed little because total energy has fallen by a similar proportion to fat intake (Figure 5.15). However, there has been a trend since 1969 towards consumption of a greater proportion of fats in non-saturated rather than saturated form (data on the fatty acid composition of the diet are available only for 1959, 1969, and 1972–97) (Figure 5.14).

Sex-specific data on individual intake showed that the trends for total energy, total fat, and percentage of energy derived from fat were similar for males and females during 1930–85 (Table 5.7).

The proportion of total energy derived from carbohydrates has declined steadily since the Second World War (Table 5.6; Figure 5.15), whereas the proportion derived from protein has remained relatively constant (Figure 5.15).

Fibre

Intake of dietary fibre has declined slowly and progressively since 1860, except during the Second World War when it increased by about 65% (Table 5.8). This increase was due mainly to an increase in cereal fibre

Table 5.6 Trends in food and nutrient supplies in the United Kingdom, 1909–50. (Modified from Greaves and Hollingsworth (1966))

	1909–13	1924–8	1934–8	1941	1944	1947	1950
Foods[a]							
Dairy products (lb)	259	261	264	314	367	361	409
Red meat (lb)	131	129	129	99	110	96	112
Poultry and game (lb)	5	6	9	6	4	7	7
Vegetables (lb)	321	335	317	311	415	428	364
Fruits (incl. nuts) (lb)	68	97	104	30	52	89	84
Cereals (lb)	237	214	211	257	253	242	223
Nutrients[b]							
Total fat (g)	98	107	131	115	124	107	133
Total protein (g)	81	79	79	83	86	89	87
Carbohydrate (g)	415	408	414	409	429	433	419
Calcium (mg)	608	646	696	707	1040	1140	1152
Vitamin A (i.u.)	2560	2950	3690	3500	3670	3640	3880
Vitamin C (mg)	81	93	96	77	102	111	95
Total energy (kcal)	2760	2810	3050	2900	3060	2940	3120

[a] per person per year.
[b] per person per day.

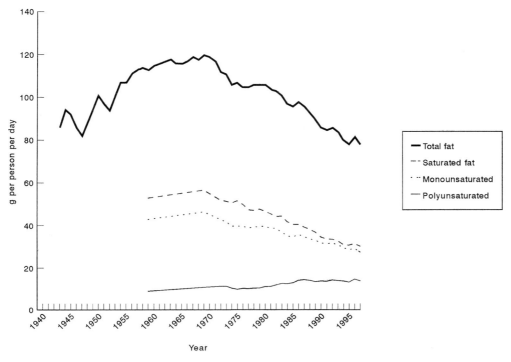

Figure 5.14   Fat consumption, Great Britain, 1943–97.

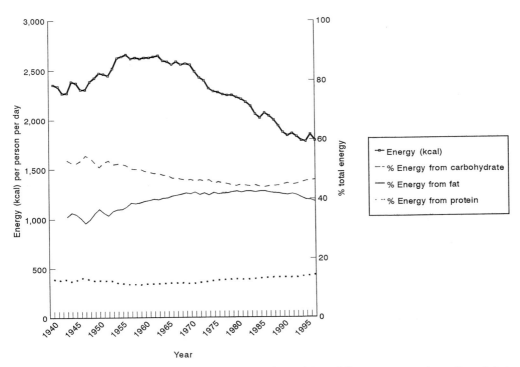

Figure 5.15   Overall energy intake, and percentages of energy obtained from different macronutrients, Great Britain, 1940–97.

Table 5.7   Mean daily intake of energy, mean daily intake of total fat, and percentage of energy from fat, for males and females aged 18–65 years, United Kingdom, 1930–85. (Data from Stephen and Sieber (1994))

Year	Males Energy (kcal)	Fat (g)	Energy from fat (%)	Females Energy (kcal)	Fat (g)	Energy from fat (%)
1930–9	3086	NA	36.9	2206	NA	38.8
1940–9	2928	105.9	34.8	2043	79.3	32.6
1950–9	3268	134.2	38.4	2447	104.6	37.3
1960–9	2833	126.0	40.9	2153	98.0	40.1
1970–9	2722	122.1	40.1	1890	84.7	40.3
1980–5	2529	104.5	38.9	1730	74.9	37.2

NA = data not available.

intake, which more than doubled from 9.2 g per person per day in 1938 to around 20 g per person per day in 1942–4, and then decreased to a level of 8.7 g per person per day in 1957. Fibre intake from other sources remained practically constant from 1860 to 1970. Data on sources of fibre are not available from 1971 onwards.

Fruit and vegetables

Fruit consumption rose markedly during 1909–97, except for a decline during the Second World War because of decreased fruit importation (Table 5.6, Figure 5.16). Total vegetable intake declined from the 1920s to 1997, except for a slight increase during the Second World War, when home production of vegetables was encouraged (Table 5.6, Figure 5.17). The post-war decline, however, was mainly due to a fall in consumption of potatoes (and to a lesser extent of fresh green vegetables). Consumption of other fresh vegetables has changed little and intake of other (non-fresh) vegetables has increased steadily since the 1940s.

Meat

Total meat consumption showed a trend similar to that for fat, with a fall in the 1940s due to rationing (Table 5.6, Figure 5.18). Meat consumption rose sharply in

Table 5.8   Trends in dietary fibre content of the British diet (g per person per day), 1860–1997.

Year	Total	Cereal	Vegetable	Fruit	Other
Estimated from food supply data[a,b]					
1860	37–47	22–32	NA	NA	NA
1880	28.6	13.9	9.6	NA	NA
1909–13	23.9	10.9	11.1	1.7	0.2
1938	22.3	9.2	10.1	2.7	0.3
1942	32.0–37.3	18.7–24.0	11.3	1.9	0.1
1944	34.1–39.6	19.1–24.6	13.2	1.8	0.1
1957	23.3	8.7	11.7	2.6	0.3
1970	22.7	8.1	11.5	2.6	0.5
Estimated from food consumption data[b,c]					
1956[b]	22.5	8.4	10.4	2.2	1.6
1961[b]	21.7	7.5	10.5	2.1	1.7
1971[b]	21.2	6.4	10.3	2.2	2.3
1976[b]	19.9	NA	NA	NA	NA
1986[c]	13.0	NA	NA	NA	NA
1992[c]	12.0	NA	NA	NA	NA
1997[c]	12.4	NA	NA	NA	NA

[a] From Bingham and Cummings (1980).
[b] From Southgate *et al.* (1978) and Bingham *et al.* (1979).
[c] From MAFF (1991*b*, 1995, 1998).
NA = data not available.

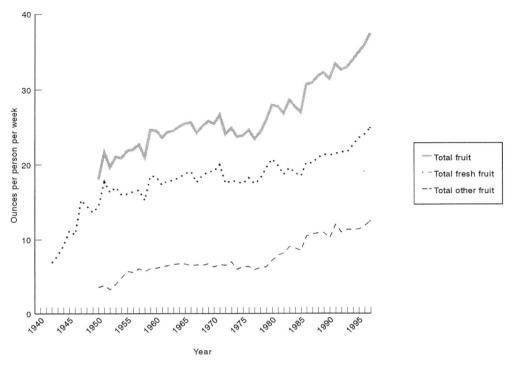

Figure 5.16 Fruit consumption, Great Britain, 1942–97.

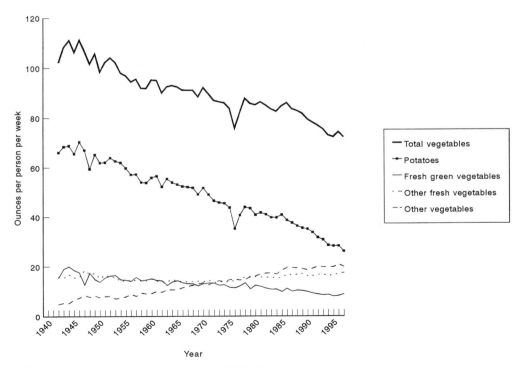

Figure 5.17 Vegetable consumption, Great Britain, 1942–97.

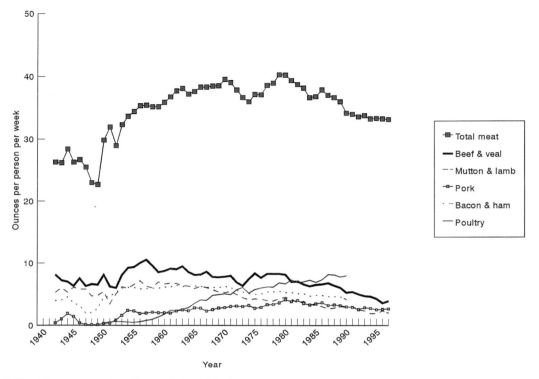

Figure 5.18   Meat consumption, Great Britain, 1942–97.

the 1950s and more slowly and inconsistently until the late 1970s, and decreased thereafter. This decline was mainly due to a fall in beef intake. In contrast, consumption of poultry has more than doubled in the last 25 years (data for bacon and ham and poultry were collected on a different basis after 1990 than previously, and therefore were not included in the graph).

Vitamins

There have also been changes over time in the amounts of vitamins present in the diet. Vitamin A intake increased from the turn of the century to the mid-1960s, particularly in the 1950s (Table 5.6, Figure 5.19), and remained steady thereafter except for a decline in the last decade. There was an increase in vitamin C intake during the twentieth century (Table 5.6, Figure 5.20), largely because of a rapid increase in the contribution made by fruits and fruit juices, which offset the decline from potatoes, the traditional main source (MAFF 1991*a*). There was a marked rise in the intake of vitamin D during the 1940s, followed by a

fall since 1951, and then a rise since the mid-1970s (Figure 5.21).

Helicobacter pylori

Figure 5.22 shows the seroprevalence of *Helicobacter pylori* in successive generations born from 1900 to 1979, estimated from samples of serum collected in Yorkshire, England, in 1969, 1979, and 1989 (Banatvala *et al*. 1993). There was a decrease in seroprevalence for cohorts born from 1920–9 to 1960–9.

Income

The gross domestic product (GDP) at constant prices and factor level is a standard measure of the income of the country as a whole, and comprises the income of individuals and the income of organizations. Over the period 1951–94, the GDP has grown at an average rate of about 2.4% per annum (Figure 5.23). There have been three substantial dips. The first occurred in the

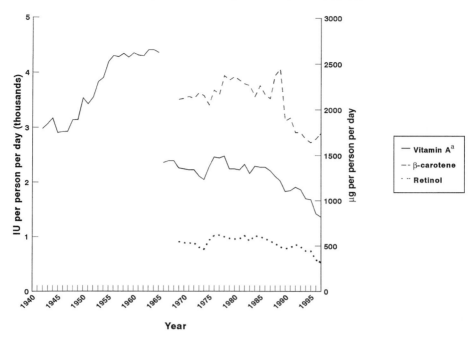

Figure 5.19 Vitamin A consumption, Great Britain, 1942–97.
[a] From 1966 onwards, Vitamin A expressed as retinol-equivalent.

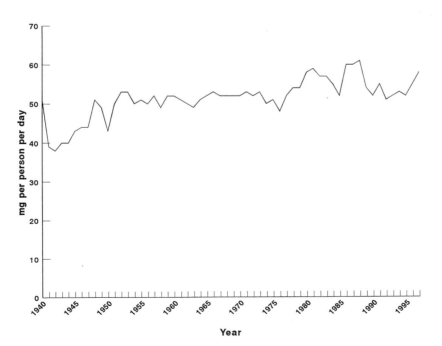

Figure 5.20 Vitamin C consumption, Great Britain, 1940–97.

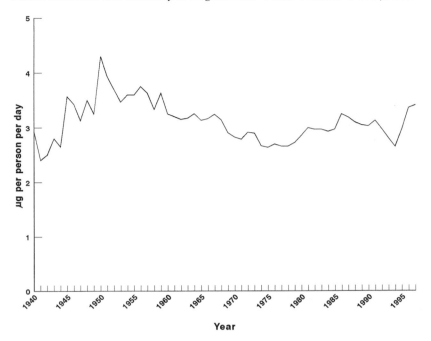

Figure 5.21   Vitamin D consumption, Great Britain, 1940–97.

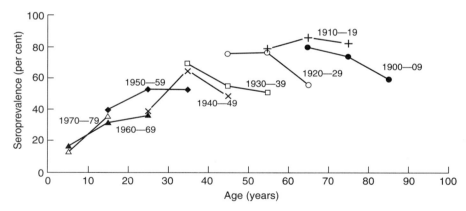

Figure 5.22   Seroprevalence of *Helicobacter pylori* in successive generations of residents in Yorkshire, England, born 1900–79. (Reproduced from Banatvala *et al.* 1993, with permission of University of Chicago Press.)

mid-1970s due to oil price rises. The other two recessions occurred in the early 1980s and early 1990s.

Disposable income is the amount of money people have available to them to spend or invest. It is equal to income from all sources, less taxes and national insurance. Figure 5.24 shows the trend in the United Kingdom since 1971. It is expressed in real terms to allow meaningful comparisons from year to year by adjusting for the effect of inflation. It increased by nearly 80% between 1971 and 1990, and then levelled off.

Data for earlier in the century are available from Bacon *et al.* (1972). Figure 5.25 shows the trend in gross national product (GNP) from 1900 to 1968, except during the two World Wars. The GNP increased slightly from 1900 until the First World War, declined

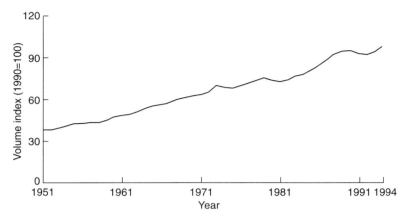

Figure 5.23 Trend in gross domestic product (GDP) at factor cost, United Kingdom, 1951–94. (Reproduced from Central Statistical Office 1996 with permission of Office for National Statistics; Crown Copyright 2000.)

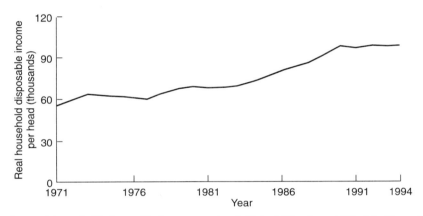

Figure 5.24 Trend in real household disposable income per head, United Kingdom, 1971–94. (Reproduced from Central Statistical Office 1996 with permission of Office for National Statistics; Crown Copyright 2000.)

during the Depression, but increased sharply after the Second World War. Further long-term data on GNP as well as other socioeconomic indicators can be found in Mitchell (1988).

Ionizing radiation

The annual collective dose from all sources of ionizing radiation, natural and man-made, to the United Kingdom population in 1993 was estimated as 150 000 mSv, and the average dose as 2.6 mSv (Hughes and O'Riordan 1993). The relative contribution to the total dose to the population from the

various natural and man-made sources is shown in Table 5.9. Natural background radiation is responsible for about 85% of exposure. The man-made contribution is largely from medical uses.

Domestic radon

There are no data on time trends in domestic radon concentrations in England and Wales, but large differences are observed between geographical areas (Wrixon *et al.* 1988). The concentrations of domestic radon are considerably raised by double glazing (Gunby *et al.* 1993), which has become much more prevalent, and to a lesser extent by draught proofing, which may also have increased. Radon concentrations

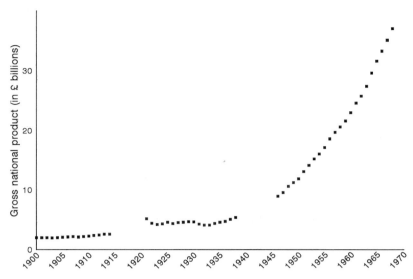

Figure 5.25 Trend in gross national product (GNP) at factor cost in current prices, United Kingdom (including Southern Ireland prior to 1921), 1900–68 (excluding World War periods).

Table 5.9 Annual ionizing radiation exposure of the population of the United Kingdom by source, 1991. (Data from Hughes and O'Riordan (1993))

Source	Annual collective dose (man Sv)	Average annual dose in μSv (% of total)
Natural		
Cosmic	15 000	260 (10)
Gamma	20 200	350 (14)
Internal	17 300	350 (11.5)
Radon	74 900	1300 (50)
Man-made		
Medical	21 400	370 (14)
Occupational[a]	430	7 (0.3)
Fallout	290	5 (0.2)
Discharges[b]	20	0.4 (<0.1)
Products	20	0.4 (<0.1)
Total	150 000	2600 (100)

[a]Some 80% from natural sources.
[b]Some 20% from natural activity.

are also affected by type of building, however, with a tendency to greater concentrations in older buildings.

Fallout radiation from nuclear explosions

The first nuclear weapon explosion in the atmosphere took place in 1945 and the amount of fallout radiation then increased until the 1962 test ban treaty. Levels in England and Wales were relatively high in the late 1950s and early 1960s (Medical Research Council 1960, 1964; Hughes *et al.* 1989; Simmonds *et al.* 1995). After the 1962 test ban treaty the level decreased, remaining low until the Chernobyl reactor accident in 1986 (Hughes *et al.* 1989).

Caesium-137

The main dietary sources of caesium-137 are milk, meat, vegetables, and cereals, with milk and meat accounting for about 60–80% of the total intake. Data on the levels of caesium-137 in milk from West Cumbria were published by Simmonds *et al.* (1995). We derived values for the United Kingdom by dividing the published figures by a factor of 1.4 in order to take into account differences in rainfall between West Cumbria and the whole country (Simmonds *et al.* 1995). The results are shown in Figure 5.26. The annual mean level of caesium-137 in milk increased in the late 1950s to a peak in 1962–4. Thereafter, it declined as a result of the 1962 test ban treaty.

Data on whole-body measurements of caesium-137 were extracted from Godfrey and Vennart (1968) for the years 1958–63 and from Newton *et al.* (1977) for the years 1964–77 and are presented in Figure 5.27. These measurements were essentially performed in residents in the south of England. The results were

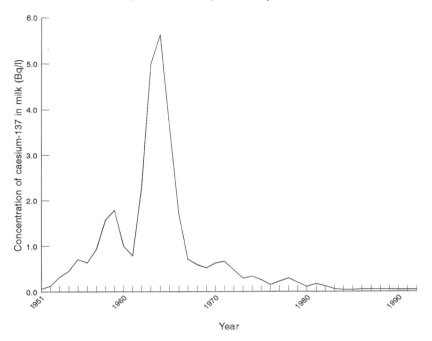

Figure 5.26 Concentration of caesium-137 in milk, United Kingdom, 1951–92.

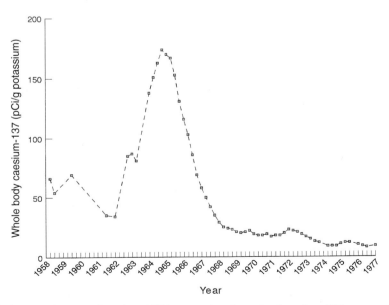

Figure 5.27 Whole-body measurements of caesium-137 (expressed as the ratio of caesium-137 to potassium) in men, south of England, 1958–77.

Table 5.10 Whole-body measurements of caesium-137 (Cs-137), south England, 1986–98. (Data from NRPB unpublished and departmental reports))
(a) Mean Cs-137 activity

Year (month)	Mean Cs-137 activity (Bq)
1986 (August)	100
1986 (November)	190
1987 (March)	175
1987 (May)	185
1987 (July)	200
1987 (September)	185
1987 (November)	140
1988 (March)	125
1988 (June)	110
1988 (September)	90
1989 (January)	75
1989 (April)	45

(b) Mean (range) Cs-137 activity

Year	Mean (range) Cs-137 activity (Bq)
1989	30 (NA)
1990	23 (NA)
1991	14 (18–34)
1992	14 (18–24)
1993	9 (9–22)
1994	NA (<7–22)
1995	NA (<7–22)
1996	NA
1997/8	21 (15–31)

NA = data not available.

expressed as the mean ratio of caesium-137 to potassium to minimize the impact of any errors that might have been introduced by the calibration procedures, as these would have affected the caesium-137 and potassium determinations similarly. Data for more recent years (and using diferent measurement units) are shown in Table 5.10. The levels of caesium-137 in the body paralleled those in the diet. The levels increased soon after the Chernobyl reactor accident in May 1986, but far less than after the 1960s tests, and fell below pre-Chernobyl levels in 1991.

Iodine-131

Iodine-131 (I^{131}) has a short half-life (8 days) and is therefore only present in the environment during periods of fallout of fresh fission products. It is deposited mainly with rain in soils and pastures, where it may be ingested by cows and concentrated in milk. Ingestion of fresh contaminated milk by man leads to concentration of I^{131} in the thyroid gland where it

delivers radiation for only a few weeks. Other foods are very minor sources of I^{131}. The highest doses are received by young children, partly because they drink so much fresh bovine milk (unless they are breastfed or fed with evaporated or dried milk) and partly because a given intake of I^{131} represents a higher dose than in adults due to their smaller thyroid glands (UNSCEAR 1977). Based on measurements of iodine in milk samples from different locations and indirect estimates for the years when levels were below the limit of detection, concentrations of I^{131} in milk from West Cumbria due to fallout have been published for the years 1951–94 (Simmonds *et al.* 1995). We divided these published figures by a factor of 1.4 (Simmonds *et al.* 1995) to estimate levels for the United Kingdom that take into account differences in rainfall between West Cumbria and the whole country. The results are shown in Figure 5.28. The highest values were during 1961–2. Only with the reactor accident at Windscale (subsequently renamed Sellafield) in 1957, was the distribution of local milk prohibited in the more heavily contaminated areas (Medical Research Council 1960). Very few determinations of I^{131} were carried out directly in human thyroids, but average doses of 6 mrad were measured in a small sample of adults in the London area during a 4-week period in 1958–9 (Robertson and Falconer 1959). The dose to the thyroid of infants from the extensive nuclear tests in 1961 and 1962 is estimated to have been about 0.1 rad (Medical Research Council 1966).

Strontium-90

Data on the levels of strontium-90 in milk from West Cumbria were published in Simmonds *et al.* (1995). Values for the United Kingdom were derived by dividing the published figures by a factor of 1.4, for the reasons given above. The results are shown in Figure 5.28.

Strontium-90 and calcium are laid down together in new bone. As a result, the amount of strontium-90 deposited in the bone depends on the ratio in which these two substances are present in the diet, not just the levels of strontium-90. Milk and milk products contributed about 60% of the strontium-90 and more than 70% of the calcium in the total diet during the period when fallout radiation was high. Other foods such as vegetables, cereals, and meat also contained appreciable levels of strontium-90 but their consumption had little overall effect on the levels deposited in the bone because they are relatively poor in calcium.

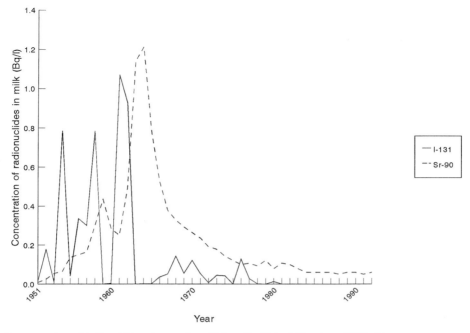

Figure 5.28   Concentration of iodine-131 and strontium-90 in milk, United Kingdom, 1951–94.

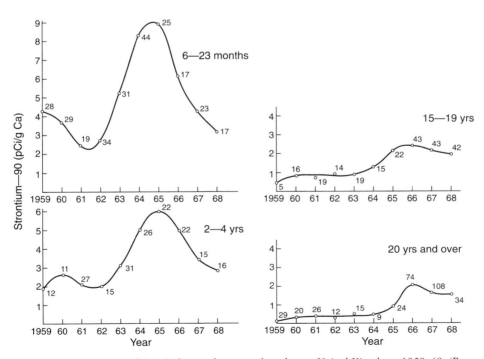

Figure 5.29   Ratio of strontium-90 to calcium in human bone at selected ages, United Kingdom, 1959–68. (Reproduced with permission from Medical Research Council 1969.) The numbers adjacent to the data points represent the numbers of samples on which the estimates are based.

Data on the mean ratio of strontium-90 to calcium in milk in England and Wales are available from Agricultural Research Council (1978) and National Radiological Protection Board (NRPB) (1980–94). These annual estimates were based on measurements in samples of milk collected throughout the year from more than 70 different depots in the country, which together handled over one-quarter of the total milk produced in the United Kingdom. The ratio of strontium-90 to calcium in milk increased in the late 1950s to a peak in 1962–4 (not shown). Thereafter, it declined as a result of the 1962 test ban treaty.

Strontium-90 levels in human bone paralleled the levels in the diet but the relationship varied by age. Young children had the highest concentrations because of the fast turnover in the bones during growth. Results of direct measurements of the levels of strontium-90 in human bones conducted in the United Kingdom from 1959 to 1968 (Medical Research Council 1960–70; Fletcher *et al.* 1966) are shown in Figure 5.29. The levels were highest at ages 6–23 months, but even at these ages, the mean levels were well below 67 pCi strontium-90/g calcium, the maximum permissible level for the general population established by the Medical Research Council (1964).

Estimated doses to the red bone marrow and the testis from nuclear weapons fallout

Estimates of annual doses to the red bone marrow and the testis from nuclear weapons fallout in Britain were extracted from Darby *et al.* (1992). The results are shown in Figure 5.30. The highest estimated doses to the red bone marrow of foetuses and 1-year-old children occurred in the late 1950s and mid 1960s. The estimated doses to the testes of adults followed a similar trend, although levels were lower than those estimated for the red bone marrow of young children.

Medical sources

The diagnostic use of X-rays in medicine involves a wide variety of techniques ranging from single radiographs of limbs to complex fluoroscopic investigations of the abdomen. Data on trends in radiation received from medical exposures in the UK are available from patient dose measurements collated by the National Patient Database at NRPB and from a national survey in 1983–5. Based on these data, it was estimated that the frequency of these examinations increased at an average rate of 2% per year between 1950 and the mid-1980s (Simmonds *et al.* 1995). A total of

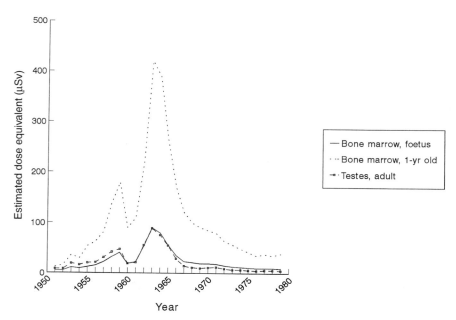

Figure 5.30   Estimated dose equivalent from nuclear weapons fallout to the red bone marrow of foetuses and 1-year-old children, and to the testes of adult men, Britain, 1951–79.

Table 5.11 Contributions to the annual collective dose from diagnostic X-ray examinations in the United Kingdom, 1991. (Data from Hughes and O'Riordan (1993))

Examination	% frequency	Collective dose in man Sv (% of total)
Computed tomography (CT scan)	2.4	4 400 (22)
Lumbar spine	3.3	3 000 (15)
Barium enema	0.9	2 800 (14)
Barium meal	1.6	2 400 (12)
Intravenous urography	1.3	2 200 (11)
Abdomen	2.9	1 600 (8)
Pelvis	2.9	1 200 (6)
Chest	24.0	400 (2)
Limbs and joints	25.0	300 (1.5)
Skull	5.6	300 (1.5)
Thoracic spine	0.9	200 (1)
Dental	25.0	200 (1)
Others	4.2	1 000 (5)
Total	100	20 000 (100)

35 million X-ray examinations per year were performed in the United Kingdom in 1983–5, representing an annual collective dose of about 16 000 man Sv from medical and dental conventional diagnostic radiology (Wall *et al.* 1986). Since then, there have been reductions in the numbers and doses of many radiological examinations, with many X-ray procedures being replaced by other diagnostic methods that do not involve ionizing radiation, such as ultrasound, endoscopy, and magnetic resonance imaging. Despite this, it is estimated that the collective dose from conventional techniques has remained unchanged at approximately 16 000 man Sv per year (Hughes and O'Riordan 1993).

This estimate of collective dose does not include a contribution from computed tomography (CT), the radiation doses from which are several times larger than those from conventional radiography. The number of CT examinations has increased markedly

since their introduction into clinical practice in 1972. In 1983 there was an average of two scanners per million population in the United Kingdom; the corresponding figure for 1993 was six (Shrimpton and Wall 1995). A total of 850 000 CT examinations were performed in 1989. It has been estimated that the collective dose from CT in the United Kingdom in 1991 was about 4400 man Sv (Table 5.11). Thus, the total collective dose from conventional radiography plus CT scans was then about 20 000 man Sv.

The number of nuclear medicine procedures has increased from 1974 to 1990 (Hughes and O'Riordan 1993). It has been estimated that 430 000 patients in the UK were administered radionuclides in 1990, yielding an average of 7.6 procedures per 1000 persons in the general population. The corresponding figure in 1982 was 6.8 per 1000. The annual collective dose from exposure to nuclear medicine procedures totalled 1400 man Sv in 1990. Thus, adding this to the dose

Table 5.12 Percentages (and numbers) of children X-rayed *in utero* by year of birth, British sample 1939–81, and Birmingham (England) 1964–81. (Data from Gilman *et al.* (1989))

Year of birth	Oxford Survey of Childhood Cancers (controls only)	Birmingham Births Register
1939–49	5.9 (113)	—
1950–9	11.9 (775)	—
1960–9/1964–9	11.3 (591)/11.7 (323)	—/9.4 (11 992)
1970–81	14.3 (233)	14.5 (26 034)
1964–81	12.7 (556)	12.4 (38 026)
1939–81	11.2 (1712)	—

— Data not available for these years.

from conventional radiography plus CT scans, the UK population received in 1990 an annual collective dose of about 21 400 man Sv from all medical exposures excluding radiotherapy. No dose estimates are available for the latter because of the complexities associated with the nature and circumstances of the exposure.

Prenatal X-rays

Table 5.12 shows data on the frequency of prenatal X-rays derived from the Oxford Survey of Childhood Cancers (OSCC) and the Birmingham Births Register (BBR) (Gilman *et al.* 1989). The OSCC was a national case-control study; the cases were all British children aged 0–15 years who died from cancer during 1953–81 and the controls were live children without cancer individually matched to the cases on age, sex, and place of residence. The information on obstetric X-rays was obtained by interviewing the mothers and examining records of family doctors, antenatal clinics, and radiologists. As the level of refusal in this study was low the controls may be regarded as a reasonably representative sample of all British children.

The BBR consisted of hospital notifications of births to residents in Birmingham (England), together with information on antenatal history (including X-rays) obtained from the records of the attending midwife or general practitioner.

The results from these two surveys are similar and show that the frequency of prenatal X-rays has not decreased over time, despite the introduction of ultrasound scans around 1970 and their widespread use since 1975 (Gilman *et al.* 1989). The only other national survey of diagnostic radiographic practices was carried out by the National Radiological Protection

Board (NRPB) during one week in 1977, and estimated the frequency of obstetric X-rays as 4.2% of all pregnancies (Kendall *et al.* 1980). This frequency is much lower than the 1977 estimates from the OSCC study (10.8%) and the BBR (17.1%). The reasons for this lower estimate are not clear, but since the NRPB survey did not specifically ask whether the woman was pregnant at the time of the radiological examination, it is possible that only examinations regarded as obstetric were counted as prenatal in this survey, whereas barium meal investigations or intravenous pyelograms, which represent a large proportion of X-rays in pregnant women, were not included. The NRPB has recently completed a survey of the frequency of X-ray examinations in Britain, which when published will give more recent data.

The timing of the X-ray examinations changed since the 1950s towards late pregnancy (Table 5.13), although there was a very low frequency during the first trimester for all the birth cohorts examined (1939–81). The average number of films per examination also declined since the 1950s. The exact average fetal dose per film is uncertain but estimates made for the period 1943–65 showed a decline (Doll and Wakeford 1997). The magnitude of the decline varied according to the assumptions underlying the various sets of estimates but at greatest it might have been from almost 20 mGy in 1943–9 to less than 5 mGy in 1960–5.

Occupational exposures

Table 5.14a shows radiation doses from occupational exposures in the United Kingdom in 1991. A total of 280 000 workers were occupationally exposed to radiation, with a collective dose of 430 man Sv. These

Table 5.13 Timing of prenatal X-rays and number of films per examination by year of birth of the irradiated children, British sample, 1939–81. (Data from Gilman *et al.* (1989))

Year of birth	% X-rayed per trimester			Total no of X-rays[a]	Mean number of films per examination in each trimester			All dated X-rays	Total no of X-rays[b]
	1st	2nd	3rd		1st	2nd	3rd		
1939–49	0.0	8.0	92.0	50	0.00	2.00	1.74	1.77	43
1950–9	1.5	9.3	89.2	536	5.50	2.65	2.00	2.10	458
1960–9	1.1	4.1	94.9	370	3.67	1.20	1.36	1.38	322
1970–81	1.1	3.4	95.4	177	5.00	1.33	1.37	1.39	163
1939–81	1.2	6.6	92.1	1133	4.90	2.19	1.67	1.73	986

[a] Only dated X-rays.
[b] Only dated X-rays with known number of films.

Table 5.14(a)　Overall radiation doses from occupational exposures, United Kingdom, 1991. (Data from Hughes and O'Riordan (1993))

Type of exposure	Total no. of potentially exposed workers	Number of workers in dose range (mSv)[a]				Annual collective dose (man Sv)
		0–5	5–15	15–50	>50	
Nuclear	44 237	42 052	2178	7	0	45.2
Defence	12 565	12 103	450	12	0	9.8
General industry	25 000	24 550	400	50	<10	11.0
Research, education[b]	10 000	10 000	0	0	0	1.0
Medicine						
Medical[b]	40 000	39 950	50	0	0	5.0
Dental[b]	20 000	20 000	0	0	0	2.0
Veterinary[b]	4000	4000	0	0	0	0.4
Natural						
Coal mines	48 669	48 600	59	10	0	28.6
Non-coal mines	1347	1019	88	237	<10	6.1
Other workplaces[b,c]	50 000	32 000	16 000	2500	<100	270
Aircrew[b]	24 000	24 000	0	0	0	50
Total (rounded)	280 000	258 000	20 000	2500	<100	430

[a] Dose ranges as in original publication

[b] Dose distribution estimated from a sample. Where a zero is indicated a few workers might receive annual doses in the relevant range.

[c] Exposures from increased radon concentrations in premises subject to regulatory practices.

Table 5.14(b)　Annual dose for classified workers with non-zero doses, United Kingdom, 1986, 1991, 1996. (Data from Health and Safety Executive (1993, 1997))

Dose category	Year 1986	1991	1996
Collective dose in man Sv	127	59.4	36.7
No. with doses >5 mSv	6579	2958	1510
No. with doses >10 mSv	3407	643	328
No. with doses >20 mSv	1032	78	132

exposures contributed 7 μSv a year to the average dose of the whole population of the United Kingdom. The most significant source of occupational exposure was natural radiation, with a collective dose of around 300 man Sv. Collective doses from other types of occupational exposure, including those in medical related jobs and in the nuclear industry, were comparatively low.

The Central Index of Dose Information held by the Health and Safety Executive holds records since 1986 of systematic ionizing radiation dose assessments made for employees who are 'classified' under the Ionizing Radiation Regulations of 1985 (HSE 1993, 1997). Table 5.14b shows collective doses for all persons on whom data were collected under the scheme, and numbers of persons exceeding certain levels of dose in 1986, 1991, and 1996. The collective dose has diminished more than three-fold, while even greater decreases have occurred in the numbers of workers receiving relatively high doses.

Medical drugs

Anti-inflammatory drugs

The total number of prescriptions (i.e. excluding preparations sold over the counter) in the United Kingdom for non-steroidal anti-inflammatory drugs (NSAIDs) other than aspirin increased from 7.6 million in 1967 to 22 million in 1985 (Walt *et al.* 1986) (Figure 5.31).

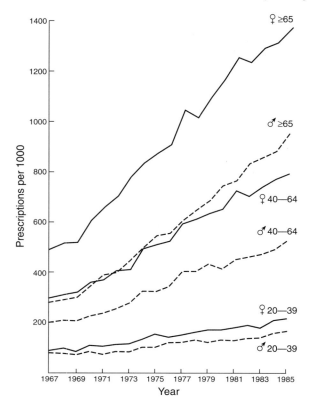

Figure 5.31   Age-specific prescription rates for non-steroidal anti-inflammatory drugs (excluding aspirin), by sex, United Kingdom, 1967–85. (Reproduced with permission from Walt *et al.* 1986. © by the Lancet Ltd.)

Hormone replacement therapy

There are no data available on national trends in the use of hormone replacement therapy (HRT) in England and Wales. The Health Surveys for England collected data on type of prescribed medicines. They noted a much greater proportion of women than men taking medicines prescribed for the endocrine system. Twenty-six per cent of women aged 45–64 were taking this group of medicines in 1995 (Prior and Di Salvo 1997), which may have been largely the result of women receiving HRT.

In a recent survey (Banks *et al.* 1996), 30% of the women aged 50–64 years attending the Oxfordshire NHS breast screening programme reported being current users of HRT, 43% being ever-users, and 14% having used HRT for five or more years. There were marked age differences in HRT use (Table 5.15), which were consistent with a possible cohort effect of increasing use among more recent generations of women.

Table 5.15   Prevalence of use of hormone replacement therapy by age among women attending the breast screening programme, Oxfordshire, 1995. (Data from Banks *et al.* (1996))

Age-group (years)	Current use % (number)	Ever use % (number)
50–54	38 (194)	51 (258)
55–59	31 (120)	46 (180)
60–64	17 (61)	28 (102)
Total	29 (375)	43 (540)

Similarly high prevalences of HRT use have been found in surveys conducted among other groups of women in England (Isaacs *et al.* 1995; Griffiths and Convery 1995).

Oestrogens taken during pregnancy

On the basis of a questionnaire sent to gynaecologists in 1973, it has been estimated by Kinlen *et al.* (1974) that about 7500 women in the United Kingdom were treated with diethylstilboestrol during pregnancy in 1940–71, mainly during the 1950s, and a further 4500 women were treated with other or unspecified oestrogens during pregnancy, mainly during the 1960s. Use decreased greatly soon after the publication of the findings on risk of vaginal adenocarcinoma in the offspring, but did not cease completely, and there was still some use until at least the mid-1980s (I. Chalmers and A. Alment personal communications).

Oral contraceptives

Statistics on oral contraceptive (OC) use were obtained from Wiseman (1984), Royal College of General Practitioners (1986), and Thorogood and Vessey (1990). OCs were introduced in the United Kingdom in 1960 and their use grew rapidly thereafter. The cumulative proportions of 'ever-users' for successive generations of women rose from about 40 per cent for women born in the 1930s, to about 70 per cent for women born in the 1940s, and 80–90 per cent for those born in the 1950s and 1960s (Figure 5.32).

In the earlier cohorts, women started using the pill late in their reproductive life, mainly for birth spacing after marriage. Only in the most recent cohorts did the pill become a popular method of contraception at young ages. As a consequence, only in cohorts born

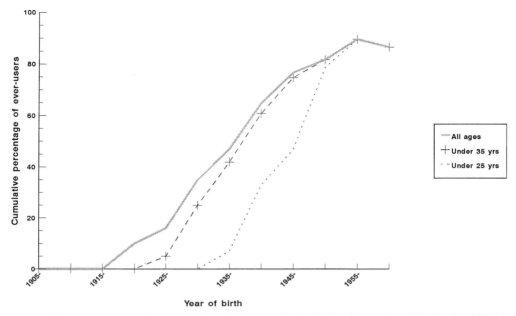

Figure 5.32 Cumulative percentage of ever-users of oral contraceptives by birth cohort and age, England and Wales.

after the 1930s were there appreciable numbers of women who were exposed to oral contraceptives early in life (Figure 5.32). The proportion of women who were OC users in the United Kingdom increased from 7% in 1972 to 28% in 1987 at ages 15–19 years and from 37% in 1976 to 45% in 1987 among those aged 20–29 (Thorogood and Vessey 1990); these increases at young ages might reflect both a rise in the proportion of women starting OC use young and in duration of use.

Mobile telephones

The numbers of cellular telephone subscribers in the United Kingdom by calendar year (Mobile Communications 1996–9) are shown in Figure 5.33. Although subscribers cannot precisely be equated with users—a person may subscribe to more than one company, and several people may use a telephone for which there is a single subscription—they give the best available data on trends in mobile telephone use.

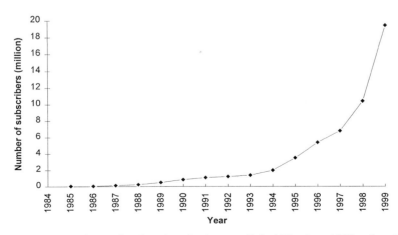

Figure 5.33 Number of cellular telephone subscribers by calendar year, United Kingdom, 1985 to June 1998.

Organ transplantation

Organ transplants at centres in England and Wales are reported to the National Transplant Database at the United Kingdom Transplant Support Service Authority (UKTSSA). The data are believed to be virtually complete since 1984, and are shown for this period in Figure 5.34.

Renal transplantation started in the United Kingdom in the early 1960s; in 1972 there were 438 transplants recorded by the UKTSSA in the United Kingdom and the Republic of Ireland, with numbers continuing to rise after this. The data for England and Wales in Figure 5.34a show an increase up to the late 1980s, but not thereafter.

Although the first cardiac transplant in the United Kingdom was in 1968, substantial numbers of heart and lung transplants occurred only after 1984. Numbers increased until 1990, but have changed little since (Figure 5.34a). The first liver transplant programme in the United Kingdom started in 1983, and numbers of transplants have increased steadily since (Figure 5.34a).

Almost all organ transplants in England and Wales are accounted for by transplantation of the organs discussed above; there have also been a few pancreatic transplants, which are not included in the Figure.

Examining trends by age (for renal, cardiac, lung, and liver transplants combined), relatively few transplants occurred in children, and very few over age

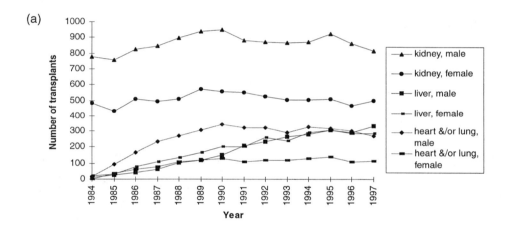

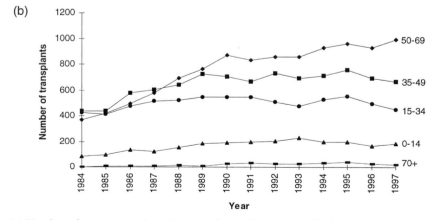

Figure 5.34   (a) Number of organ transplants by type of transplant, sex, and calendar year, England and Wales, 1984–97. (b) Number of renal, heart, lung, and liver transplants by age and calendar year, England and Wales, 1984–97.

70 years (Figure 5.34b). The number of transplants in children and at ages 50–69 has more than doubled since 1984, with lesser increases at ages 15–49, and 70 and over.

Outdoor occupations

The proportions of men and women employed in farming and of men employed in fishing from 1891 to 1991, as recorded at successive censuses, are shown in Table 5.16. Although these are not the only outdoor occupations, they are important ones whose numbers can readily be compared over time. The proportion of farmers declined markedly in men but has remained relatively stable (although low) in women. The proportion of fishermen declined (data are not presented for women because there were very few women in this occupational group).

Overcrowding

At the 1891 census, 8% of the population lived at a density of more than two people per room. This proportion declined to less than 6% in 1901, remained constant for the first two decades of the twentieth

Table 5.17   Average number of persons per room, England and Wales, 1921–91. (Data from Census of England and Wales (1921, 1931), Registrar General (1951, 1966b), OPCS (1975b, 1983c), OPCS and Registrar General for Scotland (1993a))

Year	Average number of persons per room
1921	0.91
1931	0.83
1951	0.74
1961	0.66
1971	0.59
1981	0.54
1991	0.48

century, and then fell from 1931 onwards, reaching a value of 1.5% in 1951.

Data on the average number of persons per room are available in the censuses for 1921 onwards (Census of England and Wales 1921, 1931; Registrar General 1951, 1966b; OPCS 1975b, 1983c; OPCS and Registrar General for Scotland 1993a). The number has declined markedly over time (Table 5.17).

Physical exercise

Data on physical activity have been collected by the Health Surveys for England since the first survey in 1991 (Gray 1996). The most recent data available are for 1994, so that there is as yet a very short period for which information is available. Level of physical activity was estimated from information on the time spent being active, the intensity of the activity undertaken, and its frequency. Informants were classified to one of six physical activity levels (0–5) on the basis of their reported participation in different activities in the four weeks before interview. Table 5.18 shows trends in level of physical activity. When interpreting these trends it should be noted that changes in the questionnaire were introduced in 1993, which led to a reduced proportion of people being classified to level 3 and above.

Information on involvement of adults in certain sports and other recreational physical activities has been collected by the General Household Survey (ONS 1998b) since 1987 and indicates slight increases in the proportion of adults participating in these particular activities from 1987 to 1990, but not subsequently up to 1996.

Table 5.16   Percentage of men employed in farming and fishing, and of women employed in farming, England and Wales, 1891–1991. (Data from Census of England and Wales (1893, 1911, 1924, 1934), Registrar General (1956, 1966a), OPCS and Registrar General for Scotland (1975, 1984, 1994a))

Year	Farmers (male)	Fishermen	Farmers (female)
1891[a]	11.9	0.24	0.45
1911[a]	8.4	0.18	0.64
1921[b]	8.4	0.21	0.53
1931[c]	7.6	0.18	0.34
1951[d]	6.0	0.09	0.54
1961[d]	4.4	0.08	0.42
1971[d]	3.2	0.10	0.45
1981[e]	1.5	0.04	0.26
1991[e]	0.60[f]		0.20[f]

[a] Persons aged 10+ years.
[b] Persons aged 12+ years.
[c] Persons aged 14+ years.
[d] Persons aged 15+ years.
[e] Persons aged 16+ years.
[f] Fishermen plus farmers: data not available for these occupations separately.

Table 5.18 Trends in level of physical activity (including activities at home and at work, walking, and participating in sports), England, 1991–4. (Data from Gray (1996))

Year (no. in sample)	Age (years) All	25–34	55–64
Men: Percentage in activity levels 3, 4, 5[a]			
1991 (1492)	49	59	41
1992 (1868)	48	61	45
1993 (7689)	47	58	38
1994 (7177)	49	62	40
Women: Percentage in activity levels 3, 4, 5[a]			
1991 (1750)	42	51	43
1992 (2150)	41	48	39
1993 (8880)	36	42	35
1994 (8627)	38	49	36
Men: Percentage in activity level 0[b]			
1991 (1492)	19	8	28
1992 (1868)	18	12	21
1993 (7689)	18	8	24
1994 (7177)	17	8	24
Women: Percentage in activity level 0[b]			
1991 (1750)	21	12	20
1992 (2150)	20	9	20
1993 (8880)	20	9	19
1994 (8627)	19	8	18

[a] Moderate or vigorous exercise on 12 or more occasions per week.
[b] No moderate or vigorous exercise per week.

Population mobility

Although data are not available on all movements of residence, the censuses for 1971 onwards have published data on whether individuals lived in the same local authority area or district one year before the census. The data are shown in Table 5.19. The 1961 census asked a similar question but data are not available on the same basis.

Power-frequency magnetic fields

Average population exposures in England and Wales to power-frequency magnetic fields have been esti-mated by Swanson (1996), aggregating information on exposures to various sources, the principal of which are residential background fields, appliances in homes, and overhead electricity transmission. The data show a 4.5-fold increase in population exposure over the period 1949–89 (Figure 5.35), and Swanson thought that if anything this underestimated the true increase. He considered that the same degree of increase applied to children as to the general population.

Reproductive-related variables

Age at first birth

Information on age at first birth for women born since 1920 was extracted from ONS (1997). Such data are

Table 5.19 Proportion of people aged 1 year and over who did not live in the same local authority area/district one year before the census, England and Wales, 1971–91. (Data from OPCS and Registrar General for Scotland (1974, 1983, 1994b))

Year	Living in another area in England and Wales	Living in another area of England and Wales, or Scotland or outside Great Britain
1971	5.4	6.0
1981	3.4	4.0
1991	3.3	4.0

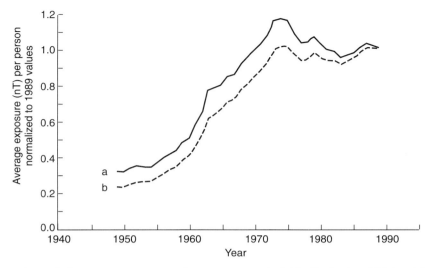

Figure 5.35 Estimated population exposure to power-frequency magnetic fields, England and Wales: (a) calculated from domestic electricity demand per consumer; (b) calculated by adding estimates of exposure from different types of exposure source (e.g. residential background, appliances), 1949–89. (Reproduced with permission from Swanson (1996).)

not available for women born earlier, and therefore as a proxy for this in cohorts born from 1875 to 1919 we calculated fertility rates of women at young ages, from cross-sectional data extracted from Registrar General (1947) and OPCS (1974*a*). For women born after 1919, cohort fertility rates were extracted from ONS (1997).

The mean age at first birth declined from 25.5 years for women born in 1920 to 23.8 years for those born in 1945, but has since risen (Figure 5.36a). The proportion of women having their first birth at ages under 25 increased from 40% for women born in 1920 to 60% for women born in 1945, but has since decreased markedly (Figure 5.36b). For first birth at ages under 20, the pattern was similar but with a later peak in 1952 and with an upturn also since 1966.

Figure 5.37 shows trends in fertility at young ages (as a proxy for age at first birth) for successive generations of women born since 1875. There was a decrease until women born early in the twentieth century, and then an increase. The subsequent pattern was similar to that described for age at first birth. Although there was a substantial increase in the rate of birth to teenage mothers among women born in the 1940s and 1950s, these represented a small group and their contribution to the overall fertility at young ages was outweighed by the declines in fertility at ages 20–29.

Age at menarche

The age at menarche of women in the United Kingdom declined considerably from 1860 to 1960 (Marshall and Tanner 1986). This decline was particularly marked among working-class women (Figure 5.38). Various surveys conducted across the United Kingdom during the first half of the nineteenth century showed that the age at menarche ranged from 14.9 to 15.6 years among working-class women and 14.0 to 14.5 years among middle-class women (Tanner 1981). However, recent surveys conducted among university students in Warwick (Dann and Roberts 1993) suggest that the downward trend may have ceased for cohorts born since the mid 1950s (Table 5.20).

Age at menopause

Age at natural menopause appears to have remained relatively constant at an average of approximately 50 years since the nineteenth century (McKinlay *et al.* 1972). The proportion of women who have had an artificial menopause has increased from about 1% for those born at the turn of the twentieth century to about 5% for those born in the late 1930s (McKinlay *et al.* 1972).

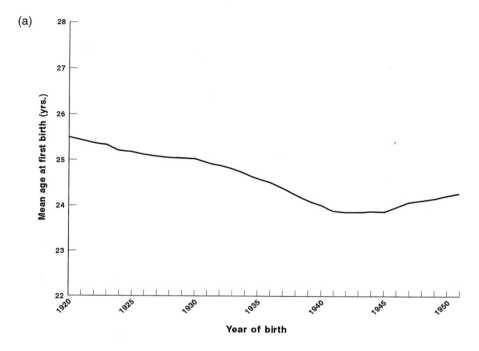

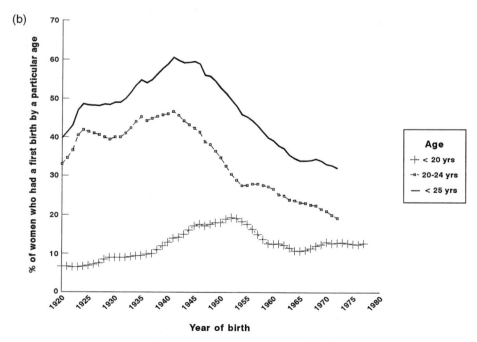

Figure 5.36   Age at first birth, England and Wales, cohorts of women born 1920–77. (a) Mean age at first birth (not available for the most recent cohorts because they have not yet completed their reproductive years). (b) Proportion of women who had a first birth by certain ages.

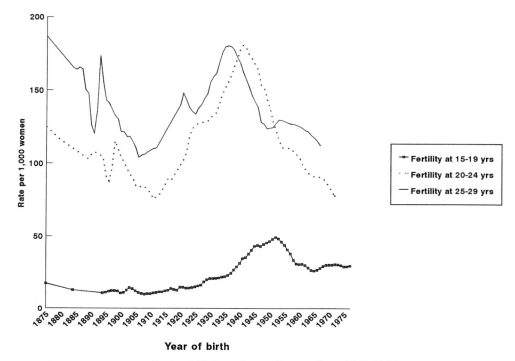

Figure 5.37 Fertility at young ages, England and Wales, cohorts of women born 1875–1977.

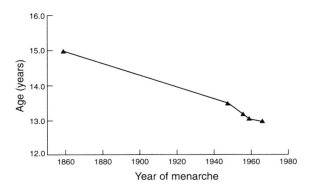

Figure 5.38 Trends in age at menarche among working-class women, United Kingdom, 1860–1960s. (Modified with permission from Marshall and Tanner (1986).)

Table 5.20 Trends in age at menarche, students at University of Warwick (England), 1971–85. (Data from Dann and Roberts (1993))

Year	Mean year of birth	Age at menarche (years) (mean (SD))
1971	1952	12.73 (1.25)
1975	1956	12.71 (1.23)
1980	1961	12.81 (1.28)
1985	1965	12.96 (1.29)

Breastfeeding

Figure 5.39 shows trends in breastfeeding practices in England and Wales in the twentieth century based on various national and regional surveys. The percentage of mothers breastfeeding at 3 months declined from 1920 to 1970, but increased markedly from 1970 to 1986.

Table 5.21 shows data from various national surveys conducted since 1946 (Douglas 1950; Davie *et al.*

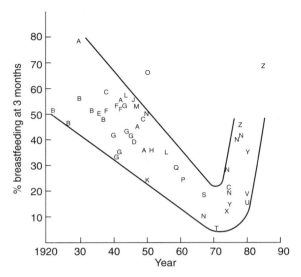

Figure 5.39 Proportions of mothers breastfeeding at 3 months in England and Wales, 1920–86. (Reproduced with permission from Whitehead and Paul (1987); see this paper for reference to individual studies indicated by letters in the Figure.)

1972; Golding and Butler 1986; Charlton and Quaife 1997). The proportion of mothers breastfeeding declined up to 1970, but has since recovered.

Family size

Data on childbearing by women in England and Wales were obtained from various sources. Average completed family sizes for successive cohorts of women born before 1920 were calculated from data on family

size (Registrar General 1960) and mean age at marriage (OPCS 1972b) for successive marriage cohorts, adjusting for the proportion of women in each cohort who remained single by age 40–44 (OPCS and Registrar General for Scotland 1993b), and who were considered as childless[2]. Average completed family size data for generations of women (irrespective of marital status) born from 1920 onwards were extracted from ONS (1997). Because the most recent cohorts were still at childbearing ages, their completed family size could not be computed, and instead we therefore extracted from ONS (1997) data on family size achieved by the age of 30 for cohorts born after 1919.

Average completed family size fell from 3.3 children per woman born in 1875 to 1.9 per woman born in 1910 (Figure 5.40). For women born from 1920 to the mid-1930s, however, family size increased from 2.0 to 2.4. Since the 1935 cohort, family size has again declined, and although the most recent cohorts are still at childbearing ages, their family size achieved by age 30 is lower than in previous cohorts.

Nulliparity

Nulliparity by age 40 for successive cohorts born before 1930 was calculated from data on the proportion of childless women and age at marriage for successive marriage cohorts (Glass and Grebenik 1954), adjusting for the proportion of women who were still single by age 40–44 (OPCS and Registrar General for Scotland 1993b) and who were regarded as childless. Nulliparity in generations of women born after 1919 (irrespective of marital status) was calculated from data in ONS (1997). Nulliparity more than halved from

Table 5.21 Percentages of mothers breastfeeding at birth and subsequent intervals, England and Wales, 1946–90. (Data from Douglas (1950), Davie *et al.* (1972), Golding and Butler (1986), and Charlton and Quaife (1997))

Time since birth	1946	1958	1970	1975	1980	1985	1990
Birth	—	68	37	51	67	65	64
4 weeks	65	43	20.9	—	—	—	—
6 weeks	—	—	—	—	42	40	39
3 months	44	—	10.9	—	—	—	—
6 months	31	—	—	—	23	21	21
9 months	12	—	—	—	12	11	12
Sample size	4669	15 360	12 981	1544	3755	4671	4942

[2] This assumption should not have affected the estimates appreciably because more than 95% of the births that occurred until the 1960s were legitimate (OPCS 1978).

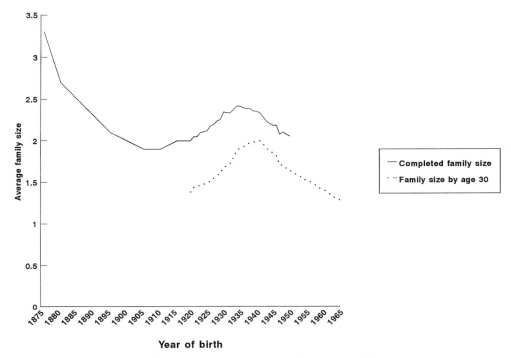

Figure 5.40 Family size by age, England and Wales, cohorts of women born 1875–1965.

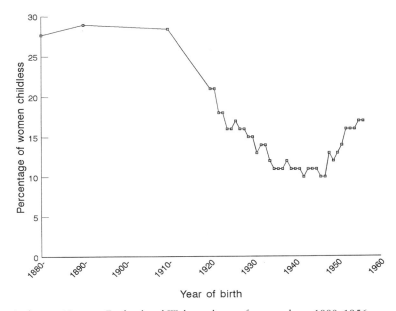

Figure 5.41 Nulliparity by age 40 years, England and Wales, cohorts of women born 1880–1956.

women born around 1910 to those born in 1935, but increased for cohorts born after 1947 (Figure 5.41). The cohorts born since 1956 are still at childbearing ages, but the proportion of women remaining childless at each age has risen progressively (Coleman 1993).

Screening

National screening programmes have been conducted in England and Wales for cancers of the breast and cervix.

Breast

The first population-based breast screening programme in England and Wales began in Guildford, Surrey as part of a trial to assess the value of this intervention in reducing mortality from breast cancer; it lasted from 1979–86 (UK Trial of Early Detection of Breast Cancer Group 1988). The United Kingdom breast screening programme was established in 1988 and aims to offer all women aged 50–64 years screening by mammography every three years. Women aged 65 years and over are not routinely invited for screening, but may attend at their own request. Results of the screening programme since 1990–1 have been published. During 1991–3, a total of 4061 402 women were invited for screening and 2865 474 accepted (acceptance rate = 70.6%) (Moss *et al.* 1995); the acceptance rate in 1996/97 was 75.2% (NHSBSP 1998). The results of the prevalent round (first screening of women) and incident rounds (subsequent screenings of the same women) of screenings performed since 1990–1 are shown in Table 5.22.

Cervix

The national cervical screening programme began in 1964. The target for the programme is that women aged 25–64 years should be screened at least once every 5 years (5.5 years before 1995). The number of smears taken in England and Wales increased rapidly at first and then more slowly, from about 0.7 million in 1965 to 2.9 million in 1980 and 4.5 million in 1995/6 (Roberts 1982; Department of Health 1994–9; Welsh Cervical Screening Office 1994–9) (Figure 5.42). The number of positive smears (classified cytologically as 'severe dysplasia/carcinoma *in situ*' or 'carcinoma *in situ*/?invasive') also increased markedly since the early 1970s (Figure 5.43).

Figure 5.44 shows the coverage of cervical screening from 1976 to 1997/8 (Central Statistical Office 1993; Department of Health 1994–9; Welsh Cervical Screening Office 1994–9). In the earlier years, coverage was expressed as numbers of smears in relation to numbers of women aged 15 years and over. Since 1989, coverage has been evaluated as the proportion of

Table 5.22   Results from the breast screening programme, women aged 50 years and over, United Kingdom, 1990–7. (Data from Moss *et al.* (1995) and NHSBSP (1998))

Year	Number screened	Referred No.	%	Biopsied No.	%	Cancers detected No.	Rate per 1000	In situ/ micro- invasive (rate per 1000)	Invasive cancer ≤10 mm (rate per 1000)
Prevalent screen									
1990–1	665 497	46 130	6.9	6038	0.9	3747	5.6	1.2	1.1
1991–2	957 946	61 796	6.5	8601	0.9	5975	6.2	1.0	1.4
1992–3	912 173	54 000	5.9	7672	0.8	5368	5.9	1.1	1.3
Total	2 535 616	161 926	6.4	22 311	0.9	15 090	6.0	1.1	1.3
Incident screen									
1990–1	12 474	528	4.2	53	0.4	43	3.4	0.6	1.2
1991–2	70 615	2112	3.1	334	0.5	242	3.4	0.6	0.7
1992–3	205 512	6159	3.0	963	0.5	813	4.0	0.7	0.9
Total	228 601	8799	3.0	1350	0.5	1098	3.8	0.6	0.8
Prevalent and incident screen[a]									
1993–4	1 209 290	63 995	5.3	9188	0.8	6695	5.5	—	—
1994–5	1 207 316	63 925	5.3	6334	0.5	6500	5.4	1.1	2.2[b]
1995–6	1 222 389	62 682	5.1	—	—	6664	6.3	1.1	2.3[b]
1996–7	1 268 236	66 333	5.2	—	—	7141	5.6	1.1	2.5[b]

[a] Not available separately for prevalent and incident in these years
[b] < 15 mm
— Data not available.

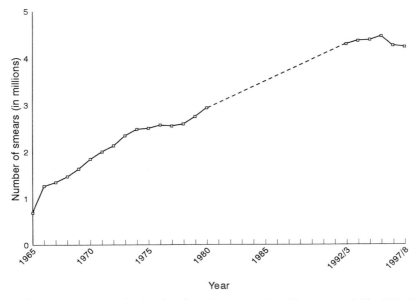

Figure 5.42 Numbers of cervical smears, England and Wales, 1965–80, 1992–8 (data not available 1981–91).

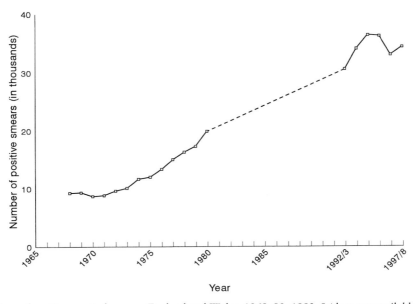

Figure 5.43 Numbers of positive cervical smears, England and Wales, 1968–80, 1992–8 (data not available 1981–91).

women aged 25–64 (minus those whose recall ceased) who have had a test at least once in the previous 5.5 years (or 5 years since 1995). Coverage increased slowly in the earlier years, from 13.3% in 1976 to 21.5% in 1989, but (on the different measure then employed) doubled from 44% in 1989 to 86% in 1993, and then stabilized.

Sexual behaviour

Data on sexual attitudes and lifestyle are available from a random sample survey undertaken among 18 896 men and women aged 16–59 years in Great Britain in 1990–1 (Johnson *et al.* 1994). By considering the responses of different age groups, one can assess

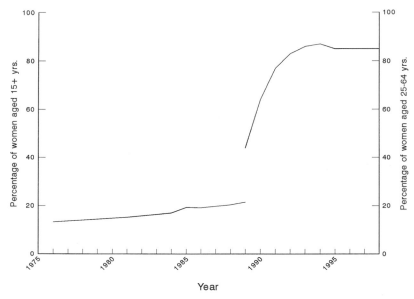

Figure 5.44   Coverage of cervical screening, Great Britain, 1976–89 and England and Wales, 1989–98.

the behaviour of different generations (although not entirely comparably, because the age at which these cohorts were questioned differed, and there may be differences between the cohorts in willingness to reveal, or in propensity to exaggerate or understate, sexual behaviour).

Age at first intercourse

The median age at first heterosexual intercourse has fallen considerably for successive generations of men and women born since the early 1930s (Table 5.23). This decline was paralleled by an increase in the pro-

portion having first intercourse before the age of 16 years (not in Table). Approximately 19% of women born in 1971–5, but fewer than 1% of those born in 1931–5, reported that they had experienced sexual intercourse before the age of 16. For men the equivalent proportions were higher—28% of men born in the most recent cohort compared with 6% of men born in 1931–5 (Johnson *et al.* 1994).

Number of sexual partners

Table 5.24 shows data from the same source on numbers of sexual partners by sex and age. Young

Table 5.23   Median age at first heterosexual intercourse for successive generations of men and women, Britain, 1990–1. (Data from Johnson *et al.* (1994))

| Age at the time of the survey | Estimated year of birth | Sample size | Median (interquartile range) age at first intercourse (years) | |
			Men	Women
55–59	1931–5	1623	20 (18–23)	21 (19–23)
50–54	1936–40	1618	19 (17–22)	20 (18–22)
45–49	1941–5	1750	18 (16–21)	19 (18–21)
40–44	1946–50	2249	18 (16–20)	19 (17–21)
35–39	1951–5	2431	18 (16–20)	18 (17–20)
30–34	1956–60	2691	17 (16–19)	18 (16–19)
25–29	1961–5	2885	17 (16–19)	18 (16–19)
20–24	1966–70	2087	17 (15–18)	17 (16–18)
16–19	1971–5	1255	17 (15–19)	17 (16–19)

people tended to report a larger number of recent partners than did older people. In part this may be a genuine age effect, with people having more partners at younger ages, but in part at least it appears to represent a generational ('cohort') effect in sexual behaviour, because the data on lifetime number of partners show greater numbers for those aged 25–44 than those aged 45–59, despite the shorter period the former have yet had to form sexual partnerships.

Sexually transmitted diseases

Since 1916, consultants in charge of genitourinary medicine clinics in England and Wales have been required to make annual returns to the Department of Health on the number of certain sexually transmitted diseases seen in their clinics. Data on numbers of new cases of gonorrhoea and syphilis were obtained from the Communicable Disease Surveillance Centre (CDSC).

Gonorrhoea

The number of new cases of gonorrhoea seen in genitourinary medicine clinics in England and Wales from 1918–97 is shown in Figure 5.45. There was a sudden increase in the number of cases seen around the Second World War followed by a rapid decline in the 1950s, probably due to the introduction and widespread use of penicillin. This downward trend was reversed in the

1960s and 1970s, probably because of changes in sexual behaviour and decreased use of barrier techniques, such as the condom, with the increased use of the oral contraceptive pill and intrauterine devices. However, it is not clear whether this increase was entirely a consequence of increased gonorrhoea incidence. During this period there were marked improvements in the services offered by the clinics, greater ability to trace sexual contacts, and reduction in the social stigma associated with sexually acquired infections; thus, people might have sought treatment who would not have done so previously. The increase in reported gonorrhoea in the 1960s and 1970s was followed by a decline in the 1980s, probably due to changes in sexual behaviour consequent on the epidemic of HIV infection and AIDS (Evans *et al.* 1993).

Syphilis

There was a large rise in the number of cases of syphilis seen at clinics during the 1940s followed by a marked decline when antibiotics became available (Figure 5.46). In the 1970s there was a small rise in men but not in women. This sex difference in trends occurred mainly because most cases of primary and secondary syphilis (58%) were in homosexual men (Evans *et al.* 1993). However, as with gonorrhoea, there has since been a decline in the number of cases of syphilis seen in clinics in England and Wales as a result of changing sexual practices with the advent of HIV infection and AIDS.

Table 5.24 Reported number of heterosexual partners by sex and age at interview, Britain, 1990–1: percentages of respondents of each age-group. (Data from Johnson *et al.* (1994))

	Men 16–24	25–34	35–44	45–59	Women 16–24	25–34	35–44	45–59
Last 5 years								
0	20.6	4.6	4.5	5.7	20.8	3.1	3.3	11.3
1–2	31.9	64.1	82.0	87.0	49.4	81.9	91.4	86.8
3–4	20.2	15.9	7.5	4.7	16.9	10.3	4.3	1.7
5–9	16.1	9.6	4.2	1.9	10.5	3.8	0.9	0.2
10+	11.2	5.8	1.7	0.7	2.5	0.8	0.2	0.04
Lifetime								
0	20.4	3.1	1.9	1.5	20.7	2.1	0.7	1.5
1–2	26.1	24.2	31.2	43.1	41.7	49.1	58.4	74.3
3–4	19.4	18.2	17.1	18.9	18.8	22.5	18.5	12.9
5–9	17.9	23.1	20.9	15.8	14.1	16.7	13.9	7.4
10+	16.2	31.4	28.9	20.8	4.6	9.7	8.5	3.8
No. of respondents	1984	2167	2051	2182	2246	2899	2576	2771

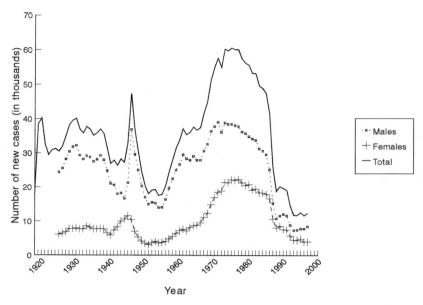

Figure 5.45   Numbers of new cases of gonorrhoea seen at genitourinary medicine clinics, England and Wales, 1918–97.

Smoking

Data on trends in smoking are available from Lee (1976), Mitchell (1988), Wald *et al.* (1988), Lee *et al.* (1990), and Wald and Nicolaides-Bouman (1991).

Secular

Consumption of tobacco by men increased slightly from 1870 to 1910, greatly from then to the mid-1940s, and has declined since (Figure 5.47a). Smoking of manufac-

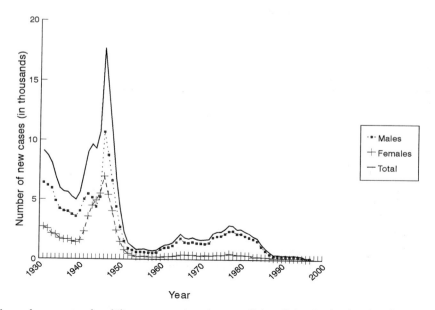

Figure 5.46   Numbers of new cases of syphilis seen at genitourinary medicine clinics, England and Wales, 1931–97.

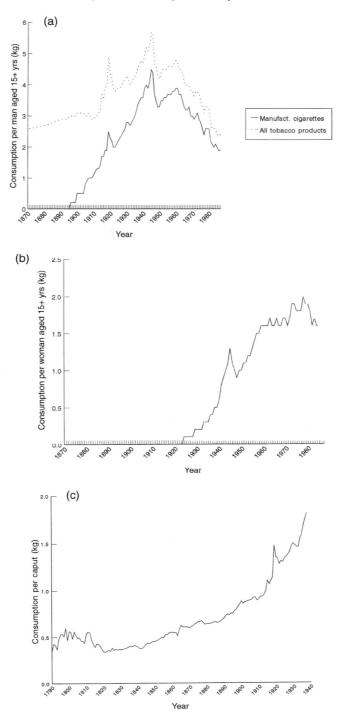

Figure 5.47 Annual consumption of tobacco goods in the United Kingdom: (a) manufactured cigarettes and all tobacco products by men, 1870–1987; (b) manufactured cigarettes by women, 1870–1987; (c) per caput (both sexes, all ages) consumption of all tobacco products, 1790–1938.

tured cigarettes by men began in the 1890s, reached a peak in 1946, and then decreased. In 1871 the tobacco was used for pipe and cigar smoking, as snuff, and for chewing, but by 1906, 30% of all tobacco consumed by men was in manufactured cigarettes. This proportion increased steadily to 80% in 1945, and has changed little since then (Wald and Nicolaides-Bouman 1991). In women, consumption of manufactured cigarettes started only in the mid-1920s and peaked in the late 1970s (Figure 5.47b). No data were collected on consumption by women of other tobacco products; very few women would have consumed them. Trends in per caput consumption of tobacco for an earlier period (1790–1938, both sexes) are shown in Figure 5.47c; these earlier trends mainly reflect consumption by men.

Comparable data to those in Figure 5.47 are not available after 1985, but since then the number of ciga-

rettes 'released for home consumption' (i.e. on which excise duty was paid) has decreased from 102.3 thousand million in 1987 to 83.3 thousand million in 1996, and there were large percentage decreases in releases of other tobacco products (ONS 1998c). In the last few years, however, there have also been substantial private imports (without duty paid) from the European Community.

Consumption of manufactured cigarettes by age is shown in Figure 5.48. The data for the years before 1946 are based on an estimation made by Lee *et al.* (1990) using an age-cohort model, because no data on age distribution of consumption had been collected at the time. In men there were marked increases in all age groups from 1891 to 1945. Consumption has since stabilized or declined at ages under 65 years, whereas at older ages the rise continued until more recently

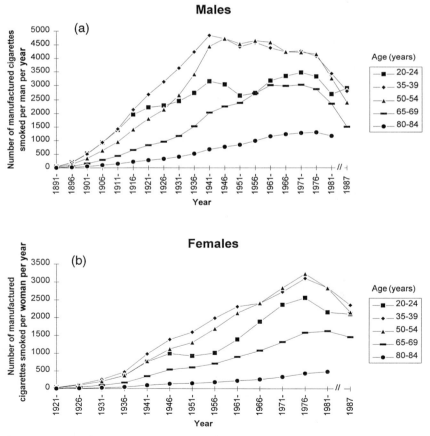

Figure 5.48 Annual consumption of manufactured cigarettes by age, United Kingdom: (a) men, 1891–1987; (b) women, 1921–87. (For clarity, only selected age groups are shown.). 1987 data not available for ages 80–84.

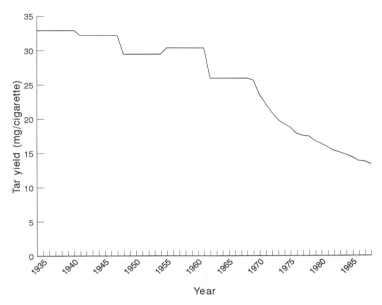

Figure 5.49   Mean per cigarette sales-weighted tar yield of manufactured cigarettes, United Kingdom, 1934–88.

before falling (Figure 5.48a). In women, consumption rose substantially from 1921 to 1976 at all ages, and declined thereafter except at ages 60 and over (Figure 5.48b). Tar yields of manufactured cigarettes declined slightly from 1935 to the early 1960s and have since fallen markedly (Figure 5.49).

The proportion of the population who were ex-smokers increased from 1956 to 1996 in both males and females, particularly in older age-groups (Table 5.25).

The percentage of men aged 16 years and over who smoked pipes decreased steadily from 14% in 1961 to 5% in 1987 (Table 5.26).

Cohort

Figures 5.50 and 5.51 show cohort trends in smoking based on data for 1891–1985 for men and 1921–85 for women from Lee *et al.* (1990). In Figure 5.50 the estimated actual numbers of cigarettes consumed are shown, and in Figure 5.51 these numbers are weighted to give constant tar estimates, allowing for decreases in tar yield of cigarettes over time. Consumption of cigarettes reached a peak in men born in about 1901–21 and has since declined, especially if the figures are weighted for tar. The peak was reached in slightly

Table 5.25   Percentages of men and women who are ex-smokers[a], by age, Great Britain[b], 1956–96 (Data from Lee (1976), Wald *et al.* (1988) and ONS (1998b))

	Males					Females				
Ages:	25–9	30–4	35–49	50–9	60+	25–9	30–4	35–49	50–9	60+
1956	9	12	11	14	14	7	9	9	7	5
1972	10	12	14	19	25	11	10	10	13	12
Ages:	25–34		35–49	50–64	65+	25–34		35–49	50–64	65+
1984	15		22	29	46	14		16	20	26
Ages:	25–9		45–54		65–74	25–9		45–54		65–74
1996	12		34		56	13		22		30

[a] Ex-smokers of any form of tobacco 1956–84; ex-smokers of cigarettes, 1996.
[b] Great Britain, 1956–84; England, 1996.

Table 5.26 Percentage of men who smoke pipes, by age. Great Britain, 1961–87. (Data from Wald *et al.* (1988) and Wald and Nicolaides-Bouman (1991))

Year	All pipe smokers					
Ages:	16–24	25–34	35–59	60+		16+
1961	5	9	14	24		14
1965	6	11	14	22		14
1968	7	11	15	21		14
1971	6	12	14	19		13
1975	4	9	12	16		11
Ages:	16–24	25–34	35–49	50–64	65+	16+
1975	4	9	11	14	16	11
1978	2	4	10	11	14	8
1981	1	6	7	12	11	7
1985	1	3	7	9	9	6
1987	1	1	5	8	8	5

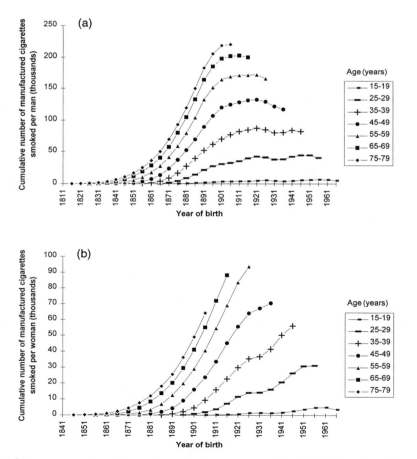

Figure 5.50 Cumulative consumption of manufactured cigarettes per adult, United Kingdom: (a) men born 1816–1966; (b) women born 1846–1966.

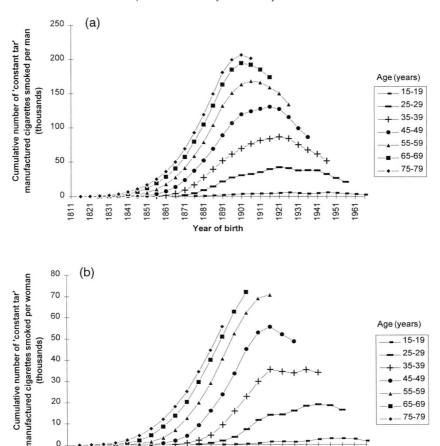

Figure 5.51 Cumulative 'constant tar' manufactured cigarette consumption per adult, United Kingdom: (a) men born 1816–1966; (b) women born 1846–1966.

different cohorts at different ages; for instance, at ages 65–69 and 75–79 the tar-weighted peak was for the cohort born in 1901, whereas at ages 25–29 and 35–39 the peak was for those born in 1921. For women, however, consumption is still increasing for the most recent cohorts, although the data available are only for smoking up to 1985.

Surgical operations

Data on certain surgical operations of potential relevance to cancer risks were extracted from the Hospital In-patient Enquiry (Ministry of Health and General Register Office 1964, 1968; Department of Health and Social Security and OPCS 1970–4; Department of Health and Social Security, OPCS and Welsh Office 1975–89), which up to 1985 collected information on a 10% sample of all discharges and deaths of NHS patients from NHS non-psychiatric hospitals in England and Wales. The data relate to episodes of hospitalization, not to individual patients (successive episodes for one individual are not linked), and therefore are most interpretable for epidemiological purposes when they relate to operations that are rare or impossible to repeat on the same person. Rates of selected operations in England and Wales for the period 1961–85 are shown in Figures 5.52–5.55. The data are presented for those, somewhat intermittent, years for which they are published. Comparable data are not available after 1985.

The rate of operations on the gallbladder, the large majority of which are cholecystectomies, increased slightly in each sex from 1961 to the late 1970s, but has since declined (Figure 5.52).

The rate of prostatectomy increased considerably from 1961 to 1985 (Figure 5.53). The proportion of prostatectomies that were per-urethral also rose markedly—they constituted 15% of all prostatectomies in 1961, 21% in 1971, 75% in 1981, and 86% in 1985. This increase in per-urethral prostatectomies occurred both at ages 45–64 years and 65 and over.

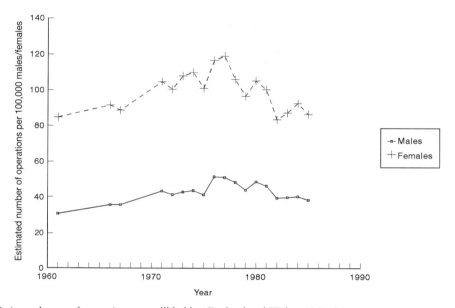

Figure 5.52   Estimated rates of operations on gallbladder, England and Wales, 1961–85.

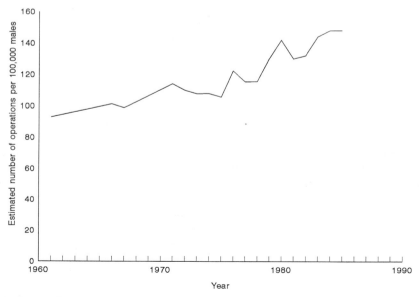

Figure 5.53   Estimated rates of prostatectomy, England and Wales, 1961–85.

The orchidopexy rate at ages under 15 years rose markedly from 1968 to 1985 (Figure 5.54). In contrast, the rate of circumcision at ages under 5 years declined during this period.

In women, the hysterectomy rate increased throughout the period, the mastectomy rate increased in the early years and was then stable, and the rate of oophorectomy decreased (Figure 5.55).

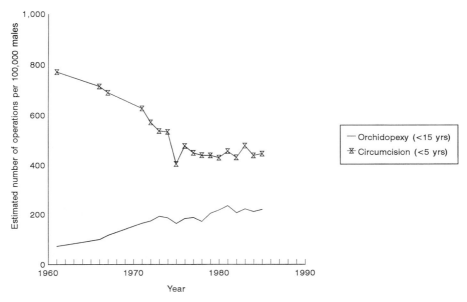

Figure 5.54 Estimated rates of orchidopexy at ages under 15 years and circumcision at ages under 5 years, England and Wales, 1961–85.

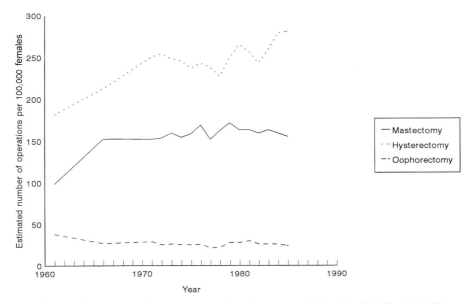

Figure 5.55 Estimated rates of mastectomy, hysterectomy, and oophorectomy, England and Wales, 1961–85.

Ultraviolet radiation (UVR)

Holidays abroad

The number of holidays abroad taken by British residents has increased markedly since 1951 (Table 5.27). Spain and France were the most popular destinations.

Hours of bright sunshine

Data on annual average daily hours of bright sunshine in England and Wales, from aggregation of measures made at meteorological stations across the country, were extracted from OPCS (1975c) for the years 1914 to 1974 and from OPCS and Communicable Disease Surveillance Centre (1995) for the years 1975 to 1993. The results are presented in Figure 5.56.

Table 5.27   Destinations of holidays abroad (in thousands), Britain, 1951–94. (Data from estimates by the Central Statistical Office (1970, 1996))

Destination	1951	1961	1971	1981	1991	1994
Spain	—	—	1 441	2 849	4 428	7 217
France	—	—	668	3 571	5 364	6 069
Greece	—	—	189	880	1 580	2 078
United States	—	—	42	722	1 414	1 558
Portugal	—	—	109	368	998	1 066
Italy	—	—	386	762	728	1 066
Cyprus	—	—	42	92	499	902
Irish Republic	—	—	—	473	624	738
Netherlands	—	—	151	315	728	711
Germany	—	—	143	341	561	547
Austria	—	—	231	328	499	492
Belgium or Luxembourg	—	—	151	289	457	—
Other countries	—	—	798	2 429	3 389	4 920
Total	1 500	4 000	4 200	13 130	20 790	27 336

— Data not available.

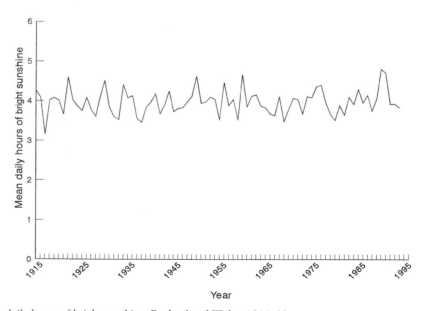

Figure 5.56   Mean daily hours of bright sunshine, England and Wales, 1914–93.

Measured ambient UVR

The National Radiological Protection Board have operated UVR monitoring stations at Leeds (latitude 54°N) and Chilton (52°N) since 1988 (as well as at Cambourne (50°N) since 1993). The available annual data for Leeds and Chilton are shown in Figure 5.57. There are, as yet, no consistent trends in annual cumulative UVR with time.

In earlier years, for which UVR measurements are not available, ambient UVR at ground level may have increased in urban areas because of decreased air pollution: it has been estimated that the reduction in atmospheric particulates after the Clean Air Acts of 1956 and 1968 may have increased UVR levels in an urban area (Bristol) by an amount equivalent to a 10% decrease in total ozone column (Leach *et al.* 1979).

Sunspots

Data on sunspot area in each month since January 1965 were obtained from htpp://science.msfc.nasa.gov/ssl/pad/solar/greenwich.htm and are shown in Figure 5.58. The data originate from observations at a network of observatories compiled by the Royal Greenwich Observatory up to 1976, and by the US Air Force and US National Oceanic and Atmospheric Administration thereafter.

Recreational exposure to UVR

Although data are not available on trends in outdoor recreational exposure to UVR, the General Household Survey (ONS 1998*b*) has collected information on involvement of adults in various recreational activities in Great Britain, which give an indication of likely trends in outdoor UVR exposures. Data on gardening are available since 1977 and on sports and other physical activities since 1986. Table 5.28 shows participation rates in the four weeks before interview for the most popular outdoor pursuits. The data suggest modest

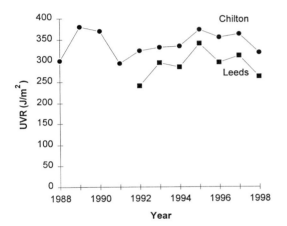

Figure 5.57 Annual total UV radiant exposure, weighted by the erythemal action spectrum, at Chilton, Oxfordshire, 1988–98 and Leeds, Yorkshire, 1992–8.

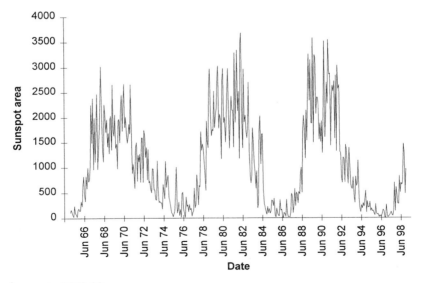

Figure 5.58 Area of sunspots, 1965–98.

Table 5.28   Percentages of adults who had participated in selected recreational activities in the 4 weeks before interview, Great Britain, 1977–96. (Data from ONS (1998*b*))

Activity	Year 1977	1980	1986	1990	1996
Gardening	42	43	43	48	48
Walking at least 2 miles	—	—	38	41	45
Cycling	—	—	8	9	11
Soccer	—	—	5	5	5
Golf	—	—	4	5	5
Running, jogging	—	—	5	5	5

— Data not available.

upward trends, in the years for which data are available, in the proportion of adults engaging in outdoor recreations; participation rates were greater for men than women (not in Table), but the increase in recreational UVR exposure appears to apply to both sexes.

Unemployment

Data on unemployment in the United Kingdom in the twentieth century were obtained from Sayer Bain *et al.* (1972) and Central Statistical Office (1971, 1975, 1977, 1990, 1995, 1996).

Figure 5.59 shows the trend in the percentage of the workforce unemployed. The values for the years 1900–21 refer to the percentage unemployed in certain trade unions; those for 1922–47 represent the insured unemployed as a percentage of the insured labour force as given by the Ministry of Labour. For subsequent years, the figures refer to registered unemployed as a percentage of the total workforce.

During the first decades of the twentieth century, unemployment was least during the two World Wars and was highest during the inter-war period, reaching a peak of 22% in 1932. After the Second World War and until 1973, the level of unemployment was relatively low and changed little. Since then, however, the level rose sharply to reach a peak in 1983 and although it has since declined, irregularly, the levels are still substantially higher than those in the 1950s and 1960s.

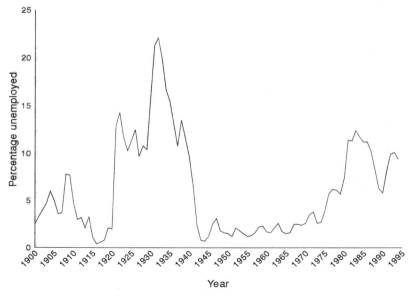

Figure 5.59   Percentage of workforce unemployed, United Kingdom, 1900–94.

6 | *Cancer trends*

Trends for cancer overall, and then for specific sites, are discussed in this chapter, as well as potential explanations for these trends and the relation to changes in levels of known risk factors. The sites presented are those which are most common or have trends of particular interest. For each of these sites, we have analysed secular and cohort trends in incidence and mortality nationally, and secular trends in mortality by region. For most sites we have systematically presented, or at least commented upon, each of these analyses[1], but for a few, where we wished simply to address one particular issue, we have only commented upon selected aspects of the data.

The sites are discussed in the order in which they are classified in the International Classification of Diseases (WHO 1978), except that cancer of unknown primary site is discussed after the sections on specific sites. Mortality data are discussed before incidence because they are available for a longer period and because for cancers with high fatality they are less likely to be affected by artefact, and hence are easier to interpret.

All malignant neoplasms (Figure 6.1)

Secular trends

Mortality from cancer has decreased substantially in males under age 70 years and females under age 50 since 1960, especially (in percentage terms) at younger ages and in males. The decreases in children have been greater than those in adults.

In women aged 50–69 years and men aged 70–84, mortality rates increased and then declined. In older women there has not been a decrease, but the mortality rate has stabilized in the last 10 years. The summation of these age-specific risks is encouraging: the all-ages[2] rate in males reached a peak in 1975–9 and has since fallen by over 10%, while the female rate reached a peak in 1985–9 and has since fallen by over 5% (Appendix C Table 1).

Cancer incidence rates[3] in males have increased moderately at ages under 35 years and at 70–84 years of age, and remained little changed at other ages. In females, there were increases of a quarter or more at ages 15–34 years, and 50 and above, and lesser increases at other ages. Overall, rates increased by 12% in men and 28% in women (Appendix C Table 1).

Mortality trends by region

Mortality in men has improved in the south of England and East Anglia, and deteriorated in most of the rest of the country. In women, Wessex was the only region in which mortality decreased, and there was no geographical pattern to the increases elsewhere, the greatest

---

[1] Because of space constraints not all of the analyses are presented as Figures. For instance, for sites with poor survival, we have generally shown the mortality but not the incidence data, although the latter are nevertheless described in the text. Similarly, although for each cancer site we analysed the full range of age categories described in the methods section, we have usually restricted the ages shown in the Figures to those at which substantial numbers of cases occurred. The full data, however, are shown in the Tables in Appendix C.

[2] Taken throughout this text to refer to ages 0–84 years (see Methods, p. 5), unless otherwise specified.

[3] Excluding non-melanoma skin cancer, because it is poorly registered (see p. 6).

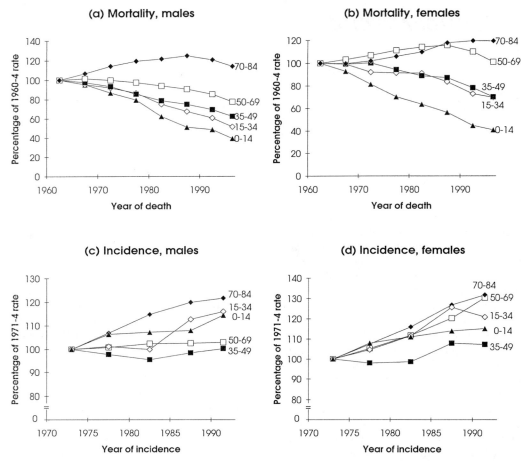

Figure 6.1   (a) (b) All malignant neoplasms, mortality, 1960–97 (ICD7 140–207, 292.3, 294; ICD8 140–209; ICD9 140–208, 238.4, 289.8); (c)(d) all malignant neoplasms except non-melanoma skin cancer, incidence, 1971–92 (ICD7 140–190, 192–207, 292.3, 294; ICD8 140–172, 173.5, 174–209; ICD9 140–172, 174–208, 238.4, 289.8).

(in percentage terms) being in Oxford region. In each sex there is now a clear north/south gradient[4] of risk, with the greatest mortality in 1990–4 in each sex in Northern region, followed by Mersey and then North Western, and the least in East Anglia and certain southern regions.

Comment

In part the increase in recorded incidence, and until recently in mortality, from cancer at older ages is real,

and reflects increases in incidence of several cancer sites, discussed individually below, but dominated by the effect of tobacco smoking. In part, however, the trend is artefactual: the change in 1984 in the Registrar General's interpretation of ICD coding rule 3 (for coding of underlying cause when both a cancer and a non-specific cause were mentioned on the death certificate—see p. 12) led to a 4.8% increase in recorded deaths from cancer at ages 75 years and above, and a lesser increase at younger ages (Grulich *et al.* 1995), but this continued only to 1993 when coding reverted

---

[4] Although we have described here and elsewhere in this book, for brevity, a 'north/south' gradient, this actually follows a pattern seen for many diseases and social factors in England and Wales, in which rates tend to divide between areas to the north and west of a line from the River Severn to the Wash, and areas to the south and east of this, with Wales resembling the north of England, and East Anglia resembling the south (maps showing this in more detail can be found in Swerdlow and dos Santos Silva (1993)).

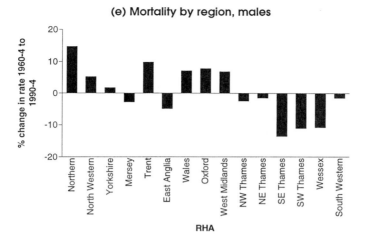

(e) Mortality by region, males

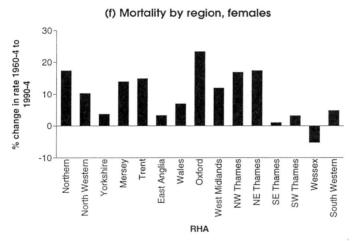

(f) Mortality by region, females

Figure 6.1 All malignant neoplasms (continued).

to the old rule. Changes in the extent to which, when cancer is mentioned on a death certificate, it is indicated by the certifier as the underlying cause of death rather than as an associated condition contributing to death, may also have increased cancer rates artefactually in recent years, by a few per cent at ages 65 and above and by less at younger ages (Grulich *et al.* 1995).

Part of the apparent increase at older ages is likely to be an artefact of better diagnosis of lymphohaemato-poietic malignancies and of solid cancers of certain internal sites, because of the introduction of more sophisticated diagnostic technologies. This is discussed by site, below.

The differences between the direction of incidence and mortality trends at younger ages, and to a lesser extent at older ages, mainly reflect improved survival for certain cancers (see Figures A3–A26) consequent on great advances in treatment, and accord with the age-specific survival trends shown in Figures A1 and B1[5]. The improvement in survival from cancer overall

---

[5] Partly because survival has improved more, in percentage point terms, at young than that at older ages, but mainly because a given percentage point improvement in survival causes a larger proportional impact on mortality at young ages, when a comparatively small proportion of cases die, than at older ages, when a greater proportion do. For instance, if 5-year survival from a cancer at young ages improved from 80% to 90%, the effect would be to decrease mortality in the 5 years by a half (all other things being equal); if at older ages a 10 percentage point improvement occurred from say 40% to 50%, however, this would only cause deaths to decrease by one-sixth.

has been less at old than at younger ages, both because treatment has been less effective at older ages and because the tumours for which the greatest increases in survival have been achieved (notably Hodgkin's disease, testicular cancer, and leukaemia) form a greater proportion of all cancers in young than in older people.

Another factor that may have contributed to divergence between cancer incidence and mortality trends (and to apparently rising incidence), is that there may have been increased registration of lesions of borderline malignancy. This may have occurred as a consequence of a greater propensity to detect and biopsy such lesions, for instance because of the introduction of screening, and/or as a consequence of changed pathological criteria for the distinction between malignant and non-malignant neoplasms. If completeness of registration has improved over time, this too would raise incidence compared with mortality, but as noted above (see p. 13), the available evidence does not indicate any appreciable improvement in the completeness of national registration since 1971.

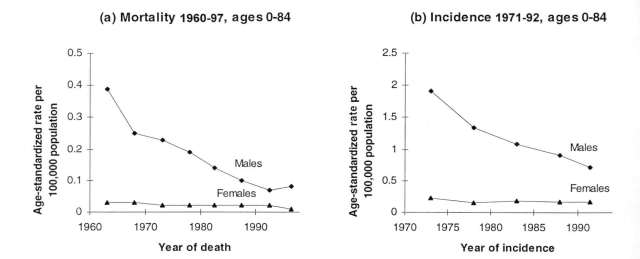

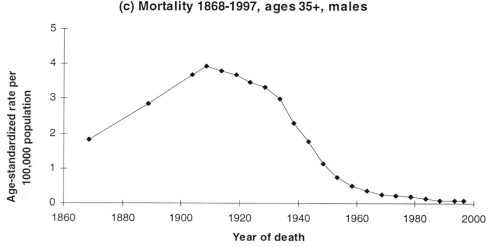

Figure 6.2   Cancer of lip (pre-ICD classifications 'Lip'; ICD2 pt. 39; ICD3 pt. 43; ICD4 pt. 45; ICD5 45a; ICD6–9 140).

Cancer of the lip (Figure 6.2)

The tumours included in this category in the ICD are those of the vermilion border of the lip, not the internal surface or the hair-bearing external surface beyond the vermilion border.

Cancer of the lip is now an uncommon tumour, but this was not always so. Rates have diminished remarkably during the twentieth century, as seen in Figures 6.2a–c. In men, the mortality rate now is a fifth of that in 1960–4 and under 5% of those in the 1920s and 30s[6], and in women there have also been several-fold decreases. Incidence data too show large decreases, of about two-thirds in males and one-third in females at ages under 85 years from 1971–4 to 1990–2 (Figure 6.2b). The known risk factors for lip cancer are chronic sun exposure, typically in farmers and fishermen, and pipe smoking[7]. Decreases in these factors (see Tables 5.16 and 5.26) are likely to account for the retreat of this tumour.

Cancers of the tongue, mouth, and pharynx (Figures 6.3 and 6.4)

We have included under this heading, those cancers of the tongue, mouth, and pharynx that are coded in ICD9 to 141, 143–6, and 148–9; these share certain epidemiological characteristics and are largely of squamous histology. We did not include cancers of the lip, salivary glands, and nasopharynx, which appear to be aetiologically distinct from the remainder of oral and pharyngeal malignancies. We have presented Figures separately for tongue plus mouth (referred to hereafter as 'oral') cancers (Figure 6.3) and pharyngeal cancers (Figure 6.4), because although these two groups show some similarities there are also differences.

Secular trends

Trends in mortality from *oral cancer* (Figure 6.3) in men have varied greatly by age. At ages 35–49 years, mortality doubled from 1970–4 to 1985–9, but has since declined. At ages 50–69 (and less consistently based on small numbers, at ages 15–34 (not shown))

there was a similar but less marked pattern. At 70–84 years of age, however, rates decreased by almost two-thirds over the study period. In women aged 35–69 there were also substantial rises from 1970–4 to a peak around 1990, and then a decline, and at older ages there was a decline of about a quarter over the study period.

Incidence of oral cancer increased considerably in adults of each sex except those aged 70–84, in whom the rate decreased by a quarter in men and was unchanged in women.

Pharyngeal cancer (Figure 6.4) death rates in men more than doubled at ages 35–49 years and increased by a third at ages 50–69; unlike oral cancer, rates were still rising in the most recent years of data available. As for oral cancer, rates decreased in the oldest age group of men, by about a half. In women, the pattern for pharyngeal cancer was very different from that for oral cancer, with a decline of four-fifths at ages 35–49 and a half at ages 50–69, as well as a decline of a third at ages 70–84. Incidence trends were in the same direction as those for mortality, with rises in men at ages 35–69 and a decrease in men at older ages and in women at all ages.

Trends by birth cohort

Mortality from *oral cancer* in men decreased steeply in successive cohorts born up to 1910–14, then increased to a peak in the cohort born in 1940–4, since which the trend has been uneven. In women there was also a decrease through to the cohort born in 1910–14, but after rising a little in the immediately succeeding cohorts, rates then showed no consistent change. Incidence data for men displayed trends similar to those for mortality. For women there was again a decrease to the 1910–14 birth cohort, but then more evidence of a recent rise than in mortality data.

Mortality and incidence data for *pharyngeal cancer* in men showed similar trends by birth cohort to those seen for oral cancer. In women, however, the pattern was different, with mortality decreasing almost throughout the span of cohorts analysed, while incidence trends were generally downward, although not entirely consistently.

---

[6] The data (Figure 6.2c) are for ages 35 and above, to allow continuity back to 1868—see p. 6. The rates before the early twentieth century are presented for historical interest, but whether the apparent increases in that period reflect changing incidence or better diagnosis and certification must be speculative.

[7] The association with pipes was first noticed in 1795 (Doll 1998), over half a century before even the earliest data in the Figure.

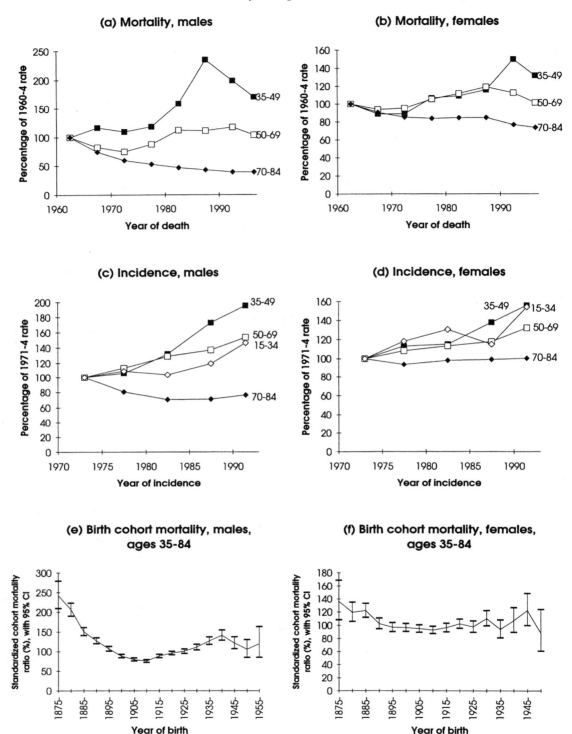

Figure 6.3 Cancers of tongue and mouth (ICD7 141, 143–4; ICD8&9 141, 143–5), mortality 1960–97, incidence 1971–92.

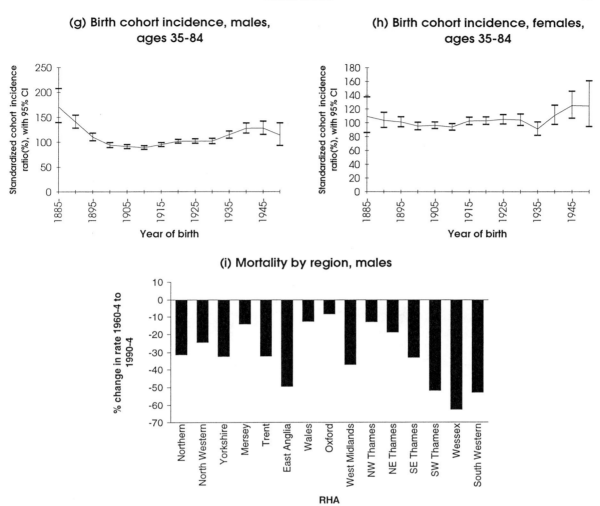

Figure 6.3   Cancers of tongue and mouth (continued)

Mortality trends by region

Mortality from *oral cancer* in men decreased in all regions, most greatly (in percentage terms) in Wessex, South Western and SW Thames regions. In women (not shown), changes were erratic based on small numbers. There is now a north/south gradient of rates in men but little regional variation in rates in women.

Pharyngeal cancer mortality in men increased in Wales and much of the north of England, while decreasing in the south. In women (not shown), based on small numbers, there were decreases of 30% or more in all regions.

Comment

The trends in oral and pharyngeal cancers must have been greatly affected by changes in smoking and alcohol consumption, which are the principal known risk factors for these tumours in Western countries. Large increases in oral and pharyngeal cancer mortality rates in men have been noted in several Western countries (Blot *et al.* 1994). The increase in rates in young men in England and Wales is of concern, although it is not as large as the increase in the same group in Scotland (Swerdlow *et al.* 1998), and it has ceased in the most recent cohorts. The increase does not appear to be due

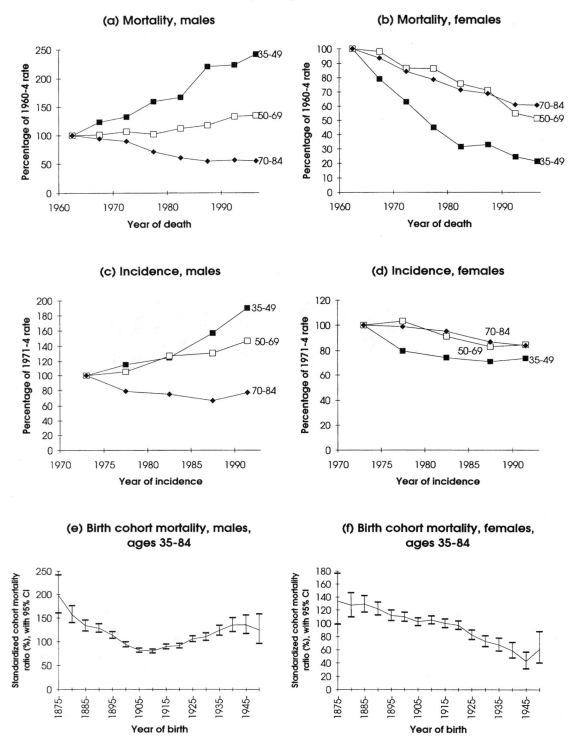

Figure 6.4   Cancer of pharynx (ICD7 145, 147, 148; ICD8&9 146, 148, 149), mortality 1960–97, incidence 1971–92.

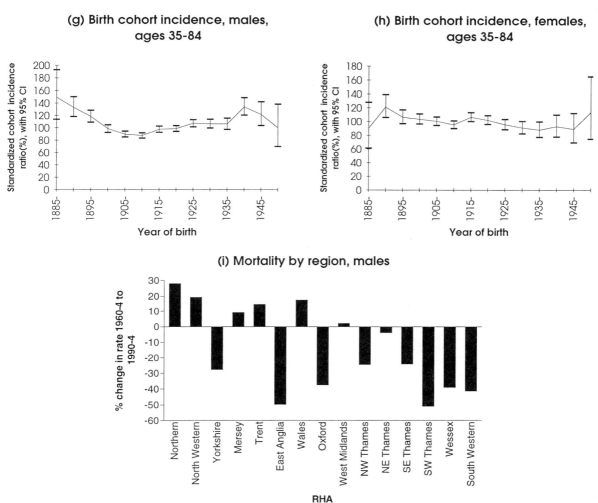

Figure 6.4 Cancer of pharynx (continued).

to changes in smoking habits, as mean tar-adjusted cigarette consumption (Figure 5.51a) and lung cancer rates (Figure 6.11) in these cohorts have been falling. It could, however, be explained by alcohol consumption. This increased greatly in both sexes combined in the 1960s and 1970s (Figure 5.3), and although such data are not available by sex, they presumably mainly reflect male consumption, as most drinking is by men. Increasing male drinking is also suggested by the large increase in cirrhosis mortality in men since 1970 (see Figure 5.5), although this may not reflect solely their alcohol consumption[8].

Taking a longer-term perspective, the trends in national alcohol consumption since 1880 (Figure 5.3), falling from high levels to a minimum in the 1930s to 1950s, then rising until 1980 and levelling off, correspond roughly with the birth cohort trends in oral and pharyngeal cancer in men lagged by about 30–40 years, i.e. the cancer rates in different cohorts of men appear to reflect approximately the drinking habits in the country when these cohorts were young adults. Although the steep decline in oral and pharyngeal cancer mortality between men born in 1875 and those born early in the twentieth century does not accord

---

[8] The only data not showing increasing alcohol consumption by men are from self-reports in surveys since 1978 (Figure 5.4, Table 5.1), which seem less likely to be reliable than the other indicators.

with the increasing tobacco consumption in these cohorts (Figure 5.51a), interpretation is complicated by the fact that these cancers, especially oral, are caused by pipe and cigar smoking at least as much as by cigarette smoking, and the former habit has decreased greatly while the latter has increased[9] (as can be deduced from Figure 5.47a, although such long-term data on pipe and cigar smoking are not available directly). A closer correlation of oral and pharyngeal cancer trends with alcohol than with smoking trends has been found in several other countries (Blot *et al.* 1994). Since oral and pharyngeal cancer risks are exceptionally high in those who both smoke and drink heavily, rates could also have risen if the proportion of young men who are heavy smokers and drinkers has increased. The trend data available on heavy smoking and drinking (Table 5.3), however, are too recent to give much illumination of the cancer trends to date.

For women, the trends in oral and pharyngeal cancer do not correspond well with smoking (Figures 5.47b, 5.48b, 5.50b, 5.51b) or lung cancer (Figure 6.11) trends, or with both-sex long-term alcohol consumption trends (Figure 5.3), although these may not reflect female consumption. Cirrhosis mortality data for women (Figure 5.5) imply that their alcohol consumption has been rising for the last 50 years, and recent sex-specific questionnaire data on alcohol consumption also suggest rises for the shorter period (since 1978) for which they are available (Table 5.1, Figure 5.4). Pharyngeal cancer rates in women have been falling, however, and the increases in oral cancer have only been appreciable at young ages and in recent birth cohorts.

Use of smokeless tobacco can cause oral cancers. Snuff taking and chewing of tobacco have not been prevalent in England and Wales in modern times[10], but a small contribution to the oral cancer rates in each sex has arisen from betel quid chewing in the immigrant population from the Indian subcontinent (Swerdlow *et al.* 1995). The growing numbers (Table 5.5) and the ageing of this population may have contributed an increasing tendency to national rates, although not large since they constitute only 3% of the national population (Table 5.4).

Consumption of fresh fruit and vegetables or of certain vitamins may be protective against oral and pharyngeal cancers. The trends in consumption of these[11] do not suggest an explanation for the cancer trends in men, especially for the rising rates in young men, although they would to some extent be compatible with the pharyngeal cancer trends in women, and improved nutrition might be the reason for the downward trend in pharyngeal compared with oral cancers in women. Per caput intakes of fresh fruit and vitamin C have increased somewhat since 1950 (Figures 5.16, 5.20), intake of fresh vegetables other than potatoes has been little changed (although potato consumption has decreased (Figure 5.17)), and vitamin A intake (Figure 5.19) has been fairly stable until a decrease in the most recent years.

The aetiology of a proportion of oral cancers may relate to sexual exposures, perhaps with human papilloma virus (Schwartz *et al.* 1998), and this may account for some of the apparently anomalous trends.

The appreciably more downward trend for pharyngeal cancer mortality than incidence in women but not in men (although not the divergence between mortality and incidence trends for oral and pharyngeal cancers overall, which has been modest and similar between the sexes—not shown) accords with the apparent improvement in survival from oral and pharyngeal cancer for women only, shown in Figure A3.

In conclusion, the trends in oral and pharyngeal cancers in men appear to be largely explicable by changes in alcohol consumption, whereas in women the trends are not clearly explained by trends in any of the known risk factors, although improved nutrition may have had an effect. It is possible that trends in the proportion of women who are heavy consumers of both alcohol and tobacco might have affected oral and pharyngeal cancer rates, but data on this exposure are not available from sufficiently long ago.

Cancer of the oesophagus (Figure 6.5)

Secular trends

Mortality from cancer of the oesophagus in men has more than doubled at ages 35–69 and increased by two-thirds at ages 70–84 since 1960. At ages 15–34 (not shown), based on small numbers, there was no clear trend. Rates in women have increased by about a

---

[9] This complication affects only the data for men, as few women have smoked pipes or cigars at any period.

[10] Although snuff taking was common in the eighteenth century (Doll 1998).

[11] The data available are for both sexes combined, so the comments regarding their relation to oral cancer trends will only apply if they are approximately applicable to the trends for each sex separately.

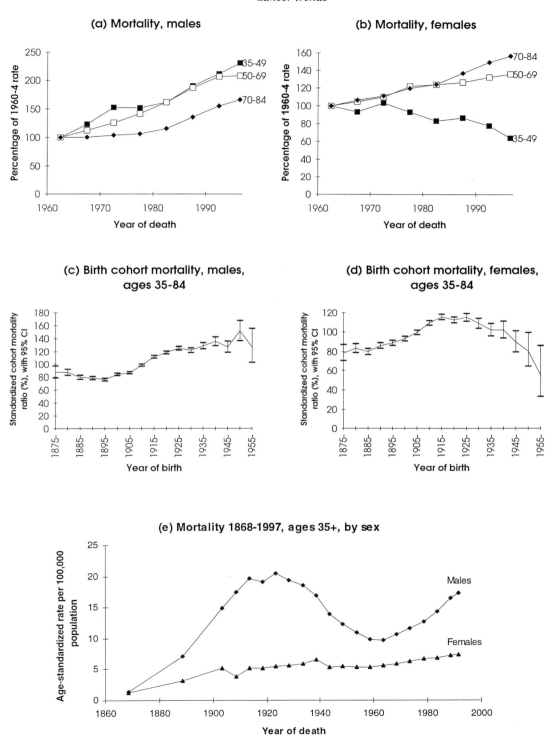

Figure 6.5 Cancer of oesophagus (pre-ICD classifications 'Oesophagus'; ICD2 pt. 40; ICD3 pt. 44; ICD4 pt. 46; ICD5 46a; ICD6–9 150: (a)–(d) mortality 1960–97; (e) mortality 1868–1997; (f), (g) mortality 1911–97; (h), (i) mortality 1960–4 to 1990–4.

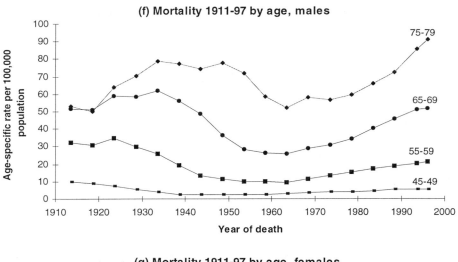

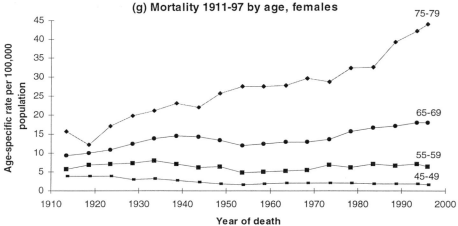

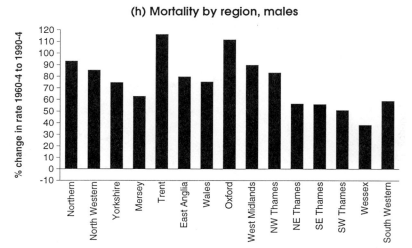

Figure 6.5   Cancer of oesophagus (continued).

(i) Mortality by region, females

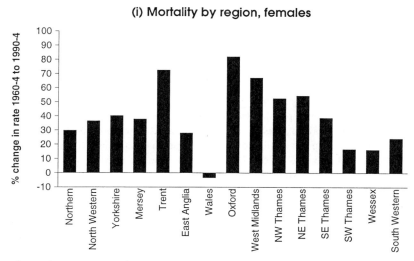

Figure 6.5 Cancer of oesophagus (continued).

third or a half at ages 50 years and above, but decreased by a third at ages 35–49. In incidence data (not shown), there were similar patterns to those for mortality in each sex.

Examining trends over a longer period, since 1868 (Figure 6.5e), oesophageal cancer rates have varied far more in men than in women. In men, a peak was reached in the late 1920s, followed by a marked decline until the late 1950s and early 1960s, and then a rise. Considered by age (Figure 6.5f), the low rates in the years around 1960 and the subsequent rise appear to have occurred at about the same time for different age-groups, whereas the peak rates in the first half of the century occurred much earlier at younger ages, i.e. approximately in a birth cohort pattern. In women (Figures 6.5e, 6.5g), the trend in oesophageal cancer mortality has generally been slightly upwards since data have been available, although with a small peak in the 1930s.

Trends by birth cohort

In males, mortality rates decreased a little for the cohorts born from 1875–9 to 1895–9. There was then a consistent increase until the cohort born in 1925–9, and a less consistent, slightly upward trend in the cohorts born since. In women, rates increased up to a peak in cohorts born during 1915–29, and have since declined markedly. In incidence data (not shown) there were similar trends.

Mortality trends by region

In men there have been considerable increases in oesophageal cancer mortality in all regions, least in the southern ones. In women there have been large regional variations in secular trends, ranging from an 80% increase in Oxford region to a slight decrease in Wales, and as a consequence regional disparity in rates has diminished.

Comment

Rates of oesophageal cancer in women in England and Wales are high compared with rates in other white populations, particularly those in continental Europe (Jensen *et al.* 1990; Smans *et al.* 1992; Parkin *et al.* 1997). Survival from oesophageal cancer is particularly poor (Figure A4), so it is unsurprising that incidence and mortality trends mirrored each other closely in the period for which data on both were available.

The main known aetiological factors for oesophageal cancer in Western countries are alcohol consumption and smoking, with a synergistic increase in risk when both exposures are combined. There appears also to be a relationship to poor diet, perhaps micronutrient deficiencies, but this is not yet well defined. In men, the rising rates of oesophageal cancer in recent years and the cohort pattern of risk do not accord with lung cancer trends as a marker of smoking (Figure 6.11)[12],

[12] Indeed comparison of Figures 6.5e and 6.12a shows that oesophageal cancer and lung cancer trends in men have been almost the mirror image of each other since early in the twentieth century.

or with recorded smoking trends (Figures 5.47a, 5.48a, 5.50a, 5.51a). Interpretation of the trends in the early cohorts is complicated, however, because risk of oesophageal cancer relates to pipe and cigar smoking, which were declining in the first half of the twentieth century (as indicated in Figure 5.47a), as well as to cigarette smoking, which was greatly increasing.

The oesophageal cancer trends do not parallel trends in fresh fruit and vegetable or vitamin A or C consumption (although data on these are not available sex-specifically) (Figures 5.16, 5.17, 5.19, 5.20). As in several other North European countries (Day and Varghese 1994), however, they would accord with trends in alcohol consumption. The peak of alcohol consumption around 1900, the low levels from the 1920s to 1960, and the subsequent rise until 1980 (Figure 5.3), each correspond approximately with oesophageal cancer trends in men around 20 years later (Figure 6.5e). They also correspond with the cohort trends in oesophageal cancer (Figure 6.5c) displaced by about 40 years from the year of birth[13]. Thus on a secular (calendar period) model of risk, the data suggest that alcohol consumption affects population rates of oesophageal cancer with a 20-year lag, while on a cohort model, the data suggest that oesophageal cancer rates reflect the alcohol consumption of men when aged in their 40s[14]. The cohort interpretation would be compatible with data from France, where rates of oesophageal cancer were low for cohorts of men who were aged 25–40 during the Second World War, when alcohol consumption in France was greatly diminished (Tuyns and Audigier 1976).

The recent trends in oesophageal cancer in men in England and Wales are similar to those in Scotland (Swerdlow *et al.* 1998), but the trends earlier in the century showed less resemblance to mortality in Scotland, where there was only a slight peak in the 1930s.

Unlike the pattern in men, both the secular and cohort trends of oesophageal cancer in women are similar to trends in lung cancer (Figure 6.11) and in smoking[15] (Figures 5.47b, 5.48b, 5.50b, 5.51b). The oesophageal cancer trends in women, however, generally do not correspond well with alcohol consumption (Figure 5.3) or cirrhosis (Figure 5.5) trends, or with

recent trends in self-reported alcohol consumption (Table 5.1, Figure 5.4). They also do not obviously parallel trends in fresh fruit and vegetable or vitamins A and C consumption (Figures 5.16, 5.17, 5.19, 5.20).

A rising incidence of adenocarcinoma of the lower end of the oesophagus has been found in the UK and several other countries (Powell and McConkey 1992; Devesa *et al.* 1998). It is not as closely related as is squamous carcinoma to cigarette smoking or the consumption of alcohol (Blot *et al.* 1991; Devesa *et al.* 1998), but it may be positively related to adiposity (which is increasing—Figure 5.6) and inversely related to *Helicobacter pylori* infection of the stomach (Chow *et al.* 1998) (which has been decreasing—Figure 5.22).

In conclusion, trends in oesophageal cancer overall in men relate better to alcohol than smoking trends and the converse is true in women. For each sex it is possible that trends in the prevalence of heavy drinking plus smoking may have been of importance, but long-term data on these are not available; in addition, there has been a contribution to the overall trends from the specific risk factors for the comparatively uncommon adenocarcinoma of the oesophagus.

Cancer of the stomach (Figure 6.6)

Secular trends

Figures 6.6a and b show stomach cancer mortality trends since 1960. Rates have decreased greatly at all ages and in both sexes. In percentage terms, the greatest decreases in men have been at ages under 70, and for all-ages the decrease has been greater in women than in men. At ages 15–34 years in each sex, the decline has diminished or ceased in recent years, and at these ages mortality rates have been similar in men and women, whereas at older ages they have been substantially greater in men. The trends in incidence (not shown) were similar to those for mortality, except that the recent cessation of the downward trend at ages 15–34 has, as yet, been less evident.

Examination of longer-term data (Figure 6.6e) shows the fall in stomach cancer to be a reversal of earlier trends. Up to the 1930s, recorded all-age mortality rates increased considerably, but since 1936–40 in

---

[13] The cohort minimum for men born in the late 1890s is essentially equivalent to the secular minimum around 1960, because men born in the 1890s would then have been aged in their 60s and 70s, the age groups that dominate all-age rates.
[14] The age-specific data since 1911, described earlier, leave it equivocal whether a secular or cohort interpretation is the more appropriate.
[15] As far as the cohort smoking peak can be judged from the available data—see pp. 63–5 and 104–6.

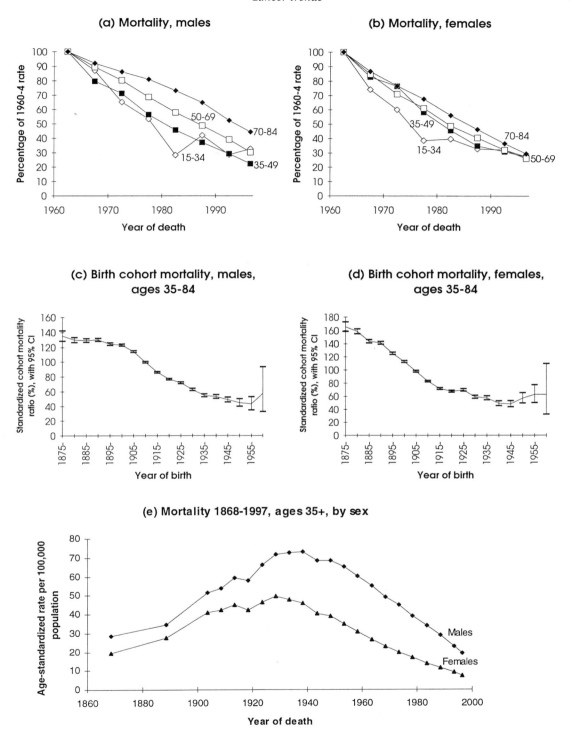

Figure 6.6 Cancer of stomach (pre-ICD classifications 'Stomach'; ICD2 pt. 40; ICD3 pt. 44; ICD4 pt. 46; ICD5 pt. 46b; ICD6–9 151): (a)–(d) mortality 1960–97; (e) mortality 1868–1997; (f), (g) mortality 1911–97; (h), (i) mortality 1960–4 to 1990–4.

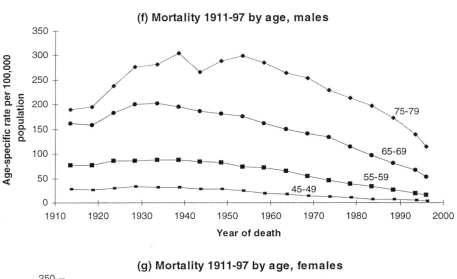

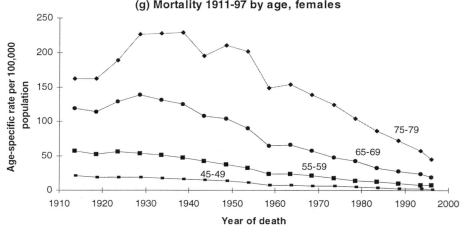

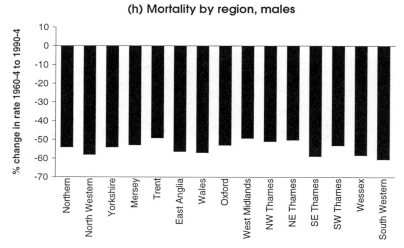

Figure 6.6   Cancer of stomach (continued).

(i) Mortality by region, females

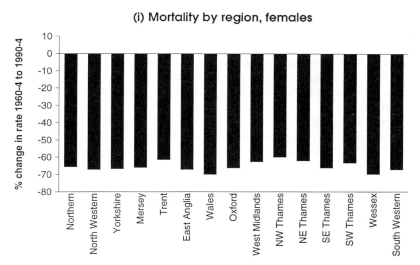

Figure 6.6   Cancer of stomach (continued).

men, and a little earlier in women, rates have been falling. When these trends are analysed by age (Figures 6.6f and g)[16], in men this pattern of rise and then fall was present at each age group, with the quinquennium of peak mortality similar at all ages except 75 years and above, at which it was later. In women, rates at most ages under 60 have diminished since the earliest period of data in the Figure (1911–15), and rates at older ages have diminished since dates that were later than this, especially at ages 75 and above[17]. In each sex and age group, there were dips in mortality rates during 1916–20 and 1941–5—the periods that included the later years of the two World Wars.

Trends by birth cohort

Mortality from stomach cancer in men decreased in successive birth cohorts born from the late nineteenth century up to 1955–9. In women there was a decrease in cohorts born before 1950, but not those born subsequently. Incidence data (not shown) revealed similar patterns, but with the downward trend interrupted in each sex by a modest peak in the cohort born in 1925–9[18].

Mortality trends by region

The decrease in stomach cancer mortality has occurred at an astonishingly uniform rate (in percentage terms) in all regions. As a consequence, the historically greater rates in Wales and Northern England than elsewhere (Stocks 1936) have persisted.

Comments

The decreasing rates of stomach cancer in England and Wales over the last 50 years form part of a pattern of decreases seen across the world. The improvements are important because stomach cancer is one of the main contributors to cancer mortality[19]. For the same reason, the cessation of the downward trend in the most recent cohorts—a pattern seen also in Scotland (Swerdlow *et al.* 1998)—is important too.

The reasons for the decrease up to recent cohorts remain uncertain. It is possible that an element of it could have been diagnostic—there may have been some transfer to more correctly localized sites of deaths that would previously have been attributed to this category—but this would not plausibly explain most of

[16] The Figures show data for selected age groups, but the comments in the text are based on examination of all ages.
[17] Although one cannot definitively decide between secular and cohort interpretations, the male data appear more explicable as a secular change and those for females are more like a cohort effect.
[18] Close inspection of the mortality data shows an indication of the same effect, but less marked.
[19] Indeed in each sex the decrease in numbers of deaths from stomach cancer over the study period (since 1960) is the largest for any cancer site.

the decline[20]. Stomach cancer is a relatively frequent diagnosis when the actual primary site is determined for deaths certified to 'primary site unknown' (Heasman and Lipworth 1966; Grulich *et al.* 1995), so that the rising proportion of cancer deaths of unspecified site (Figure 6.35) has probably contributed a small element to the downward trend in stomach cancer mortality. Changes in coding of cause of death appear to have contributed a few per cent to the downward trend[21] (see Table 4.1), but not a substantial proportion. The diminishing rates cannot be attributed to better survival (Figure A5) or to any deliberate public health measure. Improvements in food preservation methods, by refrigeration, and also the consequent decrease in use of salting, pickling, and smoking of foods may have contributed to reduced stomach cancer risks, as may the increasing availability of fresh fruits and vegetables and consequent effects on vitamin intake. As Figures 5.16, 5.19, and 5.20 show, however, although per caput consumption of fresh fruit and certain vitamins increased greatly in the years immediately after the Second World War, changes from then until the 1990s have been much less marked (although out-of-season fruit availability has improved), and fresh vegetable consumption has changed little , except for a decline in potato intake (Figure 5.17). Thus the stomach cancer trends since the War do not appear entirely explicable by contemporary trends in fruit, vegetable, and vitamin consumption, although these might have contributed. The trends might, however, have been determined by fruit and vegetable consumption in early life, as studies of migrants have suggested that it may be diet at these ages, rather than in adulthood, that is critical to stomach cancer aetiology (Haenszel 1982). The decreasing rates of stomach cancer at older ages and in earlier birth cohorts might then reflect increased consumption of fruit (with unchanged vegetable consumption) in the twentieth century before the Second World War (Table 5.6), and the cessation of improvement in mortality for post-War birth cohorts might be a consequence of the lack of

major increase in intake of these foodstuffs from 1950 to 1980 (Figures 5.16, 5.17).

In recent years evidence has emerged of an association between infection of the stomach with *Helicobacter pylori* and risk of stomach cancer. Data from Yorkshire, England, show decreasing seroprevalence of *Helicobacter pylori* in successive cohorts born from 1920–9 to 1960–9 (Figure 5.22). The decreases in the earlier cohorts parallel reductions in stomach cancer, but the continuing decreases in recent cohorts do not accord with the cessation in the fall in stomach cancer rates in these generations. They may, however, accord with the rise in the incidence of the relatively uncommon cancers of the gastric cardia, which may have negated the further fall in the erstwhile common cancers of the rest of the stomach (Powell and McConkey 1992), as the risk of cancer at this site seems to be inversely related to the prevalence of *Helicobacter pylori* infection (Hansen *et al.* 1999).

The apparent increase in stomach cancer mortality rates from 1868 to the 1930s is intriguing. A similar pattern of rise and fall occurred in data for Scotland since early in the twentieth century (Swerdlow *et al.* 1998). It is possible that these early rises in mortality reflect improved diagnosis and certification rather than changes in true incidence. On the other hand, the increase might have been real, due to changes in aetiological or preventive factors[22]. Other than during the Second World War, consumption of vegetables did not decrease appreciably and consumption of fruit increased during the first half of the twentieth century (Table 5.6), so that these would not explain contemporary increases in stomach cancer. On the other hand, increasing urbanization during the nineteenth century may have led to deteriorating fresh fruit and vegetable consumption in childhood for the cohorts whose stomach cancer rates predominated in the late nineteenth and early twentieth centuries. It may be that *Helicobacter pylori* incidence increased: certainly there were increases from the early 1920s to the early 1950s in recorded mortality from duodenal ulcer (Barker

---

[20] In Rochester, Minnesota, where diagnostic efforts and autopsy rates have been exceptionally high for many decades, large decreases in stomach cancer mortality have been found (Nobrega *et al.* 1983) as in other Western populations.

[21] Including some, but only a minority, of the drop in rates in 1941–5 compared with 1936–40, as a consequence of the introduction of ICD5.

[22] A cohort-based pattern of increase and peak would favour an aetiological/preventive explanation, whereas a secular pattern of change would be compatible with an artefactual explanation. As noted earlier, however, the actual trends were not decisively of either type. Furthermore, even when inflexion points occur later at older ages in an apparently cohort-based pattern, as occurred to some extent for stomach cancer in women, this does not definitively indicate a cohort-based origin of the trend, as these later inflexion points could also reflect a secular delay in the spread to older age groups of better diagnosis and certification.

1989), for which *Helicobacter pylori* is a major aetiological factor.

Cancers of the colon and rectum
(Figures 6.7, 6.8)

We have considered these adjacent sites together because their trends and likely aetiology are fairly similar and because cancers of the large intestine unspecified, which can include rectal as well as colonic cancers, are coded to the ICD rubric for colon cancer.

Secular trends

Mortality from cancers of the colon and rectum has decreased substantially since 1960 (Figures 6.7a,b) especially in women and at younger ages. At ages 15–34 years, rates have fallen by three-quarters in women and by two-thirds in men since 1960–4. There have been decreases too at all other ages, and if anything the rate of decline appears to be accelerating. The decreases have been greater for rectal cancer (36% in men and 44% in women at all-ages since 1960–4) than for colon cancer (decreases of 6% and 32% in the two sexes respectively).

Substantial decreases in incidence have been seen only at ages 15–34, while at older ages there have been small decreases, or increases. Unlike the mortality data, however, when decreases occurred these have been greater for colon than rectal cancers.

Table 6.1 shows trends in colorectal cancer incidence by subsite[23]. At each colonic site rates declined markedly at ages 15–34, were unchanged or declined at ages 35–49, and apart from a modest decrease for transverse colon, increased or were unchanged at older ages. The percentage decrease was generally greater for women than men. The most marked declines were for descending colon tumours in women aged 15–34, and for caecum and ascending colon tumours in both sexes at these ages. Rectal cancer rates only decreased appreciably in men aged 15–34, and in other groups rates were either unchanged or slightly increased.

The impression of decreasing incidence rates for cancers of certain subsites of the colon is somewhat exaggerated by the slightly increasing proportion of large intestinal cancers for which subsite has been unspecified: from 1971–4 to 1990–2, the proportion of colon and rectal cancers that were coded to the rubric for colon unspecified plus large intestine unspecified[24] increased from 15% to 19%[25], with larger percentage increases at young than at older ages.

Colon and rectal cancers were not entirely separated from cancers of the small intestine in mortality coding before ICD6, which was first used in England and Wales in 1950. As small intestinal cancers are comparatively uncommon, however, the data for intestinal cancers overall since 1911 shown in Figures 6.8a and b should give a good indication of colon and rectal cancer trends. It can be seen that although in recent decades mortality has been declining, as described above, this had not been the case throughout the twentieth century. At older ages rates increased from 1911 to the late 1920s, then generally changed relatively little until the 1940s, from when a steep decline began. At young and middle ages a steep decline can again be seen from the 1940s, before which rates changed relatively little.

Trends by birth cohort

In each sex, mortality has generally decreased between successive cohorts included in the analyses, but with an interruption for cohorts born in the 1920s, and a particularly large decrease from the 1945–9 to 1950–4 birth cohort in women. When examined separately for colon and rectum (not shown), the decreasing trend and the inflexion for cohorts born around 1920 were present for each site; the decrease in the 1950–4 birth cohort of women was more pronounced for colon than rectum.

In incidence data, decreasing rates have only been present in cohorts born since 1935 in men and 1925 in women. A downward inflexion for the cohort of women born in 1950–4 was present as in mortality data. Again, the overall pattern was present for colon and rectal cancers separately, and the downturn in the 1950–4 birth cohort of women was especially for colon cancer.

---

[23] The equivalent data for colorectal cancer mortality have far too great a proportion of tumours with subsite unknown in recent years for satisfactory analysis.
[24] These two unspecified categories cannot be separated in ICD coding.
[25] From 24% to 31% if these unspecified tumours are considered as a percentage of colon cancers.

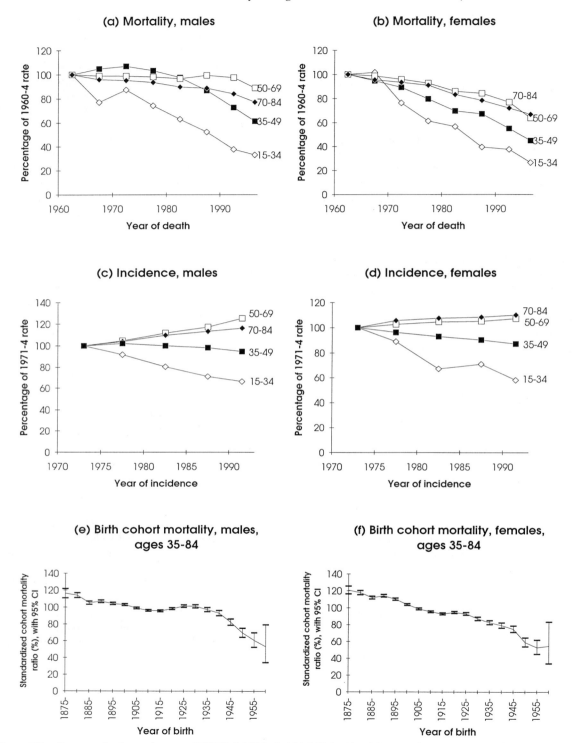

Figure 6.7 Cancers of colon and rectum (ICD7&8 153.0–8, 154; ICD9 153, 154), mortality 1960–97, incidence 1971–92.

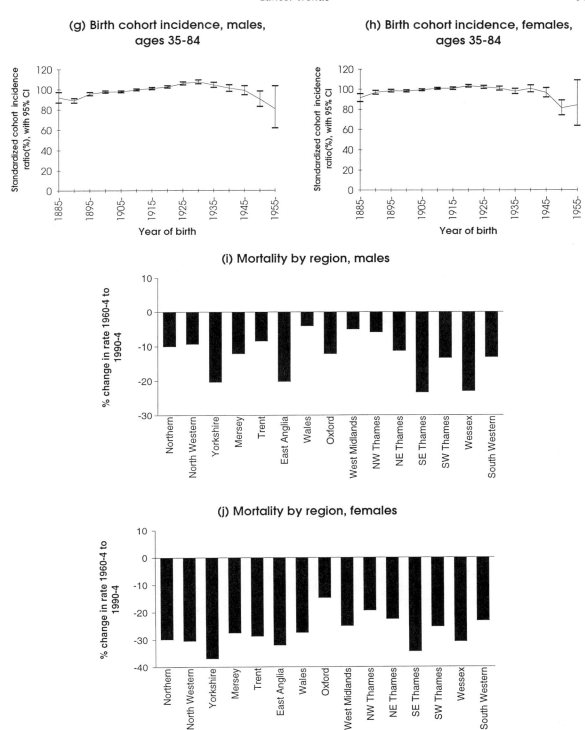

Figure 6.7 Cancers of colon and rectum (continued).

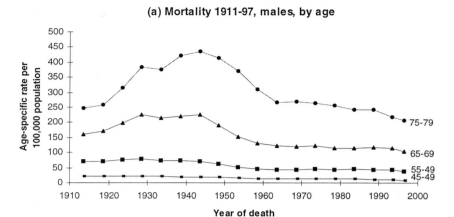

(a) Mortality 1911-97, males, by age

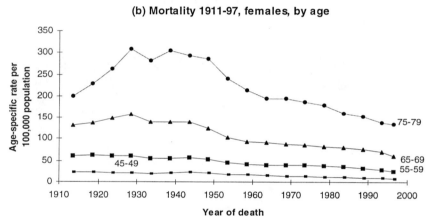

(b) Mortality 1911-97, females, by age

Figure 6.8   Cancers of small intestine, colon and rectum (ICD2 pt. 41; ICD3 pt. 45; ICD4 pts. 46; ICD5 pt. 46b, 46c, 46d; ICD6&7 152–4; ICD8 152, 153.0–.8, 154; ICD9 152–4).

Table 6.1   Trends in age-specific incidence rates of colorectal cancer by subsite: rates in 1990–2 as percentages of rates in 1971–4

Age (years)	Caecum and ascending colon		Transverse colon		Descending colon		Rectum		Colon NOS and large intestine NOS	
	Males	Females	Males	Females	Males	Females	Males	Females	Males	Females
15–34	46	39	60	54	65	36	73	97	100	93
35–49	101	88	57	62	74	72	102	96	132	111
50–69	135	112	98	83	118	98	117	105	179	139
70–84	133	117	95	87	111	101	104	105	156	135
15–84	131	112	93	83	112	97	109	105	163	135

NOS Not otherwise specified

Mortality trends by region

Mortality has decreased in all regions, substantially in women and less so in men, with modest regional varia- tion. This has not been, nor is, a tumour with marked geographical disparities in rates within England and Wales.

Comment

The more favourable trends for mortality from than incidence of cancers of the colon and rectum reflect improved survival (Figure A6), as a consequence of better surgery and perhaps earlier diagnosis (Ries 1994). A part of the most recent decrease in recorded mortality, however, is an artefact. When medical enquiries to certifiers ceased and interpretation of ICD coding rule 3 was altered in 1993 (see pp. 11–12), there was an immediate 8% decrease in recorded mortality from colorectal cancers in males and a 9% decrease in females, presumably because of these procedural changes, and in accord with the 7% decrease that we calculated in Table 4.1 these changes would be expected to bring.

Dietary factors are probably the major cause of colorectal cancers, and therefore the trends in incidence are likely to reflect dietary changes, at least to some extent, although the exact components responsible are uncertain. Several aspects of diet have been considered as possible causes of colorectal cancer, including high consumption of animal or saturated fats, lack of dietary fibre, and low consumption of raw or fresh fruit and vegetables, or of particular fruits or vegetables. Saturated fat consumption has been decreasing since about 1970 (Figure 5.14), which would accord with incidence trends since 1971 in colorectal cancer at young ages and in recent birth cohorts but not at older ages and in earlier cohorts. Total fat consumption had been rising through the century until the 1970s, except during the Second World War (Table 5.6, Figure 5.14). This would accord with the rising colorectal cancer mortality early in the century, but not the falling mortality since the 1940s.

Fibre consumption has decreased for the last hundred years (except for a temporary increase during the Second World War) (Table 5.8), so would again not explain the downward trend in colorectal cancer mortality since the 1940s or the decrease in incidence in young age groups and recent birth cohorts. Fresh fruit consumption has increased slightly since 1950, and rapidly in the years immediately before then (Figure 5.16), while fresh vegetable consumption has been little changed since 1950, apart from a decline in potato consumption (Figure 5.17); these post-war trends do not strongly accord with the colorectal cancer incidence trends. In earlier years, fruit consump-tion rose to a peak in the 1930s (Table 5.6) while colorectal cancer mortality was also rising.

Several other factors have been hypothesized to be aetiologically related to colorectal cancer, but with uncertainty on the extent (if any) of their role—sedentariness, on which we have no trend data, alcohol consumption, for which trends (Figure 5.3) were upwards in recent decades as colorectal cancer trends at younger ages have declined, and female sex hormone concentrations. It is possible that the greater decrease in colon cancer in women than men, particularly for cancers of the descending colon (a pattern seen also in Connecticut (Dubrow et al. 1993)), might relate to hormonal factors; it coincided with an increase in the use of oral contraceptives (Figure 5.32), and also with an increase in parity for cohorts of women born from early in the twentieth century to the mid-1930s, although this increase reversed for subsequent cohorts (Figures 5.37, 5.40) while the colon cancer trends did not (dos Santos Silva and Swerdlow 1996). There is evidence that colorectal cancer may be prevented by non-steroidal anti-inflammatory drugs, the use of which has increased greatly in recent decades (Figure 5.31).

Risks of colorectal cancer are increased in persons with adenomatous polyps of the colon and rectum, especially those with familial adenomatous polyposis coli (FAP). Therefore, increasing rates of prophylactic polypectomy, and, for familial polyposis, rates of colectomy, could have contributed to a decrease in rates of incidence of and death from this malignancy. FAP occurs in about 1 in 10 000 to 1 in 25 000 of the population (Bülow et al. 1986; Järvinen, 1992) and accounts for under 1% of colorectal cancers in adults (in data from Finland over a similar period to the present analyses, the percentage decreased from 0.53% to 0.14% (Järvinen 1992)). The effect of colectomy for FAP on overall rates would therefore have been slight. Since colorectal cancers occur at a particularly young age in patients with familial polyposis (in patients without prophylactic measures, the mean age of cancer incidence is about 40 years (Nugent and Northover 1994)), the impact of prophylactic colectomies will have been greater at younger ages. Even at ages under 40, however, FAP accounts for only 5% of colorectal cancer cases[26] (Bülow 1980), and therefore the effect on general population trends will not have been large.

---

[26] In Danish data for 1943–67.

Inflammatory bowel diseases lead to greatly increased risk of colorectal malignancy, and large bowel resections can reduce this risk, so that such resections might have had a minor effect on overall colorectal cancer rates[27]. Cholecystectomy appears to increase the risk of colorectal cancer, but only by about 20% (Giovannucci *et al.* 1993). The impact of changes in cholecystectomy rates will therefore have been slight, particularly as rates of the operation have themselves only changed to a small extent (see p. 66 and Figure 5.52).

Anal cancers, which are coded in the ICD with rectal cancers, share several epidemiological characteristics with cervical cancer and appear, like cervical cancer, to be caused by a sexually transmitted infection, probably by certain types of human papilloma virus. There is also an association with immunosuppression, and perhaps smoking. Since these tumours contribute only about 2% of colorectal cancers in England and Wales, however, trends in their risk factors will not have affected colorectal cancer trends materially.

The reasons for the inflexions in colorectal cancer rates in the cohorts born around 1920 and 1950 are unclear. The decrease in mortality in the 1950–4 cohort compared with its immediate predecessor was particularly marked—18% in each sex. Too few colorectal cancers are due to FAP for prevention of these cases to explain the scale of decrease, and anyway measures for identification of and prophylaxis in persons with FAP have developed gradually over the last 50 years, rather than by introduction of a screening programme at any particular date. Diet changed greatly in the years soon after the Second World War, with fresh fruit imports increasing (and other changes, such as increased fat and decreased fibre in the diet, that would be expected to have an adverse effect on colorectal cancer rates). Diet in early life would therefore have been greatly different for the 1950–4 birth cohort than its immediate predecessors, but adult diet would not.

Cancer of the pancreas (Figure 6.9)

Secular trends

Mortality from cancer of the pancreas did not change greatly in the 20 years after 1960, but more recently

rates at younger ages in women and all ages in men have started to decrease substantially. Incidence trends (not shown) were similar, although with a less marked recent reduction.

Trends by birth cohort

Trends in mortality by birth cohort have been small until recently. There were rises from the 1875–9 cohort to the 1900–4 cohort in men and the 1915–19 cohort in women[28], and subsequently decreases, especially in the most recent cohorts. Incidence trends (not shown) were similar, except that in women there was not a clear decrease in the most recent cohorts.

Mortality trends by region

In men, changes in pancreatic cancer rates have been modest. In women they have ranged from a 50% increase in Oxford region to almost no change in the southernmost regions.

Comment

Smoking is the main known risk factor for pancreatic cancer, although with a much lower attributable risk than for lung cancer. The pancreatic cancer trends would accord with this, as the highest rates were in the cohorts of men born in 1900–9 and women born in 1915–29, close to the peaks for lung cancer (Figure 6.11) and for tar-adjusted smoking[29] (Figure 5.51). The similarity of the mortality and the incidence trends for pancreatic cancer accords with the continuing poor survival from this tumour (Figure A7).

Much of the recent downturn in pancreatic cancer mortality is in years after those for which incidence data are available. Only a minority of the decrease is explicable by the changes in the Registrar General's coding procedures in 1993 (see pp. 11–12), which we estimate would have given a 3% diminution in rates, compared with the 8% decrease in men and 4% in women that occurred from 1985–9 to 1990–4, with further decreases from 1990–4 to 1995–7. Increasing rates of cancer of unspecified primary site (Figure 6.35) may also have contributed a small artefactual down-

---

[27] Only 1% of cases under age 40 in Denmark in 1943–67 were accounted for by this cause (Bülow 1980).

[28] With mortality only marginally lower in the cohort of men born in 1905–9 and of women born in 1920–29.

[29] For men, there is a close correspondence for cumulative smoking at older ages; for women there appears also to be a close correspondence, as far as can be judged from the available smoking data, although these did not give full information on the peak at older ages.

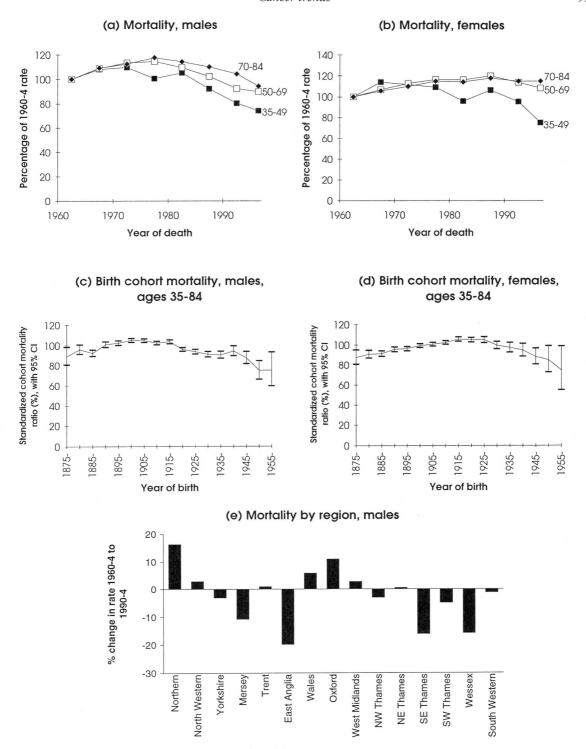

Figure 6.9 Cancer of pancreas (ICD7–9 157), mortality 1960–97.

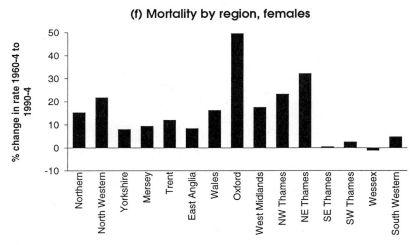

Figure 6.9   Cancer of pancreas (continued).

ward element to mortality rates for pancreatic cancer, as this cancer is relatively often the correct diagnosis for cancers certified as of unknown site (Heasman and Lipworth 1966). Autopsy leads to diagnosis of pancreatic cancers that would not otherwise have been detected (Heasman and Lipworth 1966), so that diminishing rates of non-coroner's autopsy (Figure 4.1) are likely to have contributed to the downward trend in pancreatic cancer rates. The main reason, however, for the diminishing rates of pancreatic cancer is likely to be reductions in smoking, as discussed above, although the cancer trends need to be interpreted cautiously. Because of the difficulty of diagnosis of cancers of the pancreas, and the relatively high proportion of cases in which the diagnosis is made without histological confirmation, improvements in diagnostic techniques—for instance, computed tomography, endoscopic retrograde cholangiopancreatography, and percutaneous fine-needle aspiration—have potential to increase or decrease apparent rates, either by finding cases that would not previously have been diagnosed or by correcting erroneous clinical diagnoses (Anderson *et al.* 1996).

Cancer of the larynx (Figure 6.10)

Secular trends

Laryngeal cancer mortality in men has remained little changed at ages under 50 years and decreased

moderately at older ages. In women, the pattern has been almost the opposite—rates decreased greatly at younger ages, but were little changed at older ages. Incidence of laryngeal cancer has changed little at any age in men[30], but in women has decreased somewhat at young ages and increased at older ages, especially 70–84 years.

Trends by birth cohort

Mortality in men decreased in cohorts born up to 1910–14, then did not change greatly except for a high rate in the cohort born in 1940–4. In women, mortality decreased in the earliest cohorts, then increased from the 1890–4 cohort to that born in 1920–4, and has since decreased substantially. Incidence trends were similar, except that there was no decrease in the earliest cohorts.

Mortality trends by region

Mortality in men has decreased substantially in all regions except those in the north, where there have been small decreases or an increase. In women, trends have varied from a 40% decrease in Mersey region to a 20% increase in NE Thames. There are considerable regional variations in current rates in each sex, with greatest rates generally in northern regions.

---

[30] The apparent rise and fall at ages 15–34 in Figure 6.10c is based on small numbers (Appendix C, Table 9).

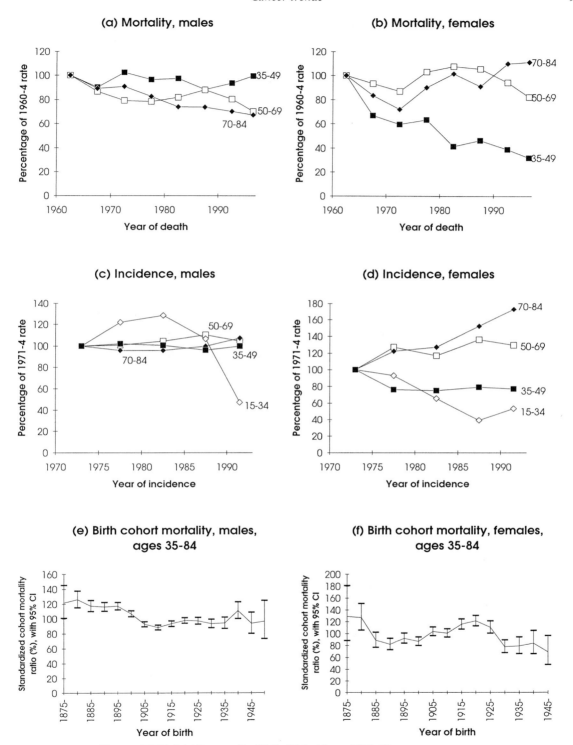

Figure 6.10   Cancer of larynx (ICD7–9 161), mortality 1960–97, incidence 1971–92.

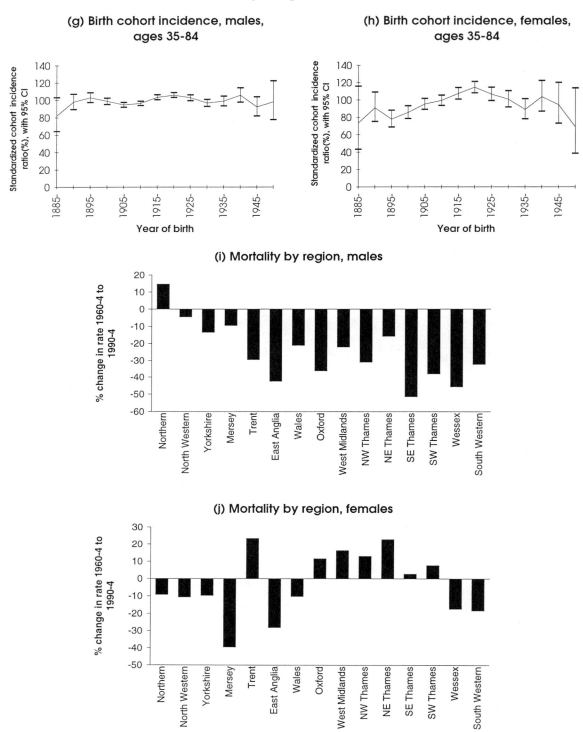

Figure 6.10   Cancer of larynx (continued).

Comment

As laryngeal cancer, like oral and pharyngeal and oesophageal cancers, is mainly attributable to alcohol and tobacco use[31] (with a multiplicative effect of both together), it is surprising that unlike these other cancers, laryngeal cancer rates have not been increasing in young men. This also contrasts with rising laryngeal (as well as oral and pharyngeal, and oesophageal) cancer rates in young men in Scotland (Swerdlow *et al.* 1998), similar trends for oesophageal and laryngeal cancers in men in France (Tuyns and Audigier 1976), and similar trends for laryngeal as for oral and pharyngeal and oesophageal cancers in men in the US (Devesa *et al.* 1990) although not in Japan (Wynder *et al.* 1991). The laryngeal cancer trends in women in England and Wales, however, resembled those for oesophageal cancer (Figure 6.5), and were less similar to the trends for pharyngeal cancer (Figure 6.4), for which decreases occurred at all ages, and unlike the trends for oral cancer (Figure 6.3).

In men, the laryngeal cancer trends bear no strong resemblance to those for smoking (Figures 5.47a, 5.48a, 5.50a, 5.51a) or lung cancer (Figure 6.11), and although the slight dip in rates for cohorts born about 1910 might correspond with low alcohol consumption (Figure 5.3) (and low cirrhosis mortality rates (Figure 5.5)) in the 1930s to 1950s, when these cohorts were young adults, the subsequent large increases in alcohol consumption and cirrhosis were not paralleled by rising laryngeal cancer rates. In women, however, the peak of laryngeal cancer incidence and mortality in the cohort born in 1920–4 corresponds with the peak of lung cancer (Figure 6.11) in this cohort, and with the peak for tar-adjusted smoking[32] (Figure 5.51b). The laryngeal cancer trends in women showed little relation to trends in alcohol consumption (Figure 5.3) or cirrhosis mortality (Figure 5.5), which have risen in recent decades.

There has been some evidence that intake of fresh fruit and vegetables, or of particular vitamins, may be protective against laryngeal cancer, but trends in consumption of these foods and nutrients (Table 5.6, Figures 5.16, 5.17, 5.19, 5.20) gave no obvious explanation for the laryngeal cancer trends. Several occupational exposures are associated with raised risk of laryngeal cancer, including work in manufacture of mustard gas, sulphuric acid mist exposure, and possibly asbestos exposure, but these cause too few cases to have affected trends materially.

Discrimination between laryngeal cancers and cancers of adjacent sites in the oro- and hypo-pharynx can be problematic (Muir 1992), so there is potential for changes in diagnostic or coding boundaries to have affected trend data.

The generally slightly more upward direction of trends for incidence than mortality from laryngeal cancer accords with evidence, although inconsistent, for a modest improvement in survival (Figure A8).

Cancer of the lung (Figures 6.11, 612)

Secular trends

Lung cancer mortality in men has decreased by a half at ages 50–69, by two-thirds at ages 35–49, and by over four-fifths at ages 15–34 since 1960. At ages 70–84, although rates increased to a peak around 1980 there has since been a diminution of a quarter. The trends in women were less favourable. Although there was a large decrease at ages 15–34, and after initial increases there have been decreases at ages 35–49 and 50–69, there has been an almost fourfold increase at ages 70–84, which continues. Overall, the peak rate of lung cancer mortality in males was reached in 1974, at 162 deaths per 100 000 men aged 15–84 per year, and in women a plateau has been reached, with the greatest rate to date, which may prove in retrospect to have been the peak of the epidemic, in 1989 at 44 per 100 000, a quarter of the peak rate in men.

Trends in incidence were similar to those for mortality except that at ages 15–34 years the decrease was considerably less than that for mortality and as a consequence the gap between incidence and mortality rates at these ages has widened. In women aged 35–49, incidence rates have ceased to improve since 1980.

The differences in trend by sex for this tumour have greatly diminished the sex ratio in rates at young ages. In 1960–4, male mortality at ages 35–49 was four times that in women; by 1995–7 it was only 1.4 times.

---

[31] For the extrinsic larynx (supraglottis), which is exposed to both inhaled and ingested agents, there is evidence that alcohol is the principal risk factor, whereas for the intrinsic larynx (glottis and subglottis), which is exposed only to inhaled agents, smoking predominates; both exposures affect each site, however (Elwood *et al.* 1984).

[32] As far as it can be judged from the available data—see pp. 65 and 104–6.

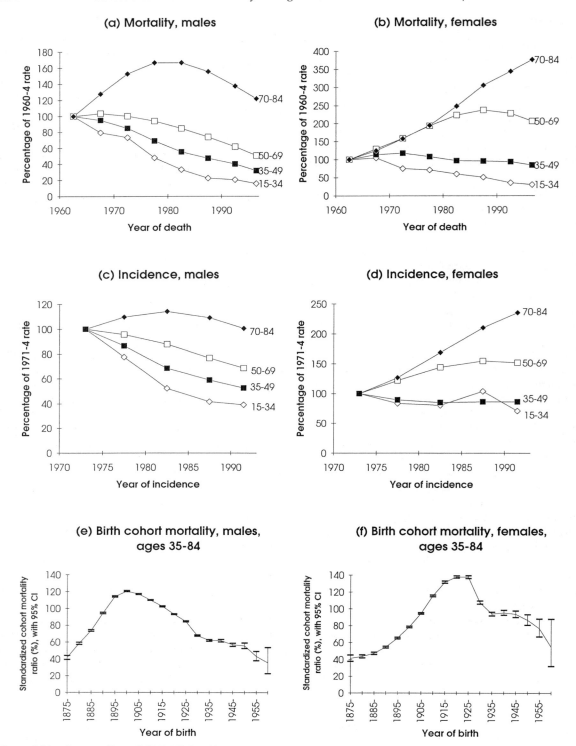

Figure 6.11 Cancer of lung (ICD7 162.0, 162.1, 162.8, 163.1, 163.3; ICD8&9 162), mortality 1960–97, incidence 1971–92.

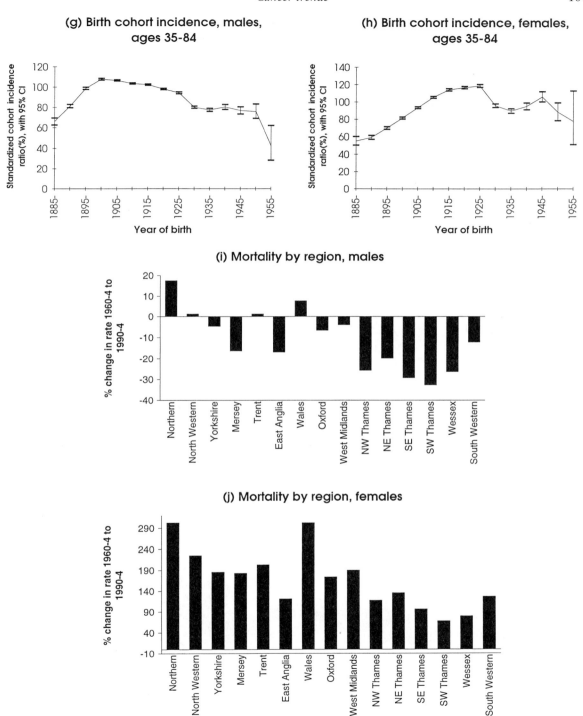

Figure 6.11 Cancer of lung (continued).

(a) Mortality 1911-97, ages 0-84, by sex

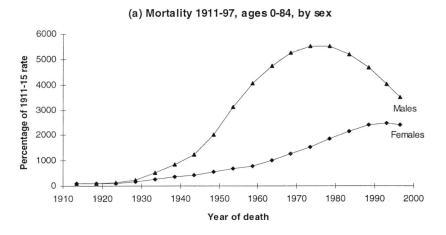

(b) Mortality 1911-97, males, by age

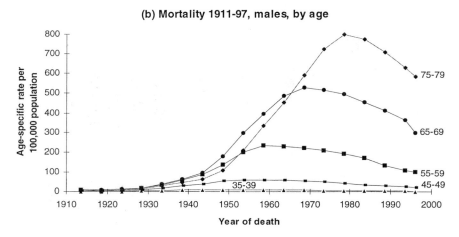

(c) Mortality 1911-97, females, by age

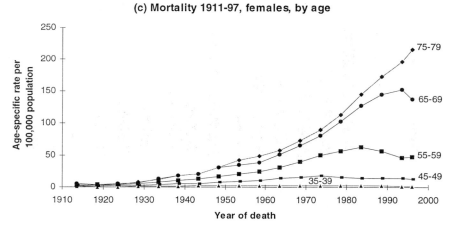

Figure 6.12   Cancers of lung and pleura (ICD2–6 as supplied by the Registrar General to Case *et al.* (1976); ICD7 162, 163; ICD8 162, 163.0; ICD9 162, 163).

Figure 6.12 shows long-term trends in mortality from lung and pleural cancers combined. ICD coding does not allow their separation before 1968 (ICD8), and although fourth digit coding added to ICD7 by the Registrar General enabled us to separate the data for the two sites back to 1960, in order to analyse trends before then we had to aggregate them. The trends displayed are virtually for lung cancer, however, as pleural cancer has been so much less common[33]. In males, recorded all-ages mortality increased over 50-fold from 1911–15 to a peak in the 1970s, before declining by a third (Figure 6.12a). In females the mortality rate has increased more gradually, but nevertheless by almost 25-fold, to a peak in 1991–5. Examining the trend in males by age (Figure 6.12b), the peak rate was reached much earlier at young ages than at older: for instance, the peak at ages 35–9 years was in 1951–5, that at ages 55–9 in 1956–60, and at ages 75–9 in 1976–80[34]. A similar effect was present for women (Figure 6.12c), but shifted about 25 years later, and with considerably lower absolute rates.

Trends by birth cohort

Mortality from lung cancer reached a peak in the cohort of men born in 1900–4 (1900 in single year of birth data) and in women born in 1920–9 (1925 in single year of birth data). The rise to the peak in each sex was progressive over cohorts born during several decades, but in women the subsequent decrease was initially extraordinarily sharp. The SCMR for women born in 1925 was 147.8 compared with 104.8 for those born 7 years later. In each sex there was a temporary halt to the decrease in rates for those born during 1940–4, and then a continued decrease for those born subsequently.

In incidence data there was a similar pattern, except that the interruption to the downward trend for those born around the time of the Second World War was longer and in women led to a marked peak in the 1945–9 cohort.

Mortality trends by region

There have been important regional differences in the progress and passing of the lung cancer epidemic in England and Wales. In men the trend in the south of England in the last 30 years has been downward, while elsewhere there has been little change or even an increase. In women there have been considerable increases in all regions, but less in the south than elsewhere. There is now a marked north/south gradient in lung cancer mortality in England and Wales, with greater rates in the north, especially in women.

Comment

The cancers included under 'lung' cancer are those of the trachea, bronchus, and lung, mainly the bronchus. Lung cancer mortality rates in men in England and Wales from 1950 to 1975 were the highest recorded in the world except for Scotland (Kurihara *et al.* 1989). The peak rate has been passed earlier in England and Wales than in most other Western countries, however, so that the recent rates in England and Wales have been less exceptional. In women, too, mortality from lung cancer has been unusually high by international standards, but less so in recent years than in the early post-war decades.

Since 1948, lung cancer has been the most common site among cancer deaths recorded in men in England and Wales[35], and since 1982 it has been the second most common in women. The large changes in lung cancer rates over time have been the dominant contribution to changes in cancer mortality rates overall for most of the period since the Second World War. The trends early in the twentieth century are likely to have included a considerable element of artefactual increase

---

[33] In 1960–4 deaths certified to pleural cancer constituted 0.2% of the total at ages 0–84 years in men and 0.7% in women; by 1990–4 this had risen to 2.0% in men and 0.8% in women, and in 1995–7 was 2.2% and 0.6% respectively. These figures slightly underestimate the proportion that are truly pleural cancers because some cases are miscertified as lung cancer: in data for 1986–91 from the GB mesothelioma register, mesotheliomas certified as lung cancer on the death certificate were just over a quarter as common as mesotheliomas certified to pleural cancer (Hutchings *et al.* 1995).

[34] It will be noted that in men the peaks at young ages are in somewhat later birth cohorts than those at older ages. There is no such discrepancy by age in women.

[35] As judged from the cancer categories then coded: the most common in that year was lung plus pleura, and the second most common was stomach plus duodenum.

from improving diagnosis[36] (Doll and Peto 1981), but at least for the period since the Second World War the trends are likely largely to have been real. The introduction of new diagnostic technologies—computerized tomography, fibre-optic bronchoscopy, and fine needle biopsy—may have affected lung cancer trends at older ages at least, but in which direction is uncertain: lung cancers could have been diagnosed that would have otherwise remained undiscovered, but also there could have been a reduction in the extent to which other lung pathologies were erroneously diagnosed as primary lung cancer (Gilliland and Samet 1994). Coding and 'medical enquiry' (see pp. 11–12) artefacts for lung cancer have been relatively slight (Table 4.1), and artefact from change in position of recording lung cancer on death certificates has probably been negligible (Grulich *et al.* 1995). Undiagnosed lung cancer is relatively frequently discovered when autopsy is performed[37], and so the diminishing frequency of non-coroner's autopsy (Figure 4.1) will have added a small artefactual downward element to lung cancer trends in recent years. The proportion of lung cancers certified after autopsy (although not necessarily first diagnosed because of it) decreased from 15% in 1972 (OPCS 1974*b*) to 9% in 1992 (OPCS 1994). Exactly comparable data are not available for earlier decades, but 25% of lung and pleural cancers were diagnosed after autopsy in both 1921–32 and 1933–8 (Kennaway and Kennaway 1947) and the proportion of all respiratory cancers that were diagnosed after autopsy was 19% in both 1954 (Registrar General 1957) and 1965

(Registrar General 1968). Lung cancer is frequently the correct diagnosis for deaths certified as of 'unknown primary site' (Heasman and Lipworth 1966; Grulich *et al.* 1995), so that rising death rates from the latter (Figure 6.35) are likely to have contributed a small decreasing tendency to the lung cancer trends.

The main cause of lung cancer is smoking, a relation first shown clearly in Britain and the US 50 years ago (Doll and Hill 1950; Wynder and Graham 1950; Doll 1998), and the secular trends in the tumour mainly reflect changes in smoking habits and the tar content of cigarettes (Figures 5.47–5.49). In cohort data, the peak of lung cancer in men born in 1900–4 accords with the cohort peak of tar-adjusted smoking cumulated to old ages[38] (Figure 5.51a), and the cohort peaks of lung cancer and tar-adjusted smoking (Figure 5.51b) in women appear also to coincide, as far as can be judged from the available data on smoking, although these did not give full information on the peak at older ages[39].

The data in Figure 5.51 on tar-adjusted numbers of cigarettes consumed do not give a completely accurate representation of the carcinogenic load of smoking sustained by different birth cohorts, however, and various facets of the data and of other aspects of smoking need consideration.

Firstly, the data available on cumulative cigarette smoking in different cohorts are imperfect in at least three respects:

(1)   The age-specific data before 1946 (and hence also the cohort-specific data) are simply retrospective

---

[36] Interpretation of the pre-war trends (Figure 6.12) is uncertain because of the large element of underdiagnosis that occurred at that time. It is difficult to know exactly how much of the pre-war increase was an artefact of better diagnosis and certification, but this can be gauged approximately from trends in women. Before the Second World War rates in women would have been negligibly affected by smoking, because few women smoked before the mid-1930s (Figure 5.47b) and occupational exposures would have been low for women at that time. One might therefore expect that the true rates in women throughout the pre-war period would have been approximately the same as those in non-smokers now. Comparison of the national mortality rates in women in England and Wales (Figure 6.12) with those in non-smokers, based on a large US cohort study (Peto *et al.* 1992), suggests that approximately complete diagnosis in women (or at least as complete as that in the US in the 1980s) was reached in the 1930s for women aged 45–69, but not until about 1950 for older age groups. If it is accepted that the rise in apparent mortality in women before the Second World War was an artefact of better diagnosis and certification, then an approximately similar extent of rise in men may have been artefactual also, and on this basis about 40% of the overall increase in men in the pre-war period was an artefact of better diagnosis, and the other 60% represented a real increase (although varying by age, as underdiagnosis appears to have been greater in older age groups).
[37] In a large study in England and Wales in 1959 (Heasman and Lipworth 1966), the effect of autopsy was to add 19% to the number of lung cancers diagnosed ante-mortem.
[38] Data on smoking cumulated to old ages are the appropriate comparison for the overall, age-standardized, lung cancer data, and our discussion has concentrated on these age-standardized rates for simplicity. The peak cohort for smoking varied by age, however, and so did the lung cancer peak in men at ages under 55 years, although not at older ages or in women (see footnote 34). The peak of lung cancer mortality in men occurred in a slightly earlier cohort at older (55 years and above) than at younger ages, which would accord with the earlier peak cohort of cumulative smoking at older than at younger ages. For women, the cumulative smoking data in Figure 5.51b leave it uncertain whether the peak of smoking shifted between cohorts at ages over 50 years. At younger ages there were certainly large shifts, and the absence of comparable shifts in the age-specific lung cancer cohort data in women may reflect the deficiencies of the tar-adjusted smoking data as a measure of carcinogenic load of smoking, discussed in the next paragraphs in this section.
[39] See note 38.

estimates, because age-specific data on smoking were not collected at that time. The estimates are based on the broadly reasonable assumption that the age distribution of smoking has been similar within different cohorts, but this may not have been entirely true; for instance the effects of the World Wars on smoking habits will have occurred at different ages for different cohorts.

(2) Tar content is not a precise measure of the dose of carcinogen available from a cigarette.

(3) Although early cohorts of men smoked far fewer manufactured cigarettes than their successors, they smoked more of other forms of tobacco (pipes, cigars), which are also causes of lung cancer, although with a lower risk than cigarettes (Doll and Peto 1976). This last argument does not apply, however, to women.

A second deficiency of the smoking data is that the dose of carcinogen received from cigarettes depends on how they are smoked, not just how many are smoked. Several aspects of the way in which cigarettes are smoked—the length of butt discarded, the depth and speed of inhalation, puff frequency and puff size—may have altered over time and affected carcinogenicity. In the 1950s, the length of butt left unsmoked was substantially less in England and Wales than the US (Doll *et al.* 1959); if butt length has increased with growing prosperity, this would have diminished the carcinogenic load per cigarette. Data from the British doctors cohort study suggest that a lower proportion of female smokers born before the First World War than of those born later inhaled, and that there was a lesser tendency in the same direction for men (Doll *et al.* 1980). (The effect of self-reported inhaling on lung cancer risk is complex, however, and not clearly deleterious (Doll and Peto 1976)).

A third reason why the smoking data do not fully represent carcinogenic effect is that risk is not proportional simply to *cumulative* dose. The pattern of accumulation of this overall dose during life is also of

importance. At one end of the smoking history, age at starting smoking is strongly related to lung cancer risk in later life (Doll and Peto 1981); at the other, lung cancer rates are also particularly dependent on smoking over the previous decade or so, and giving up smoking reduces risk of lung cancer more greatly than its contribution to decreased cumulative consumption (Doll and Peto 1976). Thus changes in the age distribution of smoking within cohorts have implications for the overall effect of cumulative doses.

Contemporary data on age at starting to smoke are not available for cohorts born in the late nineteenth and early twentieth century. Questionnaires in the British doctors' cohort study show a considerably later mean age at starting to smoke (retrospectively-reported) for women born before the First World War than those born later[40], but only slightly the same tendency for men (Doll *et al.* 1980). General population surveys in the 1960s (again enquiring retrospectively) (Wald *et al.* 1988) reinforce this conclusion for women, but for men suggested, if anything, a slight reduction in starting to smoke at young ages between cohorts born around the start of the twentieth century and those born in the 1930s. More directly, the national data available since 1946 (Lee *et al.* 1990) show increasing smoking at the youngest ages analysed, 15–19 years, until 1971–5 in men and 1976–80 in women. The implication of these trends, although one cannot quantify it accurately, is that at least in women a shift towards an earlier age at starting to smoke has occurred, which would give an influence towards the peak cohort for lung cancer being later than that for cumulative tar-adjusted cigarette consumption.

The trend towards giving up smoking in recent years has also had differing effects on different cohorts, which may again have influenced the relative carcinogenic effects of cumulative smoking for early and more recent cohorts. The growing tendency to give up smoking has occurred far more at older ages than at younger[41], and occurred in both men and women (Table 5.25)[42]. The effect of this on lung cancer rates is

---

[40] And to some extent an older age again for those born in the nineteenth century.
[41] A small part of the explanation for the greater proportion of ex-smokers at older ages is that continued smoking causes premature mortality and therefore reduces the numbers of living current smokers, but this effect is too small to be the main explanation.
[42] The position is yet more complicated because even for continuing smokers the type and number of cigarettes smoked per day will have changed over the smoker's career, in different ways for different generations. For instance, because the average tar content of cigarettes decreased greatly from 1960 onwards (and modestly before then) (Figure 5.49), a smoker born early in the twentieth century would initially have smoked relatively high-tar cigarettes, and if he changed to low tar would have done so several decades later, so that his tar consumption would tend to have been concentrated towards the early part of his smoking career. A smoker born later, but with the same lifetime cumulative constant-tar consumption, however, might well have had more of his tar consumption later in life.

complex, and difficult to predict in the absence of cohort-specific data, because the changes have varied both by age and over time. As an example, however, a large proportion of men born around the start of the twentieth century have given up smoking, but only relatively recently; this must have diminished considerably their lung cancer rates at old ages, relative to those that would have occurred, but will have had little effect on their rates at younger ages, before most of them gave up.

Finally, the smoking and lung cancer data by cohort and age may not always coincide precisely because smoking, although the predominant cause of lung cancer in England and Wales, is not the sole cause, and changes in other aetiological (or preventive) factors may also have had some effect.

A small part of the decrease in lung cancer rates may be due to the great secular reduction that has occurred in air pollution in urban areas (Figure 5.2), and to improved industrial hygiene. About 15% of lung cancers in men and 5% in women may be attributable to occupational factors, in conjunction with smoking (Doll and Peto 1981). For one component, asbestos, exposure information is discussed below under 'cancer of the pleura'. Several other occupational causes have been identified, including exposures to inorganic arsenic, chlormethyl ethers, hexavalent and possibly other chromium compounds, mustard gas production, nickel refining, and polycyclic hydrocarbons. Many of these associations have been shown at specific industrial plants in England and Wales, as described in Doll (1975), and although certain of these plants have closed and industrial hygiene in general has much improved, we do not have data on the extent to which overall occupational exposures carcinogenic to the lung have altered over time.

Exposure to radon gas in air in houses may account for about 5% of lung cancers in England and Wales (Darby *et al.* 1998), and may have increased over time with the spread of double glazing and improved draught proofing (see pp. 37–38). There is evidence that low intake of fresh fruit and vegetables can increase the risk of lung cancer, but the trends since 1950 in consumption of these foodstuffs (Figures 5.16, 5.17) have been slight compared with those in lung cancer.

The differences in lung cancer trends by region are part of a long-term process, reflecting the geographical pattern of adoption, and later cessation, of smoking. In the 1920s, lung cancer mortality rates were greatest in the area around London, and rates were relatively low in the north of England (Stocks 1936, 1939). The epidemic spread out from London, and subsequently the retreat seems to have started first in the London area, and, as for the uptake decades earlier, to have occurred sooner in men than women (Swerdlow and dos Santos Silva 1991).

The rising incidence to mortality ratio for lung cancer at ages under 35 years implies improving survival; no national data are available on survival from lung cancer at these ages, and too few cases occurred in East Anglia to assess trends. At older ages, the similar trends for incidence and mortality are unsurprising for a tumour with continuing poor survival (Figure A.9).

In conclusion, although considerable progress has been made against lung cancer since its main cause was shown 50 years ago, the preventive task is far from over. The fall in lung cancer mortality in recent cohorts represents one of the great successes of prevention in the twentieth century, albeit a success over a man-made epidemic, but the continuing rise in rates in older women, the trends in the most recent cohorts, and the narrowing gap between male and female rates, serve as a reminder that the epidemic is far from over: at its peak (in 1974 for men, 1989 for women) lung cancer accounted for 41% of cancer deaths in men and 17% in women aged under 85 years in England and Wales; in 1997 it accounted for 28% and 18%[43] in the two sexes respectively. The percentage if no one in the country had ever smoked would be about 6% in men and 5% in women[44].

Cancer of the pleura (Figure 6.13)

Secular trends

Mortality certified to cancer of the pleura has increased enormously in each sex over the past 35 years. In 1960–4 there were only 34 deaths registered per year in men aged 0–84 years in England and Wales, and 23

---

[43] Slightly greater than in 1989 because the number of deaths from other cancers in women has fallen considerably.
[44] Based on cancer rates in non-smokers in a large US cohort study in the 1980s (Peto *et al.* 1992) standardized to the England and Wales population in 1981, 6.3% of cancers in male non-smokers and 5.6% in female non-smokers at ages 35 years and above would be lung cancers. Assuming that virtually no lung cancers would occur at ages under 35 years (on which non-smoker cohort data are not available), and allowing for non-lung cancers occurring at ages under 35 years, and subtracting cancers at ages 85 and above, about 6% of cancers in male non-smokers and 5% in female non-smokers at ages under 85 would be lung cancers.

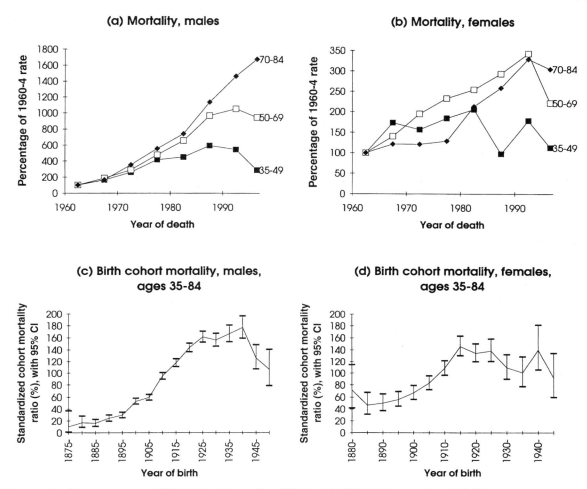

Figure 6.13 Cancer of pleura (ICD7 162.2, 163.2, 163.4; ICD8 163.0; ICD9 163), mortality 1960–97.

per year in women, but by 1995–7 there were 419 per year in men and 63 per year in women. In each sex the percentage increase has been less at ages 35–49 years than at older ages. In women the most recent trend, since 1990–4, has been downwards at all ages, whereas in men it has been downwards at ages under 70, but still rising at older ages.

In incidence data (not shown) there were steeper increases than those for mortality, with no downward trend in the most recent data, for 1990–2.

Trends by birth cohort

Mortality in men increased to a peak for those born in 1940–4 and then declined greatly. In women, there was a sharp increase up to the cohort born in 1915–19, and thereafter an inconsistent, but generally downward, trend. Incidence data (not shown) were similar, except that rates in women reached their greatest level for the cohort born in 1940–4.

Mortality trends by region

There were too few deaths in the early period to examine time trends by region for this cancer.

Comment

Pleural cancer trends reflect trends in asbestos exposure, particularly to blue asbestos (crocidolite) and brown asbestos (amosite), which are the predominant causes of this tumour, and probably also reflect improved completeness of diagnosis. The asbestos exposure has mainly been occupational, from an extraordinarily wide range of uses including shipbuilding, manufacture of asbestos goods, and construction. The induction period is typically several decades, so that it is unsurprising that the high levels of asbestos importation (Figure 5.9) and use in the 1950s to 1970s should have been followed by rising rates of pleural cancer decades later. This interpretation is over-simplified, especially as a guide to future trends, however, for two reasons. On the one hand, imported asbestos, particularly that used in construction of buildings, continues to cause exposures long after its initial use (for instance, during renovation and demolition), but on the other, protective measures for asbestos workers have greatly improved over time.

Pleural cancer mortality data have considerable scope for error from both overdiagnosis and underdiagnosis. For instance in Britain in 1967–8, 35 of 280 deaths certified to mesothelioma were found on pathological examination not to be this tumour at all (Greenberg and Lloyd Davies 1974), and in 1986–91, 41% of mesothelioma deaths recorded by the GB mesothelioma register were recorded at death with an underlying cause of death other than pleural or peritoneal malignancy (mainly as lung cancer or cancer of unspecified primary site) (Hutchings *et al.* 1995). Mesothelioma became a prescribed occupational disease, attracting financial compensation, in England and Wales in 1966 (McDonald 1979), providing a powerful incentive for more frequent diagnosis.

We have no data on trends in survival from pleural cancer because these have not been published for England and Wales, and there were too few cases in East Anglia for satisfactory analysis. The greater rate of increase in incidence than mortality rates in each sex (even before 1993—see below) are likely to reflect a degree of artefact in either the mortality or the incidence trends, however, because mesothelioma is a tumour with a dismal prognosis that as far as we know has not improved substantially.

The apparent decrease in pleural cancer mortality rates in the most recent years in Figure 6.13 is largely an artefact: rates (at ages 0–84) decreased by 16% in males and 34% in females in 1993 when medical enquiries to certifiers were stopped. The pleura had been a site for which such enquiries had been especially productive in revealing otherwise uncertified cases[45]. It has been estimated that the number of cases in men is likely to increase for the next 20 years (Peto *et al.* 1995).

Cancer of the bone (Figure 6.14)

Cancer of the bone is a comparatively uncommon tumour, which accounts for about 0.2% of cancers incident in England and Wales. We have not, therefore, presented data for this cancer site in full. Interpretation of trends at older ages is made particularly difficult by the high frequency with which the bone is a site of metastasis of cancers originating at other sites. Primary cases at older ages are often complications of Paget's disease (MacKenzie *et al.* 1961; Boyd *et al.* 1969).

Trends in bone cancer incidence are of particular interest, however, because of the raised risk in relation to ionizing radiation exposure, and in particular to radioisotopes that concentrate in the bone. As a consequence of this deposition, there is a possibility that radioactive fallout might have caused increased rates of bone cancer. Figure 6.14 therefore shows trends in incidence of bone cancer, both over time and by birth cohort. There is no consistent indication of secular increases (Figures 6.14a,b) in response to the high levels of fallout from the mid 1950s to mid 1960s (Figures 5.26, 5.28) and the high level of bone-deposition of fallout radioactivity in the mid 1960s (Figures 5.29)[46], although the incidence data only relate to the period since 1971, not the years sooner after the nuclear tests. There is also no consistent evidence of raised risk in birth cohorts who were aged under 5 years[47] in the mid 1960s (Figures 6.14g–j), when fallout radiation levels in bone reached their maximum (Figure 5.29)[48].

---

[45] A 23% decrease in 1993 would be expected (Table 4.1) from the numbers of cases that had previously been revealed by medical enquiries. Altered interpretation of rule 3 of the ICD did not affect coding of this tumour.

[46] The rise of incidence in girls aged 0–14 years to a peak in 1980–4 was not paralleled in boys, and this peak in 1980–4 was anyway largely in girls born after the peak years of fallout.

[47] The ages of maximum bone uptake—see Figure 5.29. Cohorts with exposure at young ages are also important because childhood exposures, to external ionizing radiation at least, appear to lead to far greater relative risks of bone cancer than do exposures at older ages (Tucker *et al.* 1987; Miller *et al.* 1996).

[48] The only cohort peak that was consistent between the sexes, and then with confidence intervals that would include no raised risk, was in persons born in 1951. This cohort does not appear, however, to be one that received particularly high bone radiation doses (Figure 5.28).

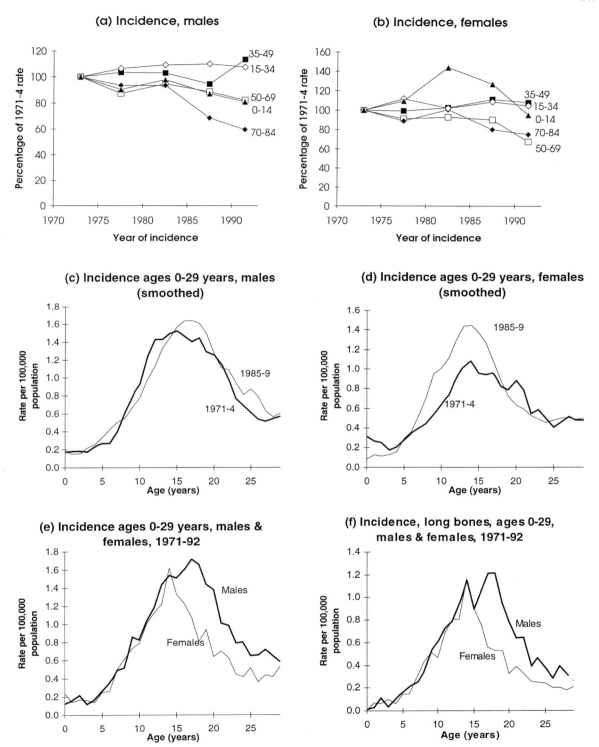

Figure 6.14 Cancer of bone (ICD7 196; ICD8, 9 170), incidence 1971–92: (a)–(e) all bones; (f) long bones.

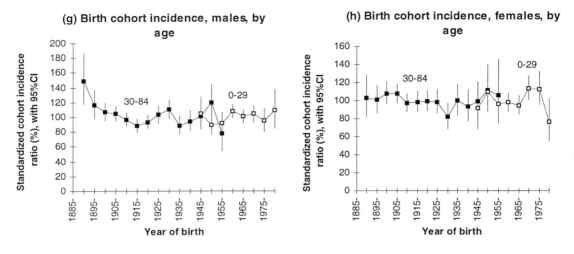

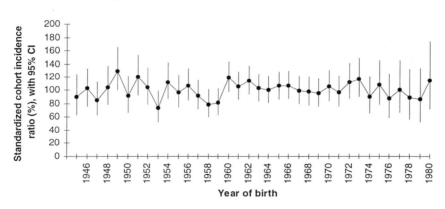

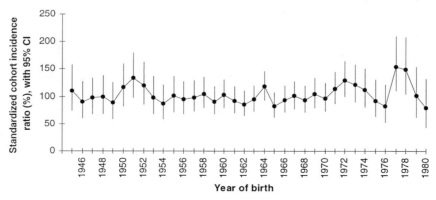

Figure 6.14   Cancer of bone (continued): (g)–(j) all bones.

Another point of interest about bone cancer is that a peak of incidence occurs in young adults, which relates to growth in adolescence (MacKenzie *et al.* 1961; Fraumeni 1967), and is accounted for mainly by tumours in the tibia and femur, the bones that grow most rapidly. As age at menarche has been decreasing over time, although perhaps with a reversal in recent cohorts (Figure 5.38, Table 5.20), and average height is increasing (Figures 5.7, 5.8), it seems of interest to determine whether the rates and age distribution of incidence of this tumour in adolescents and young adults have changed. Examination of data by single year of age (Figures 6.14c,d) shows that in males the peak does not appear to have increased substantially in magnitude, whereas in females the peak was greater in 1985–9 than 1971–4. In the Figures we have presented curves that have been smoothed by calculation of moving averages of incidence rates, rather than the rates themselves, but in unsmoothed data the same features were present, albeit more unevenly. Data by birth cohort for ages under 30 give no clear indication of upward or downward trends (Figures 6.14g,h).

Figure 6.14e compares the age distribution of bone cancer incidence at young ages in the two sexes, and Figure 6.14f shows a similar comparison for cancer of the long bones, using data for the entire period 1971–92 to give stability of large numbers. A younger and slightly lower peak of incidence is seen in females than males[49], a pattern described previously in mortality data for England and Wales for cancer of the limb bones from 1961–6 (Boyd *et al.* 1969) and in US data for incidence and mortality of osteogenic sarcoma and Ewing's sarcoma (Glass and Fraumeni 1970), and which would accord with the age distribution of growth of the long bones in the two sexes (Tanner 1989). There was not, however, a greater incidence rate for girls than boys at prepubertal ages; this contrasts with the greater rates in girls than boys at these ages noted previously in data on mortality from cancers of the limb bones in England and Wales (Boyd *et al.* 1969), and for osteosarcoma mortality in the US (Glass and Fraumeni 1970) and incidence of Ewing's sarcoma but not osteosarcoma in England and Wales in 1971–84 (dos Santos Silva and Swerdlow 1993).

Cancer of the soft tissues (Figure 6.15)

Secular trends

Mortality from cancer of the soft tissues in children decreased dramatically in the 10 years after 1970–4, but in adults, except for an unchanged rate in young women, there have been substantial increases, especially at older ages. Incidence increased at all adult ages, but in children there were decreases, although less than those for mortality.

Trends by birth cohort

Mortality rates increased until the cohort of men born in 1935–9 and of women born in 1945–9, and then decreased. Incidence increased from the earliest cohort to the most recent, with no downturn as yet.

Mortality trends by region

Mortality increased in all regions, with no consistent geographical pattern.

Comment

Soft tissue cancers include malignancies of a range of different tissues—blood and lymphatic vessels, muscle, fibrous tissue and other supporting tissue (excluding bone and cartilage), and fat. Substantial proportions of these tumours may not be coded to the ICD site code for soft tissue tumours, however. For instance, in US incidence data half of all soft tissue cancers (on histological grounds) were coded to site codes other than soft tissue[50] (Zahm *et al.* 1996), and in Denmark less than half of incident non-lymphoid extraskeletal sarcomas[51] were coded to the site code for soft tissue, with somewhat different time trends for those coded to this site and elsewhere (Lynge *et al.* 1987). Although some of the tumours coded elsewhere, for instance Kaposi's sarcoma and angiosarcomas of the liver, are ones that anyway might best be considered separately from soft tissue tumours in general, these coding variations

---

[49] More clearly for bone cancer overall than for cancers of long bones, for which the pattern was more uneven, based on smaller numbers.
[50] This included Kaposi's sarcoma, for which the correct ICD site coding category is the skin.
[51] See note 50.

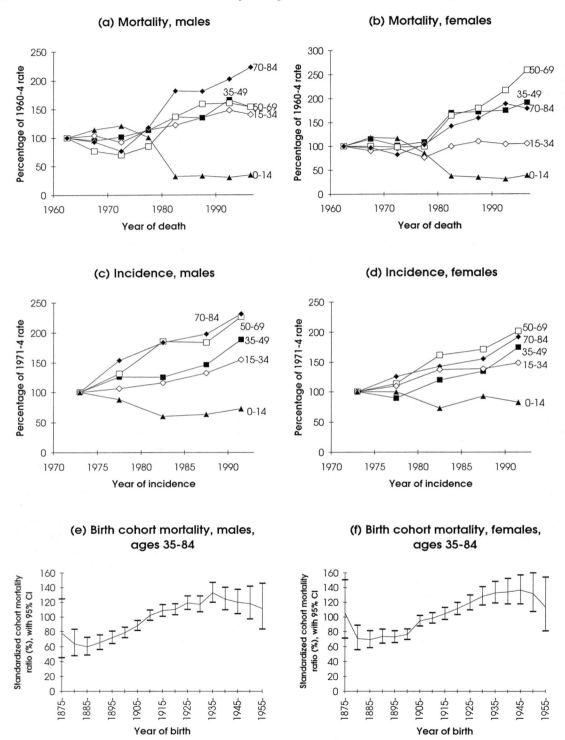

Figure 6.15 Cancer of soft tissues (ICD7 193.3, 193.4, 197; ICD8 171.0, 171.2–.9; 192.4, 192.5; ICD9 171), mortality 1960–97, incidence 1971–92.

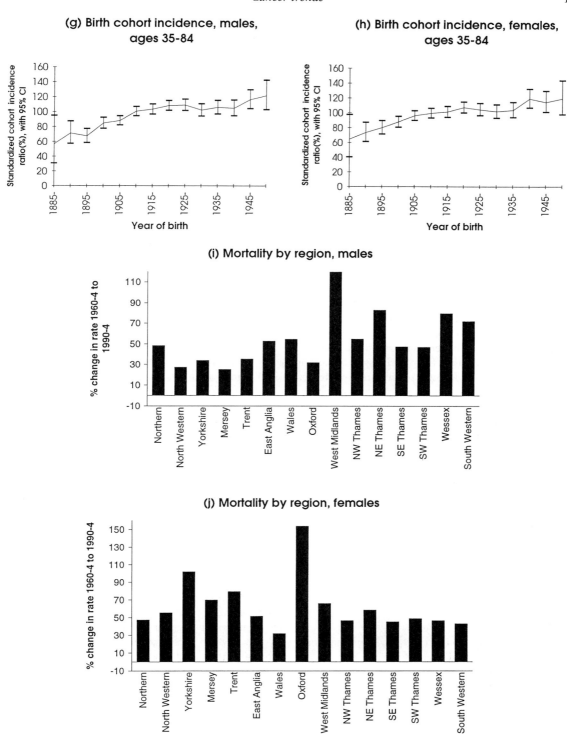

(g) Birth cohort incidence, males, ages 35-84

(h) Birth cohort incidence, females, ages 35-84

(i) Mortality by region, males

(j) Mortality by region, females

Figure 6.15   Cancer of soft tissues (continued).

nevertheless cloud interpretation of trends. Furthermore, on death certificates for patients with cancer, histology of the tumour is often not stated, which may again lead to under-assignment to the soft tissue cancer rubric. As a consequence, one cannot be sure that the apparent increases in incidence and mortality in adults are not, at least in part, due to changed reporting and coding.

Ionizing radiation exposure is a cause of a small percentage of soft tissue tumours, but too few to have affected population trends appreciably. Raised risk of soft tissue sarcomas is seen in immunodepressed subjects, including those with AIDS and patients who have received organ transplants, but the numbers of cases known to be due to these causes is small compared with the total number of cases occurring in the population. Exposure to phenoxyacetic acid herbicides, chlorophenols, and their contaminants have been found as risk factors for soft tissue tumours in some studies, but not consistently (Zahm *et al.* 1996), so that the possibility that these may have influenced trends is speculative. In summary, therefore, there have been substantial increases in recent decades in the recorded incidence of and mortality from soft tissue cancers in adults, which are not known to be due to artefact, cannot be attributed to changes in known risk factors, and need explanation.

The much greater decrease in mortality than incidence of soft tissue cancers in children accords with the large improvement in survival from childhood rhabdomyosarcoma (Figure B2)[52], which accounts for well over half of these tumours. The similarity of the trends for incidence and mortality in adults accords with the unchanged survival from soft tissue cancers at all-ages (Figure A10).

Malignant melanoma of the skin

(Figure 6.16)

Secular trends

Since 1960 (Figures 6.16a,b) mortality from malignant melanoma has increased greatly in each sex at each adult age, except that at ages 15–34 there has been little change. At ages 35–49 the most recent data show a downturn in rates, but at older ages the increase is continuing. The percentage increases have been greater in men than women, and at older than at younger ages.

Site-specific data on melanoma mortality are difficult to interpret and were not analysed, because the proportion of melanomas coded to 'other and unspecified site' has risen over 10-fold over the period, and this category now accounts for the great majority of melanoma deaths.

Cutaneous melanoma and non-melanoma skin cancer were first separated in ICD coding in ICD6, and hence from 1950 onwards in data for England and Wales. Figures 6.16n and o show melanoma mortality trends at selected ages since 1951. Although the trend in the years before those presented in Figures 6.16a and b was generally upward, it was not uniformly so, most notably at old ages in men.

Incidence of melanoma has increased more than mortality, and unlike mortality has increased greatly at all adult ages (in children trends have been erratic, based on small numbers). The increase appears to have tailed off at young ages in the most recent period of data (1990–2). When all-age rates were examined by single calendar year (Figure 6.16e), there was an indication of a peak of incidence in each sex in 1988.

The proportion of incident melanoma cases for which site was recorded has remained high (although decreasing), and we have therefore presented in Table 6.2 trends in incidence by site. There have been substantial increases in rates at each site analysed, and as the rate of melanoma of unstated site has increased, the true rates of increase of site-specific melanoma must be greater than they appear. In each sex, the percentage rises have been greatest for melanomas of the trunk and upper limb. In general, the site-specific increases have not varied greatly by age (not shown). A marked exception, however, was trunk melanoma (Figures 6.16j,k): in men the percentage increase for this site was progressively greater with older age, while in women the opposite was true. There were also variations in trend by age for melanoma of the lower limb in women, which increased more at ages 70–84 than at younger ages, and for head and neck melanoma in men, which increased more at ages 50 and above than at younger ages.

---

[52] Data on trends in childhood survival were not available for soft tissue cancers overall.

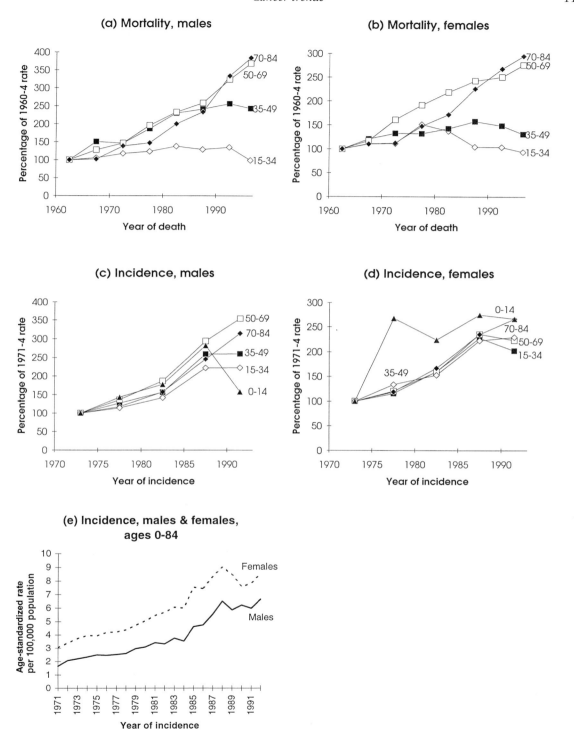

(a) Mortality, males

(b) Mortality, females

(c) Incidence, males

(d) Incidence, females

(e) Incidence, males & females, ages 0-84

Figure 6.16 Malignant melanoma of skin (ICD7 190; ICD8 172.0–.4, 172.6–.9; ICD9 172), mortality 1960–97, incidence 1971–92: (a)–(e) all skin sites.

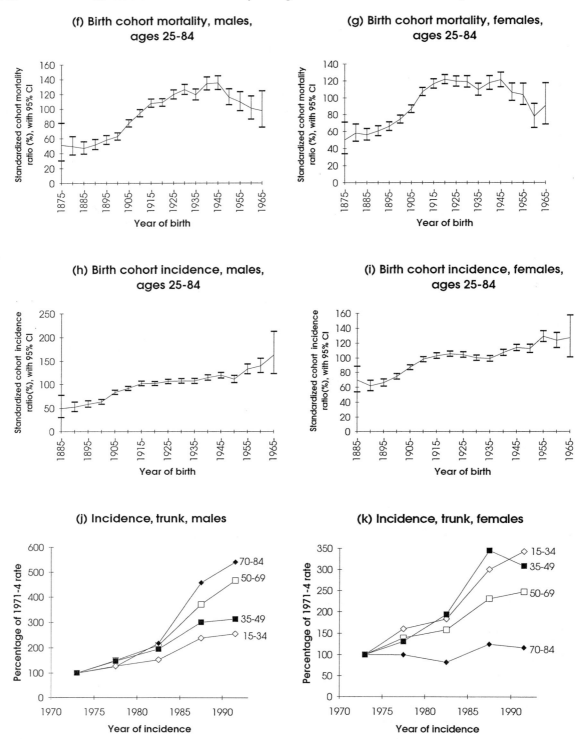

Figure 6.16   Malignant melanoma of skin (continued); (f)–(i) all skin sites; (j)–(k) trunk.

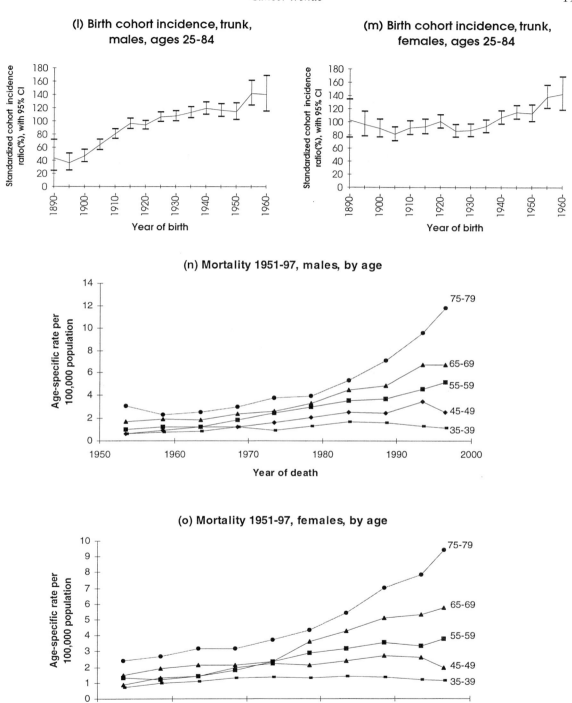

Figure 6.16   Malignant melanoma of skin (continued); (l)–(m) trunk; (n)–(o) all skin sites.

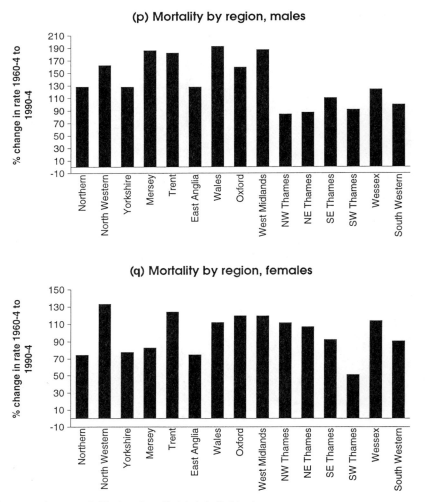

Figure 6.16   Malignant melanoma of skin (continued): (p), (q) all skin sites.

Table 6.2   Incidence of melanoma of the skin at ages 15–84 years by site, 1971–4 and 1990–2

Site	Males 1971–4		1990–2		1990–2 rate as % of 1971–4 rate	Females 1971–4		1990–2		1990–2 rate as % of 1971–4 rate
	No.	Rate[a]	No.	Rate[a]		No.	Rate[a]	No.	Rate[a]	
Head and neck	401	0.62	878	1.62	261	545	0.66	788	1.13	171
Upper limb	271	0.39	642	1.12	288	519	0.65	1086	1.70	262
Trunk	510	0.70	1604	2.77	397	450	0.56	889	1.39	250
Lower limb	473	0.69	762	1.34	193	1973	2.43	3030	4.71	193
Other and NK site	124	0.19	595	1.05	560	115	0.14	726	1.12	793
All sites	1779	2.59	4481	7.90	305	3602	4.44	6519	10.04	226

[a] Rate per 100 000 per year.

Trends by birth cohort

There were large increases in melanoma mortality in cohorts born up to the 1920s in women and 1940s in men, but in generations born since 1950 there have been substantial declines in each sex.

Incidence of melanoma in each sex increased strongly in the cohorts born before 1920, and has increased less consistently but nevertheless substantially in the cohorts born since then. Examination of site-specific cohort trends revealed no major deviation from this pattern except that for head and neck melanoma (not shown) there was no consistent change in risk beyond the cohorts of women born in 1910–14 and men born in 1920–4, and for trunk melanoma (Figures 6.16l,m), while the pattern for men was similar to that for cutaneous melanoma overall, in women an increase occurred only in cohorts born from the mid 1930s onwards.

Mortality trends by region

There were large increases in melanoma rates in all regions, with greater percentage increases for men than women in all regions except West Midlands, but no consistent geographical pattern of the extent of increase. In each sex, rates are now greatest in the south of England and lower further north.

Comment

The large increases in melanoma rates in England and Wales, greater for incidence than mortality, are part of an increasing trend in white populations worldwide, observed as far back as data have been available. In men the increases in incidence and mortality have been much larger (in percentage terms) than for any other cancer site included in this book except pleura; in women, the increases have been the third or fourth largest[53]. Although diagnostic artefacts may account for part of the increase, there is little doubt that it is mainly real. There may have been an increasing tendency to biopsy borderline-malignant melanocytic lesions, and some change in pathological criteria for diagnosis of malignancy in such lesions, but an international study of melanoma, which included one centre in England, concluded that such changes in criteria for

malignancy could not account for more than a small proportion of the increasing rates (van der Esch *et al.* 1991). Furthermore, while such changes may have influenced recorded incidence rates, and the disparity between the rates of increase of incidence and mortality, they would not explain the rising mortality from melanoma until recent cohorts.

An artefactual increase in mortality occurred in 1993, when medical enquiries by the Registrar General for imprecisely certified deaths were stopped and the 1984 change in interpretation of ICD coding rule 3 was reversed. The extent of the increase caused is uncertain. On the basis of the previous effects of these certification and coding procedures a 4% increase would be expected (Table 4.1), but the actual changes in recorded mortality rates from 1992 to 1993 were an 18% increase in males and 28% in females; melanoma is a tumour, however, for which year to year fluctuations in rates have anyway been appreciable.

The increases in melanoma incidence are probably due mainly to changes in sun exposure behaviour (NRPB 1995), especially the rise in recreational (intermittent) sun exposures of untanned skin, both from outdoor leisure in Britain (Table 5.28) and from the great increase in holidays in countries with greater UVR fluxes (Table 5.27). A small contribution to rising melanoma rates may also have occurred from increases in ambient UVR levels in urban areas in the 1950s and 1960s as a consequence of diminished air pollution (see p. 69 and Figure 5.2). In the more recent years for which direct UVR measures exist, however, there has been no clear trend in ambient UVR levels in England and Wales (Figure 5.57), and hours of sunshine in England and Wales do not appear to have altered systematically for many decades (Figure 5.56). There may have been some effect on melanoma rates from increasing exposure to tanning lamps and sunbeds, now used by a quarter of the young adult population in England (Bulman 1995), although their relation to melanoma risk remains uncertain.

Melanomas of the head and neck (and lentigo maligna melanomas, which tend to occur at these sites) appear to relate aetiologically to cumulative exposure to the sun, and typically occur in elderly male outdoor workers. While rates of head and neck melanoma have increased less rapidly than melanoma rates at most

---

[53] Third after pleura and non-Hodgkin's lymphoma (NHL) for incidence, fourth after lung cancer, pleura and NHL for mortality; this comment excludes Kaposi's sarcoma, which is briefly discussed on page 195, but for which we do not have data for a comparable period to the other sites. (Curiously, the largest percentage *decrease* in incidence and mortality in each sex was also for a UVR-associated site, the lip.)

other anatomical sites, they have nevertheless increased substantially, contrary to the decrease in outdoor work indicated in Table 5.16. This suggests an aetiological effect of recreational UVR exposures on incidence of these tumours, even though they are on skin sites conventionally considered as 'permanently' rather than 'intermittently' exposed to UVR.

In the absence of objective data on trends in recreational sun exposure of different parts of the body it is all too easy to devise subjective, *post hoc* explanations of site-specific melanoma trends; with this proviso we note that the differing birth cohort trends between the sexes for melanoma of the trunk, with increases occurring in far earlier cohorts in men than women, might accord with changes in beachwear exposures of the trunk by the two sexes over the twentieth century.

Houghton *et al.* (1978) showed an intriguing correlation between sunspot activity and melanoma incidence 0–2 years later in Connecticut, New York, and Finland, and similar relations were shown also in certain Canadian provinces (Wigle 1978) and Denmark (Houghton and Viola 1981) although not Norway (Houghton *et al.* 1978). Comparing the England and Wales rates in Figures 6.16e with yearly sunspot areas (a better indicator of sunspot activity than sunspot numbers, although with similar timing of the peaks) in Figure 5.58 showed no suggestion of such a relation; indeed the only apparent peak in melanoma rates, in 1988, occurred just *before* a peak of sunspot activity (or about 7 years after the previous sunspot peak)[54].

Raised risk of melanoma has been found in certain immunosuppressed groups, but the effect is too small to have affected national melanoma trends materially. Rates of melanoma are far greater in whites than non-whites, so the increase in the proportion of the population of England and Wales who are non-white (Table 5.5) must have had a slight restraining influence on the upward trend of melanoma in the population overall[55].

The greater increase in melanoma incidence than mortality is due at least in part to improved treatment and a tendency towards earlier presentation, at tumour stages when treatment is more successful[56]. To some extent it may be due to an increasing tendency to biopsy borderline-malignant lesions, and to changed pathological criteria for malignancy of borderline lesions, although as discussed previously these are unlikely to have had large effects. All of these explanations would be compatible with the improved survival seen in Figure A.11.

The reversal of the increase in mortality rates in recent birth cohorts accords with trends in other white populations (Thörn *et al.* 1992; Roush *et al.* 1992; Giles *et al.* 1996), and may reflect better results of treatment, for the reasons discussed above, and/or a cessation of the rise in true incidence.

Cancer of the breast in women
(Figure 6.17)

Secular trends

Breast cancer mortality in women at postmenopausal ages (taken to be 50 years and above) increased by more than 20% from 1960–4 to 1985–9, but has since declined, by 20% at ages 50–69 and 10% at older ages. At premenopausal ages too there was an initial increase, but the peak was reached earlier, in 1970–4, and there has since been a decline of 25%.

Incidence of breast cancer in women at postmenopausal ages has increased throughout the period for which data are available, but particularly in recent years at ages 50–69; the recorded rate in this age-group increased by 29% from 1988 to 1991, but was then unchanged in 1992 (Figure 6.17d). At premenopausal ages, there was a small decrease until 1980–4, and then an increase to a rate 10% above that in 1971–4.

Figure 6.17g shows breast cancer mortality rates at ages 35 years and above since 1868. Rates at pre- and postmenopausal ages separately since 1911 are shown in Figure 6.17h. The most notable feature of these long-term trends is the relatively small changes in rates that have occurred over long periods, compared with the scale of secular variation for many other cancer sites. At premenopausal ages there was an increase until 1971–5, and then a decrease, especially in the 1990s. At postmenopausal ages there was a general

---

[54] The yearly trend and the 1988 peak were also not obviously related to recent year to year variations in hours of sunshine (Figure 5.56) or, for the limited period for which data were available, measured annual ambient UVR (Figure 5.57).
[55] Within white populations, rates are raised in persons with fair complexion and those with many or atypical naevi, but we have no evidence on whether the prevalence of these characteristics has altered over time.
[56] A trend toward thinner tumours at presentation has been reported from several centres internationally, including one in Bristol, England (van der Esch *et al.* 1991).

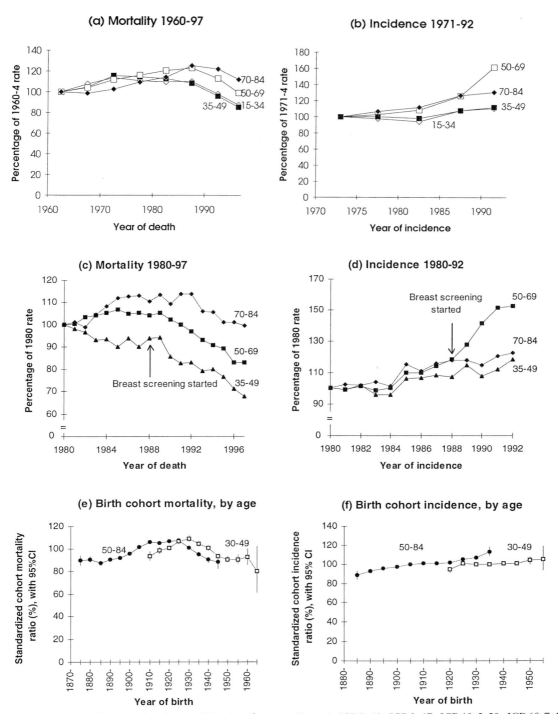

Figure 6.17 Cancer of breast, female (pre-ICD classifications 'Breast'; ICD2 43; ICD3 47; ICD4&5 50; ICD6&7 170; ICD8&9 174): (a), (e) mortality 1960–97; (b) incidence 1971–92; (c) mortality 1980–97; (d) incidence 1980–92; (f) incidence 1971–87; (g) mortality 1868–1997; (h), (i) mortality 1911–97; (j) mortality 1960–4 to 1990–4.

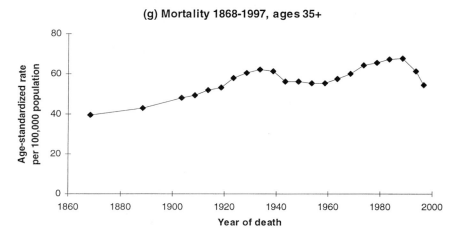

(g) Mortality 1868-1997, ages 35+

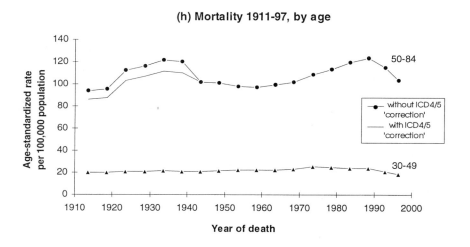

(h) Mortality 1911-97, by age

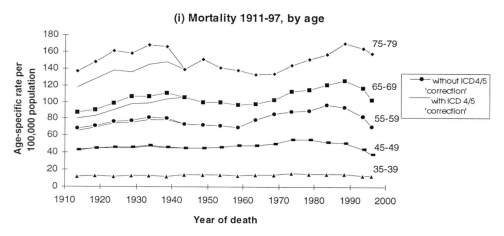

(i) Mortality 1911-97, by age

Figure 6.17   Cancer of breast, female (continued).

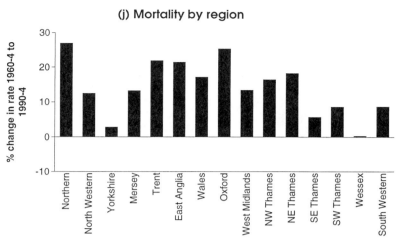

Figure 6.17   Cancer of breast, female (continued).

increase up to 1990, although interrupted in mid-century (lowest in 1956–60), and there was a sharp decrease in the 1990s. Examined by finer age group (Figure 6.17i), the postmenopausal peak in the 1930s and subsequent minimum did not clearly follow either a cohort or a secular pattern: the peak occurred at a similar period in each age-group, but the subsequent minimum occurred later at older ages, although not as much as would be observed in a purely cohort-based change. Because these trends include an appreciable artefact in 1940, when the basis of coding of underlying cause of death altered with the introduction of ICD5, we have presented in Figures 6.17h and i, in addition to rates calculated from the actual coded data, also rates for 1911–40 'corrected'[57] for the ICD change. After making this correction, the peak in postmenopausal breast cancer around the late 1930s was less pronounced and was less consistent in date at different ages, but nevertheless was still present and followed by a dip in the late 1950s and 1960s. Over the whole period from 1911–15 to 1986–90, after correcting for the ICD4/5 change, there was a 42% increase in breast cancer mortality at postmenopausal ages.

Trends by birth cohort

Mortality from breast cancer in women at postmenopausal ages rose from the cohort born in 1885–9 to that born in 1910–14, there was then a slight dip before a peak in the cohort born in 1925–9, after which rates declined (Figure 6.17e). At younger ages, mortality increased to a peak in the 1930–4 birth cohort and then declined.

Breast cancer incidence[58] showed a generally increasing trend. At postmenopausal ages there was a consistent rise from the earliest to the latest cohorts, interrupted only by a slight dip for those born in 1915–24, while for women at premenopausal ages, rates were almost unchanged from the cohort born in 1925–9 to that born in 1945–9, with rises before and after this.

Analyses of mortality and incidence by single year of birth, for pre- and for postmenopausal ages (not shown), did not illuminate further the results shown for 5-year periods of birth. In particular, the dip in postmenopausal breast cancer rates, compared with the prevailing trend, for women born in 1915–24 was not confined to those born during the First World War and

[57] The correction was conducted by multiplying the actual rates by correction factors published by Case *et al.* (1976) that were derived from death certificates double-coded to ICD4 and 5.
[58] Analysed only for 1971–87 because the data for 1988–92 were heavily influenced by the introduction of the national breast screening programme (see below), with large increases in recorded rates for cohorts who were aged 50–69 during the years when screening started.

was not the consequence of decreased risk in women born in any one or two particular years.

Mortality trends by region

Regional trends in mortality varied from no change in Wessex to a 27% increase in Northern region, with no geographical pattern. Although rates are now slightly lower in the north of England than the rest of the country, the variation is slight. Examining the regional trends by age (not shown), at 50–84 years of age the changes were similar to those for women overall, while at ages under 50 they ranged from decreases of 18% in NE Thames region and 14% in NW Thames region to increases of 8% in Oxford region and 7% in North Western and East Anglia regions, with no geographical pattern.

Comment

Breast cancer is the most common cancer in women in England and Wales, and since 1951 has been the most common cause of cancer death[59]. The mortality rates in the country are exceptionally high by international standards (Kurihara *et al.* 1989). The trends in breast cancer, although small in percentage terms, are important numerically because the tumour occurs with such frequency. Annually over 25 000 cases occur and over 10 000 women die from the cancer in England and Wales; it accounts for 29% of all cancers incident and 19% of all cancer deaths in women[60]. There are indications of differences in aetiology between breast cancers occurring before and after the menopause, and we therefore conducted many of the analyses separately for these two age-groups.

Interpretation of trends is probably more complex for breast cancer than for any other cancer in this book. The trend data show several features likely to have different causes from each other, and information is available on a particularly large number of risk and protective factors. Many of these factors, however, are indirectly related to aetiology, and several may simply be partial surrogates for the same, underlying hormonal factors, for which no direct data are available.

We will discuss separately the reasons for the breast cancer trends before the last few years, for which aetiological and artefactual factors are the prime considerations, and the abrupt changes recently, for which the effects of treatment and screening need mainly to be examined.

Possible artefacts

The long-term increases in pre- and postmenopausal breast cancer mortality are unlikely to be due principally to diagnostic artefacts: the tumour is of an easily accessible site, and its diagnosis as a cause of death is not dependent on sophisticated, recently available technology.

At older ages, artefacts of death certification and coding have had some effect on apparent rates. As noted above, the introduction of ICD5 in 1940 led to an abrupt artefactual decrease in postmenopausal breast cancer mortality (a 6% decrease at all-ages (Table 4.1), comprising 14% at ages 75 and above, 8% at ages 65–74, and far smaller decreases at younger ages (Case *et al.* 1976)), and accounted for about half of the postmenopausal decrease from 1936–40 to 1941–5 (Figures 6.17h,i). There is evidence that a quarter or more of the increase in recorded mortality rates at ages 75–84 in recent years, but far less at younger ages, may have been due to change in the position of recording of breast cancer on death certificates (Grulich *et al.* 1995). The change in 1984 to the Registrar General's interpretation of ICD coding rule 3 caused a 4% increase in recorded breast cancer mortality (10% at ages 75 and above, but only 1% at ages younger than this (OPCS 1985)). The reversal of this rule 3 interpretation in 1993, however, along with the cessation of medical enquiries for ill-specified causes of death, caused a 4% decrease in mortality in that year (Table 4.1)[61]; this accounted for one-sixth of the total decrease in recorded breast cancer mortality that has occurred since the peak rate in 1989.

In summary, artefacts of certification and coding have affected breast cancer trends appreciably, and have had a greater impact than for most other cancer sites, but they do not primarily explain either the

---

[59] Previously, cancers of the large intestine (colon plus rectum) were the most common.

[60] Mortality at ages 0–84 in 1995–7; incidence at ages 0–84 in 1990–2, ignoring incident cases of non-melanoma skin cancer.

[61] Again with a much greater effect for older ages than young. The expected consequence of reversal of the rule 3 interpretation would be a 9% decrease at ages 75 and above and a 1% decrease at younger ages (OPCS 1985). Medical enquiries for this site had previously revealed only 0.5% extra cases, so cessation of these enquiries would have had little additional effect.

upward trend in breast cancer mortality rates over much of the twentieth century or the recent downturn. The long-term rise is likely to reflect increasing incidence. The data on incidence, for the relatively recent period for which they are available, showed a considerable continuing increase at postmenopausal ages and a less marked, less consistent increase at premenopausal ages. These incidence data would not have been affected by the artefacts discussed above (although they could have been affected by changes in completeness of registration). The extent of histological verification of breast cancers recorded in the cancer registration data appears to have remained unchanged, at around 80%, over the period investigated (based on data from several of the English regional cancer registries, published in *Cancer Incidence in Five Continents* (Waterhouse *et al.* 1976; Muir *et al.* 1987; Parkin *et al.* 1997)).

A small effect on breast cancer rates will have occurred from the rise in mastectomy rates in the 1960s (Figure 5.55), which will have reduced the numbers of breasts at risk of malignancy. To the extent that women undergoing this operation (often because of malignancy) remain alive, rates of breast cancer in relation to breasts-at-risk will have risen slightly more than is apparent from the rates calculated with denominators of women-at-risk.

Age at menarche and height

Young age at menarche and tall adult height are risk factors for breast cancer (perhaps as indicators of growth and nutrition in childhood) that have increased for the past hundred years or more (Figures 5.38, 5.7, 5.8) and would accord with the long-term rising rates of breast cancer. There is evidence that the trend in age at menarche may have reversed for women born since the mid-1950s (Table 5.20), but these cohorts are too young as yet for stable estimates of their breast cancer incidence to be available. There is no indication of diminished height in the 1915–24 birth cohort, whose postmenopausal breast cancer risk was below the trend in the surrounding cohorts, nor was there any parallel in the breast cancer data with the decreased average

height of women born during 1936–40 that is shown in Figure 5.8.

In Norway, where fat, meat, and calorie consumption decreased markedly during the privations of the Second World War, a lower than expected incidence of breast cancer has been found in the cohort of women who reached the age of puberty during these years (Tretli and Gaard 1996). The lack of any dip in risk for the corresponding cohort in England and Wales (and also in data from Scotland (Swerdlow *et al.* 1998)) may reflect the fact that the War had much less ill-effect on nutrition in Britain than Norway (and indeed generally led to improved nutrition for poorer people—see footnote 87). The comparatively low rate of breast cancer in women born in 1915–24 (seen similarly in Scotland for incidence in women born in 1915–19 (Swerdlow *et al.* 1998)), however, is in a group who reached puberty, or ages immediately before it, in the Depression of the early 1930s, when there were food shortages for the poor[62].

Reproductive factors

Several reproductive factors are associated with risk of breast cancer. Risk is raised in women who remain childless or first give birth relatively late in life, and to a much lesser extent is raised in those who have few compared with many children. The trends in these factors (Figures 5.36, 5.37, 5.40, 5.41), however, especially nulliparity and age at first birth which are the most important, often do not parallel the breast cancer trends. Although the decreasing fertility at young ages in cohorts born from 1875–9 to 1905–9 accords with the increasing mortality from and incidence of breast cancer in these cohorts, the lack of change in nulliparity between these cohorts does not accord with the breast cancer trends, and subsequently age at first childbirth decreased (Figures 5.36, 5.37) and the rate of nulliparity more than halved (Figure 5.41) from the cohort of women born in 1910–14 to that born in 1930–4, whereas breast cancer incidence rates increased between these cohorts at postmenopausal ages and to some extent, for the shorter period for which data were available, at premenopausal ages[63].

---

[62] We do not have direct data on year by year changes in nutrition at that time, but Figure 5.59 shows unemployment trends that indicate the severity of the downturn and hence of circumstances for the poor.

[63] This contrasts with results from Canada and the US, where cohort trends in mortality from breast cancer paralleled those for late age at first birth, as indicated by nulliparity/fertility at ages 20–24 (Wigle 1977; Blot 1980). It is similar, however, to the conclusion reached by Hems (1980), comparing breast cancer mortality in England and Wales from 1911–75 with cohort-specific measures of child-bearing (birth rate at ages 20–4 and family size by age 45 years) for cohorts born up to 1910.

For cohorts born in the first 15 years after the Second World War, age at first birth and nulliparity increased, which would accord with the rising incidence of breast cancer.

Risk of breast cancer is increased by older age at menopause, but there was little change in age of menopause in women in England and Wales in the twentieth century (see p. 51).

Lactation has been reported to reduce the risk of breast cancer. Prevalence of breast feeding decreased from 1920 until 1970, but then increased (Table 5.21, Figure 5.39). The decrease was for cohorts in whom breast cancer incidence generally increased, while the subsequent upturn in breast feeding will largely have affected women who are as yet too young for stable estimates of their breast cancer incidence to be available.

Oral contraceptives and other hormonal drugs

Current evidence suggests that oral contraceptives have only a small effect on breast cancer risk, which is to increase it in current and recent users (CGHFBC 1996). Oral contraceptive use increased greatly in women born since the late 1920s, and use from a young age increased in women born from about 1940 (Figure 5.32); premenopausal breast cancer incidence trends in the earliest of these cohorts were stable, but for those born in the 1940s and 50s incidence has been rising.

The effect on breast cancer rates of increasing use of postmenopausal hormone replacement therapy (HRT) is likely to have been slight (Ursin *et al.* 1994), given the levels of HRT use found in surveys in England (see p. 46 and Table 5.15) and the small increase in breast cancer risk that occurs with usual durations of use (CGHFBC 1997). Treatment with diethylstilboestrol in pregnancy can increase the risk of subsequent breast cancer, but this treatment was relatively little used in the UK (see p. 46). Tamoxifen treatment of breast cancer leads to a substantially decreased risk of contralateral breast cancer[64], so that a factor militating slightly towards lower breast cancer incidence in recent years must have been decreasing numbers of contralateral cancers as the use of tamoxifen has spread. Tamoxifen has been marketed for breast cancer treat-

ment in the UK since September 1973, and has been widely used in postmenopausal women since the mid 1970s and in premenopausal women since about 1983. There has been some subsequent increase in prevalence and duration of use.

Obesity and exercise

At postmenopausal (but not premenopausal) ages obesity is a risk factor for breast cancer, probably because adipose tissue is the main source of oestrogens in women after the menopause. Data on obesity are available only since 1980, and show an increasing prevalence of overweight in postmenopausal women (Figure 5.6) as breast cancer incidence has increased.

Vigorous physical activity is associated with a reduced risk of breast cancer, in young women at least (Bernstein *et al.* 1994), so changing levels of exercise may have influenced trends in incidence. Data on exercise trends are only available since 1991 (Table 5.18); if the decreasing trend seen since then applied in earlier years, it would accord with the increasing rates of breast cancer incidence, although more limited information on sports activities, from 1987–96, would suggest a slight increase in exercise (see p 49).

Diet and alcohol consumption

High fat consumption has been suggested as a cause of breast cancer, mainly on the basis of correlations between fat consumption levels in different countries and their levels of breast cancer (Armstrong and Doll 1975; Gray *et al.* 1979). On a secular basis, the continuing increase in premenopausal breast cancer over a long period until about 1975, but interrupted by a dip in risks from about 1936 to 1945, shows similarities with the trends in fat consumption shown in Tables 5.6 and 5.7 and Figure 5.14, in which against a background of increasing consumption until the late 1960s, there was a decrease in fat intake during and soon after the Second World War[65]. For postmenopausal breast cancer, the low rates in the decades soon after the Second World War, and higher rates in the 1970s and 80s, occurred about 10–20 years after relatively low fat consumption during and just after the war and a rise thereafter. Fat consumption per caput in England

---

[64] Rates are about halved, at least during the first few years of treatment (EBCTCG, 1998). (About 5% of breast cancers in general are contralateral.)

[65] This similarity, however, is with no lag period.

and Wales reached a peak in 1969, before declining (Figure 5.14), while registered postmenopausal breast cancer incidence rates continued to increase for more than 20 years after this, with no sign yet of a downturn. The cancer trends after 1987 are difficult to interpret, however, because of the impact of screening (see below). Phyto-oestrogen consumption (e.g. from soya products) has been suggested as preventive of breast cancer, but we have no data on trends in consumption of phyto-oestrogens.

In several studies, alcohol intake has been found associated with an increased risk of breast cancer, and the evidence overall suggests an aetiological relationship. Alcohol consumption by women has probably increased in the post-war years up to the 1980s (Figures 5.3, 5.5); for most of this period at younger ages, and the later part at older ages, breast cancer rates rose.

Prenatal factors

There has been growing interest in the last few years in the possibility that prenatal factors may be aetiological for breast cancer (Trichopoulos 1990). In the England and Wales data, there was no change in breast cancer risk for cohorts of women born in the Depression of the early 1930s (Figure 5.59) or during the Second World War[66]—periods when living conditions in Britain changed abruptly. There was a slightly decreased risk for women born around the time of the First World War[67], when living conditions were poor, but this cohort is also the one that reached puberty during the years of the Depression, so if early life factors were of importance either (or both) of these events could have been of relevance.

Several studies have shown a relation of raised risk of breast cancer to high birthweight (Michels *et al.* 1996; De Stavola *et al.* 2000). The proportion of births in England and Wales that were of high birthweight probably decreased from 1958 to 1977 (although this information was based on sample studies), and there was an increase thereafter (Figure 5.12); these cohorts of

women are too young at present, however, to gain stable information on their risks of breast cancer.

Other aetiological factors

Certain benign breast lesions are risk factors for breast cancer, but to our knowledge there are no data on trends in incidence of these lesions. Genetic factors are important in the aetiology of breast cancer, particularly at young ages, and as specific genes are discovered, prophylactic measures in high risk women with these genes may affect breast cancer rates. The identification of breast cancer genes is too recent, however, to have affected the rates in this book.

Treatment and screening

The decrease in breast cancer mortality at premenopausal ages since 1970–4 and at older ages since 1985–9 is mainly a consequence of better survival (see Figure A12), due to more effective treatment by tamoxifen and other new therapies (EBCTCG 1992, 1998). In the most recent years, however, it may also reflect the benefits of screening. The national screening programme started in 1988, and aims to screen women aged 50–64 years every 3 years and older women on demand (see p. 56 and Table 5.22), so that it might explain at least part of the decrease in mortality at ages 50 and above. The expected effects of screening would be an initial increase in recorded incidence, as cases are detected earlier than they would otherwise have been, and then a decrease in mortality as the benefits of screening take effect. A large increase in incidence at ages 50–69 was seen from 1988 onwards, which ceased in 1992, the most recent year for which data were available. The screening programme detected 2900 invasive cancers in 1990/1, 5000 in 1991/2, and 4400 in 1992/3 (Moss *et al.* 1995)[68], which is somewhat more than the 3260 extra cancers registered at ages 50–69 in 1991 and 3250 extra in 1992 compared with 1987, the last year before screening started (and a time when trends in incidence were already upward)[69].

---

[66] Nor was there any change for these cohorts in Scottish data (Swerdlow *et al.* 1998).

[67] For postmenopausal breast cancer, at least, compared with immediately surrounding cohorts.

[68] Although the data on screen-detected cancers were not published by age, we estimate that at least 95% of the cancers were detected at ages 50–69. Ninety five per cent of cancers detected by the screening programme in 1991/2 were in women *invited* for screening (Chamberlain *et al.* 1993), and 97% of invited women were under age 65 at the time of screening (the remaining 3% were probably invited at age 64 but screened a few months later, so that their tumours too were probably diagnosed at ages 50–69).

[69] By implication, it seems likely that not all of the cases detected by screening were successfully registered in the incidence data.

The trend in mortality from breast cancer at ages 50–69, which had been upward, altered direction in 1986, before screening was introduced, but the extent of decrease from 1985–89, 2%, was far less than that subsequently: from 1989–96 there was a 21% decrease (but no further reduction in 1997). This compares with a 29% decrease after 7–10 years of follow-up in pooled results of published trials of screening, which had compliance rates of 61–89%[70] (Day 1991).

At ages 70–84 years, incidence did not show the marked rise after 1988 seen for the 50–69 years age-group, but mortality turned down sharply after 1992, with an 11% decrease from 1992–5 and little change thereafter. Much of the decrease, however, was due to the changes in the Registrar General's coding procedures in 1993, discussed on p. 124. Screening at ages 50–64 would be expected to have had some effect on mortality at ages 70 and above, after a lag period, simply because the later follow-up of the screened women will have been at these ages. In addition, the screening programme was open to women aged over 64 years, on demand.

The screening programme is not intended for women aged under 50 years, and so would not explain the decline in mortality at these younger ages, which anyway began well before the screening programme started[71]. It is notable, however, that the downward trend in mortality at ages 35–49 has accelerated in recent years, and indeed the percentage fall from 1989–96 was exactly the same as that at ages 50–69 (21%)—a reminder that the improvements at older ages in this period might not have been due mainly to screening and do not provide strong evidence that screening has been effective.

In summary, improvements in treatment have reduced mortality from breast cancer in recent years, and screening has clearly led to an abrupt increase in recorded incidence since 1988, but it is far more uncertain what effect, if any, screening has had on mortality, because similar reductions in death rates have occurred at screened and certain unscreened ages. It is too early to judge this fully, however, as screening was introduced progressively over several years; mortality data for the years immediately after 1997 will therefore be of particular interest.

Cancer of the breast in men
(Figure 6.18)

Secular trends

Breast cancer mortality in men has decreased over the study period, more at young than at older ages, and particularly in the most recent years examined. Age-specific incidence rates were inconsistent, with some decrease at young but not older ages over the period as a whole.

Trends by birth cohort

The greatest mortality rates were in cohorts of men born late in the nineteenth century, and in subsequent cohorts there has been, although not entirely consistently, a decline. Cohort trends in incidence were also inconsistent, but mainly downward in recent cohorts.

Mortality trends by region

Regional trends (not shown) were erratic, based on small numbers.

Comment

Insufficient is known about the aetiology of breast cancer in men to be able to explain the trends in incidence by changes in risk factors. One study found that risk was substantially increased in men with greater weight in young adulthood, perhaps because of greater bioavailable oestrogen levels in heavier men (Casagrande *et al.* 1988). Obesity in men has increased since 1980, when national data were first available (Figure 5.6 and pp. 24–5), while breast cancer incidence has not risen.

Another study found raised risk associated with undescended testis (Thomas *et al.* 1992), the prevalence of which appears to be increasing (John Radcliffe Hospital Cryptorchidism Study Group 1992).

---

[70] i.e. reasonably similar to the England and Wales compliance rates—see p. 56. There is a difference, however, in mean length of follow-up, as it took several years for all of the England and Wales screening units to open, and it then took time for the prevalent screening round to be completed; in addition the trials only included women free of breast cancer at entry, whereas the England and Wales mortality data have no such exclusion.

[71] Furthermore, even if the formal screening programme has 'spilled over' to give *ad hoc* screening activity for younger women, this is unlikely to have had much impact on mortality rates because screening at these ages is relatively ineffective: just under a 5% reduction in breast cancer mortality was found in aggregated results of trials (Day 1991).

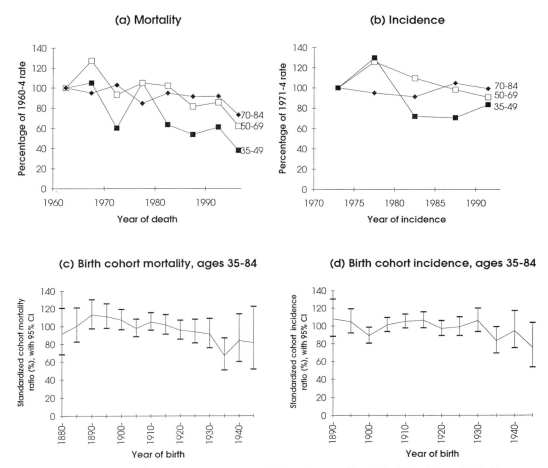

Figure 6.18 Cancer of breast, male (ICD7 170; ICD8 174; ICD9 175), mortality 1960–97, incidence 1971–92.

Gynaecomastia has also been found a risk factor, but its secular trends are unknown.

A small artefact in incidence trends will have occurred with the introduction of ICD9, in 1979, for an unusual reason. Because breast cancer is so much less common in men than women, even a small percentage error in cancer registry recording of the sex of women with breast cancer can have an appreciable effect on apparent rates in men (but will have a negligible effect on the much larger total in women). The Ninth Revision of the ICD, unlike previous revisions, included separate three-digit codes for breast cancer in men and women, so that undetected miscoding was much less likely[72]. Examination of England and Wales cancer registrations coded to male breast

cancer under ICD8 showed 3% who were probably women (Swerdlow and dos Santos Silva 1993), and thus a 3% artefactual decrease in rates probably occurred in 1979.

Cancer of the cervix uteri (Figure 6.19)

Secular trends

Mortality from cancer of the cervix at age 35 years and above decreased by a half or more since 1960, but at younger ages the pattern has been very different. From 1960–4 to 1985–9 the rate at ages 15–34 more than

---

[72] The cause code and the sex code would both need to be incorrect for the error not be found at validation checks.

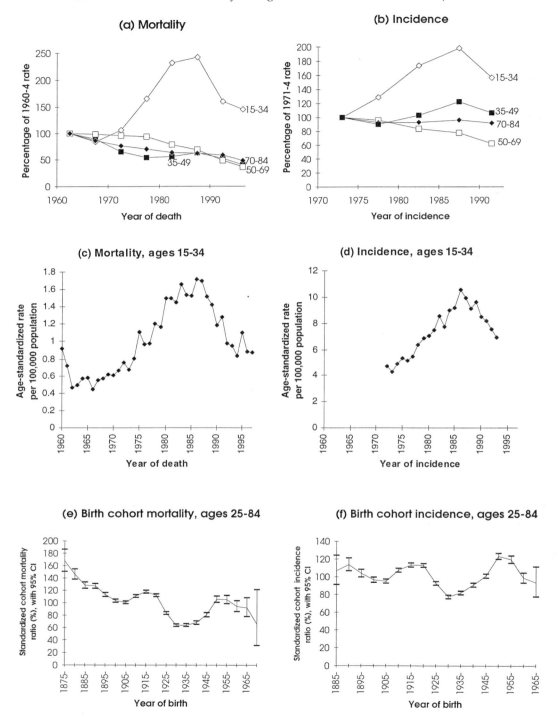

Figure 6.19 Cancer of cervix uteri (ICD7 171; ICD8&9 180): (a), (c), (e) mortality 1960–97; (b), (d), (f), (g) incidence 1971–92; (h) mortality 1941–97; (i) mortality 1960–4 to 1990–4.

(g) Birth cohort incidence, by age

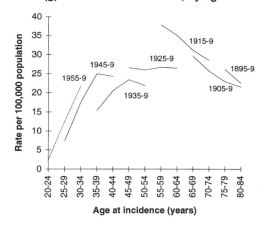

(h) Mortality 1941-97, by age

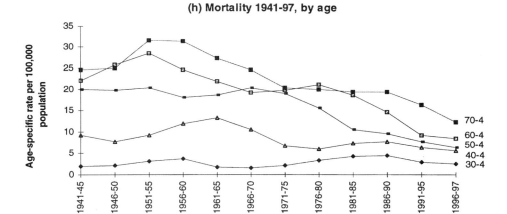

(i) Mortality by region

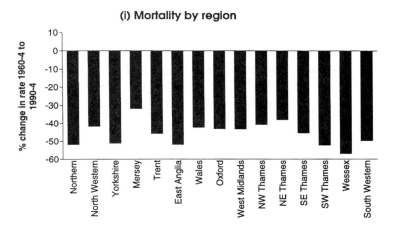

Figure 6.19 Cancer of cervix uteri (continued).

doubled, but it has since diminished rapidly, halving from 1987 to 1994.

Incidence at ages 15–34 doubled from 1971–4 to 1985–9, and at ages 35–49 increased by 20% between these years; at ages 50–69 there was a decrease and at ages 70–84 a slight decrease. In the last period of data available, however, compared with the penultimate one, there was a downturn in rates at all ages, which on examination by single calendar year (not shown) occurred largely from 1990 to 1992: the incidence rate of cervical cancer at ages 0–84 in 1992 was 78% of that 2 years earlier, with the greatest and most abrupt declines at ages 35–49 and 50–69.

Figure 6.19h shows mortality over a longer period, since 1941–5[73]. At ages 30–4, a peak can be seen in 1956–60 as well as the peak in the 1980s noted above. At ages 40–4, the first peak occurred 5 years later and at 50–4 it occurred a further 5 years later. At older ages the peak can be seen at yet later dates[74], but there was also an earlier peak which did not vary appreciably in date with increasing age, but instead occurred in 1951–5 for all ages from 55 to 79 years.

Trends by birth cohort

Mortality decreased in cohorts born from 1875–9 to 1905–9, although with a perturbation for the cohort born in 1890–4, and subsequently there were two peaks, in women born in 1915–19 and in 1950–4. The trend in the most recent cohorts has been downward. In incidence data, too, there were peaks in the 1915–19 and 1950–4 cohorts, and a less-certain peak in the cohort born in 1890–4.

Examination of the age distribution of cervical cancer incidence within birth cohorts (Figure 6.19g) shows that although the absolute rates varied considerably between cohorts, the age/incidence distribution was fairly consistent, with rates ceasing to increase beyond age 49 years, and declining beyond age 64 years.

Mortality trends by region

Decreases in cervical cancer mortality occurred in all regions, with no geographical pattern; the least improvement was in Mersey region, the greatest in Wessex. Because of the variation in trends by age, we also examined regional mortality data separately for ages under 50 years and older than this (not shown). In the younger age group, there were decreases of a quarter to a half in each region, with the largest decrease in Mersey region. At older ages, decreases of at least a third occurred in each region, with the greatest decreases occurring in Wessex, SW Thames, and Yorkshire regions.

Comment

The main reasons for the trends in cervical cancer are the effects of aetiological factors and screening, as discussed below, but several potential artefacts also need consideration. Apparent rates of cervical cancer are dependent on the extent to which cancer registrations and death certificates for uterine cancers specify whether the tumour is located in the cervix or corpus uteri. For incidence, and for mortality under age 50 years, cervical cancer trends will have been little affected by imprecision of anatomical specification because under 9% of uterine cancers were of unspecified subsite throughout the study period, with changes of only a few per cent. For mortality at ages 50–84 years, however, the proportion of uterine cancers that were not further specified increased from 5.3% in 1951–5 and 6.5% in 1960–4 to 22.5% in 1995–7. Although most of the unspecified tumours at these ages will have been malignancies of the corpus not the cervix (Swerdlow 1989), the decreasing precision of certification may nevertheless have been a contributor to the apparently falling mortality from cervical cancer at older ages. The data for 1941–50 in Figure 6.19h must be interpreted cautiously because uterine cancers of unknown subsite were not coded separately from those of the corpus uteri at that time, and hence their contribution to the trends cannot be assessed.

Another potential artefact in cervical cancer incidence rates is that diagnostic and coding boundaries between cervical malignancy and cervical intraepithelial neoplasia (dysplasia and cancer *in situ*) may have altered over time, particularly as screening has

---

[73] Cervical cancer was first categorized separately in mortality data in 1940.

[74] The extent of delay with increasing age is not quite as would be expected from a purely cohort-based pattern, in which the peak would be 5 years later for each extra 5 years of age. The amplitude of variation, in proportional terms, also diminished with age, which may indicate a diminishing effect of sexual behaviour at young ages on cervical cancer risk as women grow older.

revealed more cases of early disease. We have no data on whether these boundaries have altered, but note that it is implausible that such a change could explain the large variation in trends by age, and it would not explain the mortality trends, which showed a similar pattern by birth cohort to that for incidence.

A further source of artefact[75] arises from changes over time in rates of hysterectomy, as this operation will have affected the number of uteruses at risk of cervical cancer whereas the incidence and mortality rates are perforce calculated in relation to numbers of women. Hysterectomy rates in England and Wales increased considerably over the period for which data are available, 1961–85 (Figure 5.55), which will have contributed a downward element to the incidence and mortality rates, particularly at older ages. Alderson and Donnan (1978) estimated that cumulative hysterectomy rates by age 70 were 6% for women in England and Wales born around 1900, increasing to a projected 19% for those born in 1946.

Despite the need to take account of these potential artefacts, the main influences on cervical cancer rates have been trends in screening (discussed below), and in the sexual behaviour of successive cohorts of women. There is strong evidence that certain types of human papilloma virus (HPV), sexually transmitted, are an aetiological factor in most cases of cervical cancer. Young age at first intercourse and large numbers of sexual partners are risk factors, probably in the main because they influence risk of HPV infection, but they may also have smaller independent associations (Schiffman *et al.* 1996). Survey data indicate that age at first intercourse has been decreasing in cohorts born from 1931–5 to 1971–5 (Table 5.23), and that the average number of sexual partners has been increasing for much, at least, of this span of cohorts (Table 5.24). This would accord with the trends in cervical cancer up to the 1950–4 cohort, but not subsequently. There may also have been a small effect of parity on the trends, as high parity has been found to be independently associ-

ated with risk of cervical cancer in some studies. Trends in parity have only intermittently corresponded with those for cervical cancer, however: for cohorts born from 1875–1909, parity (Figures 5.37 and 5.40) and cervical cancer mortality decreased in parallel, but for cohorts born since, the peaks and troughs in parity do not correspond with those for cervical cancer.

Beral (1974) showed for mortality up to 1971 a close similarity between trends in cervical cancer by birth cohort and trends in incidence of gonorrhoea, as a marker of sexually transmitted diseases, when these cohorts were aged 20 years (the age of peak incidence of gonorrhoea). With the addition of 26 further years of mortality data, and on examination of incidence data, this is still true. As comparison between Figure 5.45 and Figures 6.19e and f shows, cervical cancer rates reached a peak in cohorts born about 20–25 years before peaks in gonorrhoea rates[76]. The steep increase in cervical cancer incidence in cohorts born from 1930–4 to 1950–4 reflects the rise in opportunity for oncogenic sexual infections consequent on freer sexual behaviours in the generations who grew up using the oral contraceptive pill (which may also itself have had an independent effect in increasing risk). As the increase in rates occurred for mortality as well as incidence, it cannot have been the result of better case-finding, through screening, or changed diagnostic criteria for borderline malignant lesions. The reversal of the upward trend in the most recent cohorts, who were young adults at a time when gonorrhoea rates were lower, may reflect more cautious sexual behaviour (including increased use of barrier contraceptives) with the advent of AIDS, and possibly also an effect of screening (although this is intended to be for older women). A similar reversal, since a peak for the 1955–9 birth cohort, has been seen in Scotland (Swerdlow *et al.* 1998) but has not, to our knowledge, been reported from elsewhere.

As well as these cohort-based peaks and troughs in cervical cancer rates, there has been an underlying secular decrease in mortality rates, which is likely to be due to

---

[75] Whether this is considered an artefact or real is somewhat arbitrary, depending on whether one is interested from an aetiological or public health perspective.

[76] Peaks of gonorrhoea occurred in 1946 and 1975, while corresponding peaks of cervical cancer occurred in the cohorts born (in analyses by single year of birth, not shown) in 1919 (incidence and mortality) and 1953 (incidence) or 1954 (mortality). The older age of the 1919 cohort in 1946 than of the 1953/4 cohort in 1975 may reflect the exceptional circumstance of the return home of men after the Second World War, and also perhaps a secular decline in age of peak sexual experience: Table 5.23 shows that age of women at first intercourse, at least, has declined by several years over recent generations. The inflexion in incidence and mortality from cervical cancer in the cohort born in 1890–4, shown in Figures 6.19e and f, reflected a peak of mortality in the 1890 cohort and of incidence in the 1893 cohort, which would correspond with the peak of gonorrhoea in 1920, after the First World War.

The age distribution of cervical cancer incidence shown in Figure 6.19g also accords with an aetiology primarily determined by exposures in young adulthood, leading to malignancies incident over the next 20-30 years of life and then somewhat diminishing at older ages. It should be noted, however, that age-specific incidence rates within cohorts could reflect secular as well as age-related influences: in particular, lower rates with older age in a cohort might in part reflect the growing coverage of the screening programme over time.

the national screening programme. This programme started in 1964 and has since increased its activity considerably (Figure 5.42). The larger decrease for mortality than incidence at ages 35 and above may have occurred because screening, as well as detecting and preventing the progress of premalignant lesions, will have detected and led to the registration of borderline malignant lesions that otherwise might not have been detected. Corresponding with the unusual feature that incidence and mortality rates have diverged only at ages over 34 years, survival (Figure A13b) showed no change at ages 15–34 but a substantial improvement at ages 35–69 (the data presented in the Figure are for East Anglia, but the survival data for England and Wales (not shown) are similar for the more limited period for which they are available). The decrease of a quarter in the incidence rate of cervical cancer at ages under 70 from 1990 to 1992 would accord with a rapid effect of the great increase in coverage of the cervical screening programme at ages 25–64 that occurred from 1989 onward (Figure 5.44).

An association has been found in several studies between smoking and risk of cervical cancer, although it is not clear that this association is causal rather than due to confounding by sexual infections (Doll 1996; Schiffman *et al.* 1996). The peak of cervical cancer in the cohort of women born in 1915–19 was a little before that for lung cancer (1920–9) (Figure 6.11), as a marker of smoking; trends in these two malignancies in more recent cohorts showed no resemblance, and the cervical cancer rates did not follow cohort trends for tar-adjusted smoking, except to some extent in cohorts born from the 1930s onwards (Figure 5.51b).

Although most cervical cancers are of squamous histology, with the above risk factors, about 5–10% are adenocarcinomas, which as well as sharing these risk factors with squamous cancers, also share aetiological features with cancers of the corpus uteri (see p. 136). *In utero* exposure to diethylstilboestrol (used to treat threatened abortion and other conditions in pregnancy) is a rare cause of cervical adenocarcinoma in young women, but this treatment was not used commonly in England and Wales (see p. 46) and so its effect on trends (if any) should have been negligible.

Cancer of the corpus uteri (Figure 6.20)

Secular trends

Mortality from cancer of the corpus uteri has decreased since 1960 by one-third or more at each adult age-group under 70 years, and by a fifth at ages 70–84. Incidence rates have not changed greatly, although there have been small increases at old ages.

Trends by birth cohort

Mortality increased until the cohort born at the beginning of the twentieth century, but has since decreased continuously. Incidence increased to a peak in the cohort born in 1925–9 and has since decreased somewhat unevenly.

Mortality trends by region

Mortality has decreased in all regions, by between 20% and 50%, with no consistent regional pattern.

Comment

Cancers of the corpus uteri occur mainly in its surface lining, the endometrium[77], and histologically are largely adenocarcinomas. As noted when discussing cancer of the cervix, uterine cancers not further specified are mainly cancers of the corpus uteri, except at the youngest ages, and hence we have combined corpus and unspecified uterine cancers in the analyses presented[78].

Apparent trends in mortality from cancer of the corpus uteri (aggregated with cancers of the uterus unspecified) at old ages have been affected appreciably in recent years by coding artefact. The 1984 change in the Registrar General's interpretation of ICD coding rule 3 (see p. 12) increased recorded mortality from endometrial cancer by 5% (OPCS 1985) (9% at ages 75 years and above, but only 2% at younger ages). In 1993, however, an artefactual downward element was contributed to mortality rates by the reversal in this

---

[77] We have therefore followed common practice in referring on occasion to cancers of the corpus uteri overall as 'endometrial cancers'.

[78] In case the proportion of unspecified tumours that are cervical has changed over time, as it appears to have done in the US (Percy *et al.* 1983), however, we also analysed trends for tumours specifically coded to uterine corpus (not shown). For incidence these analyses showed virtually the same trends as for corpus plus unspecified uterus. For mortality, the trend in cancers specified as corpus was more downward than that for these tumours plus those of the uterus unspecified (at all ages, the decrease from 1960–4 to 1995–7 was just over a half for the former category whereas it was a third for the latter).

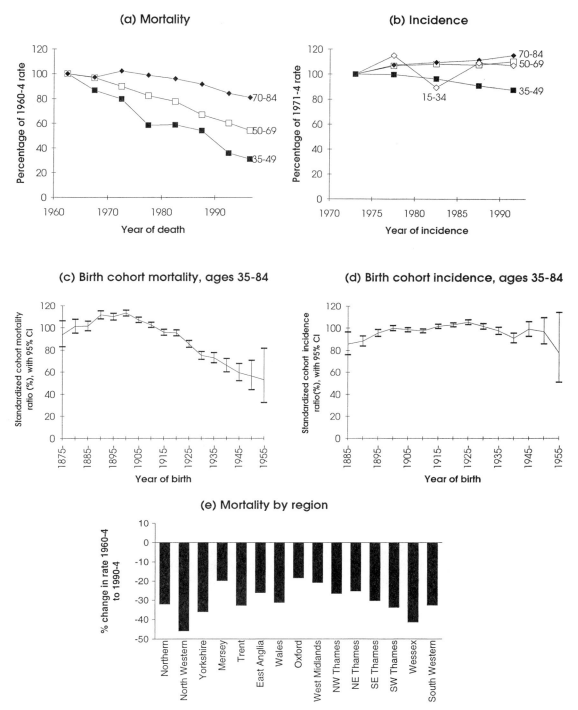

Figure 6.20   Cancer of corpus uteri plus uterus unspecified (ICD7 172, 174; ICD8 182; ICD9 179, 182), mortality 1960–97, incidence 1971–92.

interpretation of coding rule 3, and to a small extent by the cessation of 'medical enquiries' for ill-specified death certificates (see p. 11), which together would be expected (on the basis discussed on p. 12) to give a 6% decrease in rates.

A factor leading to an underestimation of the decrease in mortality at older ages is the deterioration in specification of the subsite of uterine cancers in mortality data in recent years (see p. 132). Although most of the unspecified tumours at these ages will have been cancers of the corpus[79], and therefore correctly allocated by combining corpus and unspecified tumours in the analysis, some will have been cervical cancers, and thus the true fall in corpus cancer mortality is likely to have been greater than that shown in Figure 6.20, although less than would be shown by analysis solely of cancers specified as located in the corpus.

Hysterectomy rates affect the trends in cancer of the corpus uteri, as the rates of the cancer are calculated with women rather than uteruses as the denominator. The rising frequency of hysterectomy (Figure 5.55) will therefore have contributed a downward element to the cancer rates.

Risk of cancer of the corpus uteri is increased by nulliparity, early menarche, late age at menopause, obesity, and oestrogen replacement therapy (similar risk factors to those for breast cancer, with which it shares several descriptive epidemiological features). The common pathway of these aetiological factors is an increased exposure to unopposed oestrogen (i.e. oestrogen in the absence of progesterone).

Trends in incidence of cancer of the corpus uteri since 1971 have been slight, perhaps reflecting the countervailing effects of different risk factors. In the absence of strong trends or inflexions in risk, it is easier to decide which risk factors fail to accord with the trends than to conclude which factors are likely to explain them. Nulliparity, which is associated with raised risk of the cancer, decreased in cohorts of women born up to the 1940s and has since increased (Figure 5.41), while the peak of endometrial cancer was for women born in the 1920s, with an inconsistent decrease since. Parity, which has been found in some studies to be inversely associated with risk of endometrial cancer, has had trends approximately the converse of those for nulliparity, for cohorts born in the twentieth century (Figure 5.40); again these trends

do not correspond substantially with those for endometrial cancer.

Risk of endometrial cancer is increased by early menarche and late menopause: age at menarche decreased in cohorts of women born until the mid-1950s (Figure 5.38, Table 5.20), but may have stabilized since (Table 5.20), whereas incidence of endometrial cancer was little changed between cohorts born at the start of the twentieth century and those born recently, in whom it may have decreased. Age at menopause has changed little over the last century, except for an increasing, but small, percentage of women with artificial menopause (see p. 51).

The raised risk of endometrial cancer in relation to obesity appears to occur particularly at old ages, and is primarily in relation to severe obesity rather than being a linear relation of risk to weight-for-height (Grady and Ernster 1996). The attributable fraction may be large (Grady and Ernster 1996). It is consonant with this that while the prevalence of obesity has risen (Figure 5.6), endometrial cancer rates have increased somewhat at older but not younger ages.

Use of unopposed oestrogen replacement therapy raises the risk of endometrial cancer, and was the cause of a sharp rise in incidence of (but not mortality from) the tumour at menopausal ages in the United States in the 1970s, which was followed by a decline when rates of prescription of the drug diminished (Walker and Jick 1980). No such epidemic can be seen in the England and Wales data despite widespread use of HRT in recent years (see p. 46 and Table 5.15). The US epidemic was consequent on the use of high-dose unopposed oestrogens. Prescriptions of hormone replacement therapy in the US increased again after 1980, without a concomitant rise in endometrial cancers, probably because oestrogen doses were lower and progestins were added, with a consequent reduction or abolition of risk (Persky *et al.* 1990). The lack of an epidemic of endometrial cancer in the UK implies that use of unopposed oestrogens (on which we have no data) was not frequent in the UK.

Risk of endometrial cancer is raised in users of sequential oral contraceptives, which were withdrawn from the market in the mid-1970s (Grady and Ernster 1996), but is reduced by about 50% in users of combined oral contraceptives. The latter would accord with the decreasing trend in endometrial cancer incidence at

---

[79] At young ages most are cervical, but a relatively low proportion of uterine cancers at these ages are of unspecified subsite (see p. 132).

ages 35–49 after 1979, but based on modest numbers there was not a clearly downward trend at ages 15–34. Considered by birth cohort, there has been a generally downward trend in endometrial cancer incidence across the span of cohorts in whom oral contraceptive use became common (Figure 5.32). An increased risk of endometrial cancer occurs in breast cancer patients treated with tamoxifen, a non-steroidal hormone which has both anti-oestrogenic and oestrogenic effects. Its use in England and Wales has been widespread at post-menopausal ages since the mid 1970s and at pre-menopausal ages since around 1983 (see p. 126). Patients with breast cancer are a small proportion of the population, however, and hence the effect on the endometrial cancer trends in the general population will not have been large—we estimate that tamoxifen-induced endometrial cancers have accounted for about 2% of the national total in recent years.

There is some evidence, including results of international correlation studies (Armstrong and Doll 1975), for an association of risk of endometrial cancer with fat consumption. Trends in fat consumption (Figure 5.14), which increased until 1969 and then decreased, do not obviously accord with the endometrial cancer trends, however. Risk of endometrial cancer incidence (but perhaps not mortality) has been found to be decreased in smokers in almost all studies, possibly because of an anti-oestrogenic effect of smoking. The cohort trends in endometrial cancer, and the secular trends, however, are far from being the inverse of those for lung cancer (Figure 6.11) or of smoking (Figures 5.47b, 5.48b, 5.50b, 5.51b).

The decreasing rates of mortality from endometrial cancer, while incidence rates have fallen less or have not decreased, are likely mainly to reflect better survival due to better treatment or earlier detection. Figure A14 indicates a small improvement in 5-year survival.

Cancer of the ovary (Figure 6.21)

Secular trends

Mortality from ovarian cancer at adult ages under 50 years has decreased by about a half since the early 1970s, and in children there has been a greater decrease. At ages 50–69, however, mortality has not diminished, and at ages 70–84 it has increased by 50%.

Incidence rates have changed little or decreased moderately at adult ages under 50, and have increased at older ages. Trends in children have been erratic, based on small numbers.

Trends by birth cohort

Ovarian cancer mortality increased between the cohorts born in the nineteenth century and that born in 1920–4, and has since decreased greatly, except in the most recent cohorts.

In incidence data by birth cohort there was a similar pattern, except that the decrease, from a peak in the 1925–9 cohort, was smaller.

Mortality trends by region

Ovarian cancer mortality changed by less than a third in each region. In general there were increases where rates were initially lowest and little change where they had been highest ($p < 0.001$ for the inverse correlation between the 1960–4 rate and the absolute change in rate from 1960–4 to 1990–4). There is now a gradient, although not large, of higher rates further south in the country.

Comment

The three-digit ICD category for ovarian cancer also includes cancers of the Fallopian tube and other uterine adnexa, but these non-ovarian sites comprise under 2% of the total. Ovarian cancer mortality and incidence trends at younger ages have diverged substantially since 1971 as a consequence of the introduction of chemotherapy. At older ages, however, there has been a lesser divergence, implying that at a population level survival has not been as beneficially affected. Figure A15 shows that the improvement in survival for all-ages has been modest, and comparison of Figures B3 and A15 shows a much greater improvement for children than for all-ages. Examination of age-specific survival data for adults in East Anglia and in England and Wales (not shown) did not reveal greater improvements in survival at young than at older adult ages, however.

The ovary is situated deep within the abdomen, and diagnosis of ovarian malignancy can be difficult. The regional pattern of greater increases in rates where they were initially lower would be compatible with improvements in diagnosis having greatest effect where there was greatest scope for this to occur. Deaths of women coded to cancer of unspecified primary site are relatively often due to cancer of the ovary (Heasman and Lipworth 1966; Grulich *et al.* 1995), so that the

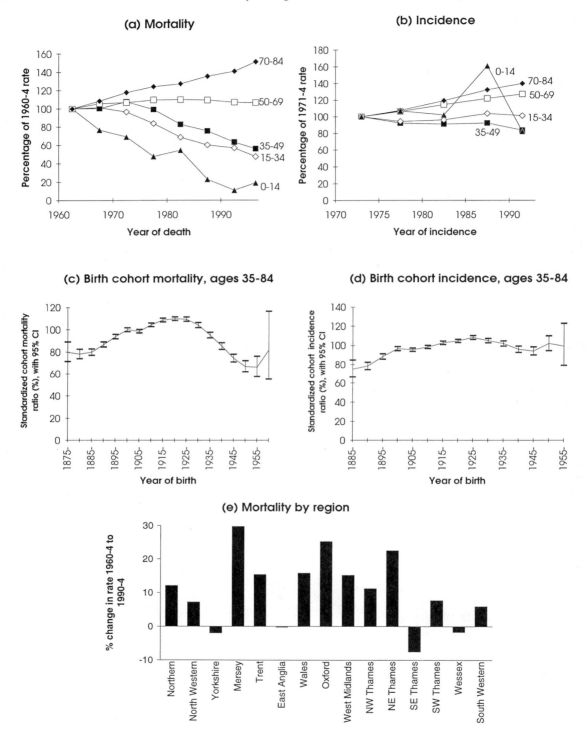

Figure 6.21   Cancer of ovary (ICD7 175; ICD8&9 183), mortality 1960–97, incidence 1971–92.

rising rates of mortality from cancer of unspecified primary site may have added an artefactual downward element to ovarian cancer mortality rates. A decreasing tendency may also have been contributed by the diminishing rates of non-coroner's autopsy (Figure 4.1), as post-mortem examinations substantially increase the number of ovarian cancers diagnosed (Heasman and Lipworth 1966). Ovarian cancer mortality rates were little affected by changes in the Registrar General's interpretation of ICD coding rule 3 (Grulich *et al.* 1995) or the cessation of medical enquiries to certifiers in 1993; we estimate that the changes to OPCS procedures in 1993 (see pp. 11–12) resulted in a 3% decrease in rates.

Risk of ovarian cancer, especially in younger women (Whittemore *et al.* 1992), increases with decreasing parity. The trends in incidence of the tumour for the earliest cohorts in the analysis were the inverse of the trends in family size (Figure 5.40)[80], but for subsequent cohorts this was not generally so. Ovarian cancer risk is reduced by use of oral contraceptives. Oral contraceptive use increased rapidly in the cohorts born from 1925 to 1949 (Figure 5.32), which accords with the downward trend in ovarian cancer incidence in these cohorts. In cohorts born from 1950 onwards, prevalence of ever-use of oral contraceptives has increased relatively little (although age at first use may have declined and duration of use increased—see pp. 46–7), and declining parity may have been the predominant reason for the small increase in ovarian cancer.

There has been recent evidence that clomiphene, a drug used to induce ovulation for treatment of infertility, might increase the risk of ovarian cancer (Rossing *et al.* 1994), but at most it can have accounted for only very few cases in England and Wales.

The great majority of ovarian cancers are epithelial, for which the above risk factors apply, but a small percentage are of germ cell histology[81]. These, it has been hypothesized (Walker *et al.* 1988), may have an aetiology related to prenatal hormone exposure (i.e. similar to the hypothesized aetiology of testicular germ cell cancers), but firm evidence of such a relationship is lacking. Like testicular cancer, incidence of ovarian germ cell cancers has been rising at younger ages (under age 45 years) and decreasing at older ages in England and Wales (dos Santos Silva and Swerdlow 1991).

Rates of ovarian cancer are also affected by rates of oophorectomy, and of hysterectomies that involve removal of the ovaries, because these operations reduce the number of ovaries at risk of malignancy. Risk may also be reduced, although it is far less certain, by hysterectomy without oophorectomy. In the period for which data are available, the rate of oophorectomy decreased while that of hysterectomy (not all of which will have included oophorectomy) increased (Figure 5.55), so that the net effect is unclear.

Cancer of the prostate (Figure 6.22)

Secular trends

Mortality from cancer of the prostate at ages 50 years and above has been rising substantially since 1970–4, although with a downturn in the most recent data, for 1995–7. At ages 35–49, prostatic cancer is uncommon and trends have been less consistent, but there is evidence of a rise in recent years. Incidence trends at ages 35 years and above have been upward, especially at ages 50 and above. At each age-group shown in the Figure[82], the increasing trend has been somewhat steeper for incidence than mortality.

Trends by birth cohort

Mortality from prostatic cancer increased sharply in cohorts born from 1895–9 to 1915–19 and slightly in cohorts born subsequently. Incidence increased through virtually the entire span of cohorts analysed.

Mortality trends by region

Mortality from cancer of the prostate increased somewhat in all regions, most greatly in those where it had initially been lowest (inverse linear correlation between initial rate and absolute increase, $p<0.001$).

Comment

Similar increases in incidence and mortality rates for prostatic cancer to those in England and Wales have

---

[80] The same was true in mortality data for England and Wales for 1931–75 examined by Beral *et al.* (1978).
[81] Although a larger proportion at younger ages—germ cell tumours constitute about 30% of cases at ages under 30 years in England and Wales (dos Santos Silva and Swerdlow 1995).
[82] At ages under 35 years, prostatic cancer is rare and rates are unstable.

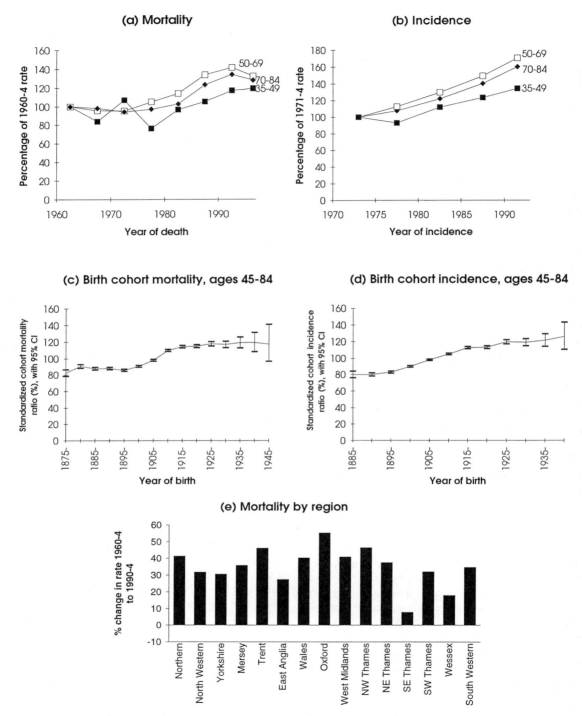

Figure 6.22   Cancer of prostate (ICD7 177; ICD8&9 185), mortality 1960–97, incidence 1971–92.

also been recorded in many Western countries, for mortality particularly at ages over 65 years (Ross and Schottenfeld 1996). Increases in mortality internationally have been greater where rates were initially lower (Ross and Schottenfeld 1996), and the same pattern can be seen in the comparison of trends between the regions of England and Wales. Much of the apparent increase in incidence in recent decades is probably a diagnostic artefact. Asymptomatic prostatic carcinoma is common in older men (Breslow *et al.* 1977), and there is therefore great scope for increasing detection. Histological examination of curettings from transurethral resections of the prostate (TURP) leads to incidental diagnosis of prostatic cancer in a substantial proportion of cases[83], and the rising use of TURP to treat benign prostatic hypertrophy has increased detection of early, asymptomatic prostatic cancers (Potosky *et al.* 1990; Levy *et al.* 1993). A Canadian study (Levy *et al.* 1993) has suggested that more intensive pathological scrutiny of tissue obtained from TURP may also have raised the rates of diagnosis. The use of transrectal ultrasound, too, may have increased detection. In England and Wales, the use of TURP increased particularly during 1969–79, although there were also increases before and after then (see p. 66). Corresponding with this pattern, there were considerable increases from 1970 to 1980 in the proportion of registered prostatic cancers for which histological verification was obtained, with less if any increase from 1980 to 1990 in most regions for which data were available (Table 6.3). The rate of increase in registered prostatic cancer incidence in Figure 6.22b, however, was no greater from 1971–80 than subsequently.

In the US, the introduction around 1990 of prostate-specific antigen screening appears to have greatly increased, or at least accelerated, the diagnosis of early tumours (Corder *et al.* 1994). The England and Wales data are suggestive of the same effect: the registration rate of prostatic cancer at ages 15–84 increased by 15% from 1990 to 1992, compared with an average of 3% per annum from 1971 to 1990.

In addition, there has now been a marked decline in mortality rates in US whites and blacks since around 1991 (Tarone *et al.* 2000) and in the European Union overall since 1992 (Levi *et al.* 2000), and a similar, if less pronounced, decline can be seen in the mortality data for 1995–7 at all-ages in England and Wales, which might be due to prostate-specific antigen screening or better treatment.

Although greater detection rates in life might to some extent have affected the diagnosis of cause of death, the effects of the diagnostic artefacts above are likely to have been much less for mortality than for incidence data. The greater increase in recorded incidence than mortality, a pattern seen also in the United States (Brawley 1997), would accord with rising detection of earlier, good prognosis, tumours. The apparent improvement in survival (Figure A16) would be consonant with this.

Autopsy can reveal 'latent' prostatic cancers that would otherwise have remained undetected, but as noted on pp. 8–9, the number of cancers detected by autopsy has probably been falling over the last 30 years: in 1972, 9% of prostatic cancer deaths in England and Wales were certified after autopsy (although not necessarily detected because of it) (OPCS 1974*b*) compared

Table 6.3 Percentage of registrations of prostatic cancer with histological verification, selected regional cancer registries in England and Wales, around 1970, 1980 and 1990[a].

Registry	% histologically verified		
	1970	1980	1990
Birmingham and West Midlands	53	76	—
Mersey	44	48	81
North Western	—	68	72
Oxford	57	78	74
South Thames	51	83	67
South Western	56	71	73
Trent	45	69	—

[a] Periods of data and data sources as in Table 4.2.
— Data not published.

---

[83] Fourteen per cent of cases in an intensive scrutiny of prostatic tissue from TURPs conducted at an average age of 70 years in the US (Rohr 1987).

with 4% in 1992 (OPCS 1994). Part of the increase in recorded mortality—perhaps a half or more at older ages in recent years—may be an artefact of changed certification practice (Grulich *et al.* 1995); there has been a rise in the extent to which, when prostatic cancer is entered on the death certificate it is stated as the underlying cause of death rather than as a mentioned but non-underlying cause. There was also an artefactual increase in mortality of 6% in 1984 due to changes in OPCS interpretation of ICD coding rule 3 (see pp. 11–12). When this change was reversed, in 1993, and medical enquiries to certifiers ceased, we estimate a 6% artefactual decrease resulted (Table 4.1)[84].

As well as the rises due to the various artefactual factors above, it seems likely from the size of increase in recorded rates that has occurred, encompassing mortality as well as incidence, that an element of the increase is real. It is therefore encouraging to note that the rise in mortality rates has slowed greatly for cohorts born since 1920. Insufficient is understood about the causes of prostatic cancer to assess how the trends in rates of the cancer relate to those for known aetiological factors. Internationally, prostatic cancer mortality rates correlate strongly with fat consumption (Armstrong and Doll 1975), and several individual-based studies have supported such an association, although it is not well-established (Ross and Schottenfeld 1996). Per caput fat consumption reached a peak in 1969 before decreasing (Figure 5.14), while the trend in prostatic cancer incidence was still upward in the most recent data available (for 1990–2), and mortality rates increased until the mid-1990s, before falling.

Cancer of the testis (Figure 6.23)

Secular trends

Mortality from cancer of the testis has decreased substantially at all ages since the early 1970s, most greatly at young ages and least at 70–84 years. Incidence at adult ages under 70 years has increased by about a half or more. Figure 6.23c shows that the increase has been limited to the ages at which the peak incidence occurred (30–34 years) and neighbouring age-groups.

Longer-term data (Figure 6.23g) show that mortality at young ages had been rising for 60 years (at least) before the decrease started in the 1970s, whereas rates at ages 50–84 have been falling since early in the century, although this fall has accelerated in the last 20 years. It took over 50 years, from 1911–15 to 1976–80, for rates at ages 50–84 to halve, while they halved again from 1976–80 to 1995–7. As Figure 6.23h shows, the peak of testicular cancer in young adults that is now characteristic of this tumour developed during the twentieth century, and virtually did not exist when the century began, whereas the reverse process has occurred at old ages.

Trends by birth cohort

The trend in mortality from testicular cancer at ages 50–84 was generally upward in cohorts born before 1905, and then decreased steeply in men born up to 1934 but not in those born subsequently. Mortality in younger adults showed no consistent trend in cohorts born before 1935, but has since decreased greatly.

Trends in incidence of testicular cancer at ages 50–84 were inconsistent in early cohorts, but have been rising since those born in 1920–4. At ages 15–49, there was a steady increase from the cohort born in 1925–9 to that born in 1960–4, but a less clear trend for those born subsequently. Trends in children (not shown) were erratic, based on small numbers. Cohort data for testicular cancer incidence at young adult ages by single year of birth (Figure 6.23f) showed deviations from the prevailing trend for some individual cohorts born in the early 1930s, 1964, and the early 1970s, but no appreciable deviation for cohorts born during the Second World War and no consistent diminution for those born during the worst of the Depression (Figures 5.25, 5.59).

Mortality trends by region

Testicular cancer mortality has decreased greatly in all regions, but generally by a greater percentage in the south of England than in the north and Wales.

Comment

Testicular cancer is much the most common cancer in men aged 15–34 in England and Wales, and at these ages the tumours are almost all of germ cell histology. There are differences in epidemiology between testicular cancers occurring at the young adult peak (up to

---

[84] The actual percentage changes from 1983 to 1984 and 1992 to 1993 were similar to those predicted from the effects of the coding changes.

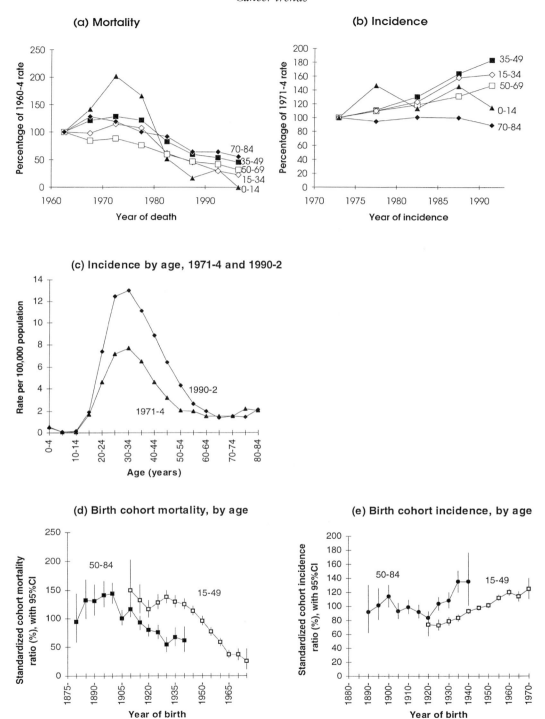

Figure 6.23 Cancer of testis (ICD2 pt. 45; ICD3 pt. 49; ICD4 pt. 51; ICD5 pt. 51c; ICD6&7 178; ICD8&9 186): (a), (d) mortality 1960–97; (b), (c), (e), (f) incidence 1971–92; (g) mortality 1911–97; (h) mortality 1911–70; (i), mortality 1960–4 to 1990–4.

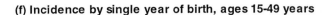

(f) Incidence by single year of birth, ages 15-49 years

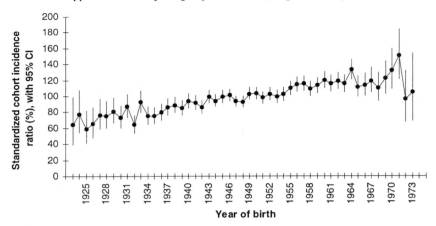

(g) Mortality 1911-97

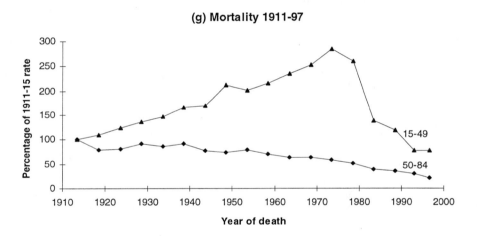

(h) Mortality by age, 1911-15, 1936-40, 1966-70

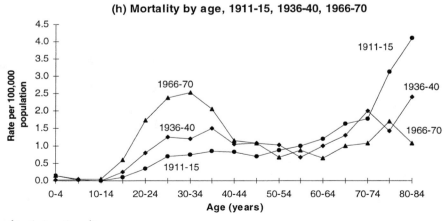

Figure 6.23   Cancer of testis (continued).

(i) Mortality by region

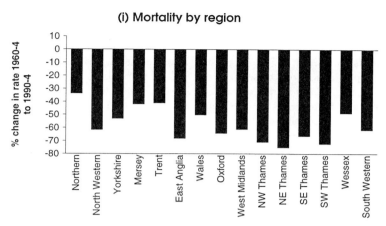

Figure 6.23   Cancer of testis (continued).

about age 50 years) and those at older ages. The increasing incidence of testicular cancer in young men in England and Wales, which the mortality data indicate has been occurring at least since early in the twentieth century, corresponds with increases in incidence seen in white populations around the world as far back as data have been available. It cannot be accounted for by diagnostic changes, as cases can usually be identified from clinical symptoms and examination, and its scale is too large plausibly to be due to better registration. The reason for the increase is not known. The rising rate parallels a rising incidence of undescended testis (John Radcliffe Hospital Cryptorchidism Study Group 1992)[85], the main known risk factor for testicular cancer, but as only 10% of testicular cancers occur in undescended testes this does not in itself explain the increase in the cancer rate.

It has been hypothesized that *in utero* exposure to high concentrations of free oestrogens in the first trimester of pregnancy may be aetiological for testicular cancer (Henderson *et al.* 1983). Prescription of exogenous oestrogens to treat threatened abortion was comparatively uncommon in the UK (see p. 46). It has been suggested that *in utero* exposure to environmental oestrogenic chemicals or dietary oestrogens ingested by the mother might be of importance and have increased over time (Sharpe and Skakkebaek 1993), but their aetiological role, if any, and relevant time trends are uncertain. Another possibility is that bioavailable endogenous oestrogen levels in mothers may have

altered over time, perhaps because of changing nutrition, but again it is not known whether this has occurred.

Many other prenatal factors have been investigated as possible risk factors for testicular cancer that might be associated with maternal hormone concentrations. Two that have shown associations in some studies are primogeniture and dizygotic (DZ) twinship. The proportion of livebirths in England and Wales that were firstbirths decreased from 1938 to 1964 (Figure 5.11), however, while testicular cancer incidence in these cohorts was increasing. Dizygotic twinning is too uncommon to itself have had an appreciable influence on rates of testicular cancer, but its trends are of interest in comparison with those for testicular cancer because there is evidence that DZ twinning may be a marker for gonadotropin and sex hormone levels in the mother, and hence perhaps DZ twinning rates might be a marker for hormone levels in mothers generally at a population level. DZ twinning rates, however, showed no consistent trend from 1938 to 1954 (Figure 5.13) and decreased markedly from 1955 to 1980, while the cohorts born in the earlier period showed substantial increases in the incidence of testicular cancer, and there was an uneven (but not a decreasing) trend for cohorts born since.

In some studies but not all, risk of testicular cancer has been associated with low birthweight, a risk factor for cryptorchidism. The percentage of births in England and Wales that were of low birthweight

---

[85] There has also been a rise in orchidopexy rates (Figure 5.54), although interpretation of the effect of this is difficult. On the one hand it may reflect a rising prevalence of undescended testes, which are at raised risk of testicular cancer; on the other hand, but uncertainly, orchidopexy may reduce the risk of malignancy in testes that are brought down into the scrotum.

(≤2.5 kg) remained unchanged from 1953–72 (Figure 5.12)[86], while in the cohorts born in the early part of these years testicular cancer incidence was upward and in the later ones inconsistent. Since 1978 low birthweight has increased in prevalence, but these cohorts are as yet too young to assess their testicular cancer incidence at adult ages, and their trends in testicular cancer at childhood ages have been inconsistent.

In several studies, risk of testicular cancer has been raised in men who were first-born to women having this pregnancy at a relatively late age. Although this factor could not explain testicular cancer trends fully, it could contribute to them. Henderson *et al.* (1997) noted in Los Angeles County that testicular cancer incidence rose to a peak in the late 1980s, probably in the cohort of men born about 1955–60, and then declined. This pattern coincided approximately with a fall in mean age at first full-term pregnancy (FFTP) for women born from 1910 to 1940, who would have been giving birth about 1930–60, and a rise in age at FFTP for women born subsequently. In England and Wales, the pattern showed similarities: age at FFTP decreased for women born from 1920 to the early 1940s, and then rose (Figure 5.36), while testicular cancer incidence increased strongly for men born from 1940 to 1960, but may since have levelled off, although these cohorts are still too young to be sure about this.

Assessment of testicular cancer incidence by single year of birth gave no indication of the temporary cessation in the increasing trend for men born during and soon before the Second World War, that has been observed in Denmark, Norway, and Sweden (Bergström *et al.* 1996), although not in Finland, East Germany, Poland (Bergström *et al.* 1996), and Scotland (Swerdlow *et al.* 1998). The UK, unlike Denmark and Norway (but also Poland), was not occupied during the war, and although the war affected food supplies, it did not lead to malnutrition[87]. Perhaps of more significance in the UK context, there was also no dip in risk for men born during the Depression of the 1930s, when the living circumstances including nutrition of the poor were badly affected; it should be noted, however, that the data analysed on testicular cancer in these cohorts did not cover the peak ages of incidence of the tumour.

Height, which is probably strongly related to childhood nutrition, has been found to be associated with risk of testicular cancer in some but not all studies. Height of men has increased (Figures 5.7, 5.8) through the period for which testicular cancer rates have increased. The apparent interruption of this rise in height for the cohort born in 1936–40 (Figure 5.8), however, had no counterpart in the testicular cancer data.

Decreasing age at puberty, increasing sedentariness, and lack of exercise (UK Testicular Cancer Study Group 1994) have been put forward as possible causes of the increasing rates of testicular cancer, but insufficient quantitative data are available to test their contribution to the trend in incidence.

A potential artefact in testicular cancer data at older ages is that lymphomas of the testis, which are relatively common at old but not younger ages, are coded in the ICD to lymphoma if the histology is stated, but to cancer of the testis if it is not. Thus, apparent trends in testicular cancer could be affected if there has been a change over time in the specificity of histological information available about these tumours. This makes it particularly difficult to interpret the trends in rates at old ages, when many of the testicular cancers recorded in the England and Wales data may actually be lymphomas (Pike *et al.* 1987).

The decreasing mortality from testicular cancer since the early 1970s, while incidence has risen at ages under 65 and remained unchanged at older ages, reflects the great impact on survival from teratoma and late stage seminoma of the introduction of chemotherapy in the 1970s, and from seminoma of intensive radiotherapy before that (Figures A17, B3).

Cancer of the penis (Figure 6.24)

Cancer of the penis is uncommon in Britain, but its trends are of interest because there is evidence that it may have a closely similar aetiology, from a sexually transmitted infection, to that of cancer of the cervix in

---

[86] Low birthweight babies are at greater risk than others of dying soon after birth, but the percentage of persons in these cohorts surviving beyond the neonatal period who had been of low birthweight also remained unchanged (e.g. 5.72% in 1953, 5.75% in 1971, calculated from Alberman (1974)).

[87] Indeed for the poor and for nutritionally vulnerable groups, rationing and specific wartime nutritional measures led to improved nutrition, in the later war years at least (Baines *et al.* 1963).

(a) Birth cohort mortality, ages 35-84

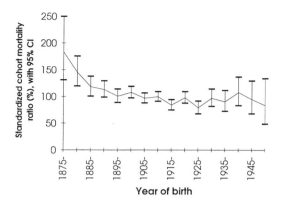

(b) Birth cohort incidence, ages 35-84

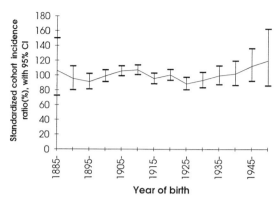

Figure 6.24   Cancer of penis (ICD7 179.0; ICD8 187.0; ICD9 187.1–.4), mortality 1960–97, incidence 1971–92.

women. For instance, rates of cervical cancer have been found to be increased in wives of men with penile cancer (Martinez 1969; Graham *et al.* 1979; Smith *et al.* 1980). Figure 6.24 therefore shows penile cancer trends by birth cohort. In mortality data there is no evidence of the large peaks and troughs seen for cervical cancer (Figure 6.19), and indeed no substantial change since cohorts born late in the nineteenth century. In incidence data by birth cohort, however, there was evidence of a pattern analogous to, but less marked than, that for cervical cancer, and occurring, although not entirely consistently, in cohorts born about 5 years earlier. This would accord with the generally younger peak age of incidence of most sexual infections in women (at ages 16–19) than men (at ages 20–24) (Simms *et al.* 1998). There was a fall in both penile and cervical cancer incidence in successive cohorts born in the late nineteenth century, reaching a minimum for men born in 1895–9 and women born in 1905–9, then a rise to a peak for men born in 1910–14 and women born in 1915–19, a second minimum for men born in 1925–9 and women in 1930–4, and then a rise which in women reached a peak in the cohort born in 1950–4 and in men is of uncertain peak, with wide confidence intervals for the highest SIR, in the cohort born in 1950–4.

Cancer of the penis is much less common in circumcised men, particularly those circumcised at birth, than in uncircumcised men. Data on circumcision rates in England and Wales are available only since 1961 (Figure 5.54), i.e. only for more recent birth cohorts than those in Figure 6.24, and show a decline; these data will have excluded religious circumcisions conducted at home, but it seems unlikely that the number of these has increased.

Cancer of the scrotum (Figure 6.25)

Figure 6.25 shows the decline since 1911–20, the earliest years for which data were published[88], in mortality from cancer of the scrotum—a tumour which has had particular historical connections with England. The mortality rate at ages under 85 years in 1995–7 was less than a tenth of that early in the century. Incidence too has declined—by a half in the period since 1971–4.

An occupational cause of this tumour was first recognized over 200 years ago by Percival Pott (Pott 1775), a surgeon at St Bartholomew's Hospital in London, who noted the high risk in English chimney sweeps. Several other occupational causes have been identified in the country in more recent times—in workers exposed to pitch and tar (Butlin 1892), mule-spinners in the cotton industry (Southam and Wilson 1922), tool-setters, tool-fitters, and machine operators exposed to lubricating oils (Cruickshank and Squire 1950), and workers in coal-gas and coke production (Doll *et al.* 1972). The declining rates of scrotal cancer over time reflect a decrease in occupationally-caused cases, as these are the majority (Waldron *et al.* 1984).

---

[88] Data for years before 1960 were extracted from the annual review volumes of the Registrar General. Data for 1911–20 were available only for these years in aggregate. No data were published for 1921–2 and 1950–7.

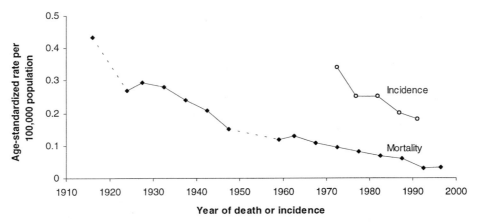

Figure 6.25   Cancer of scrotum (ICD2 pt. 44; ICD3 pt. 48; ICD4 pt. 51; ICD5 51a; ICD7 179.1; ICD8 172.5; ICD9 187.7), ages 0–84, mortality 1911–20, 1923–49, 1958–97, incidence 1971–92.

Cancer of the bladder (Figure 6.26)

Secular trends

Bladder cancer mortality in men aged 35–69 years has decreased substantially. At ages 70–84 years a peak was reached in 1975–9, with a subsequent decline. In women, there has been a large decline at ages 35–49 years, but at ages 50–69 rates have decreased only since 1975–9, and at older ages rates increased until the early 1990s. Mortality from bladder cancer at ages 15–34 is rare; rates have varied considerably over time and are discussed separately below.

In each sex, incidence of bladder cancer at ages 50 and above increased substantially until 1985–9 and then tended to level off. At ages 35–49 there was a small peak in each sex in 1985–9, but rates were not greatly changed over the study period overall.

Rates of bladder cancer at ages 15–34 were based on much smaller numbers than at older ages, and the mortality trends could not satisfactorily be presented in Figures 6.26a and b. There were interesting trends in this age group, however, and these are therefore shown separately in Figures 6.26e and f. In males, mortality and incidence trends were generally downward, with an interruption for mortality in the 1980s, based on small numbers, and for incidence in 1985–9, based on larger numbers. In females, there was an evidence of a small epidemic in the 1970s and 1980s: the mortality rate increased from 0.1 per million in 1960–4 and 1965–9 (based on 4 and 2 deaths respectively), to 0.3 in 1970–4 and 1975–9 (9 and 10 deaths) and 0.4 in

1980–4 and 1985–9 (14 and 15 deaths), before declining to 0.3 in 1990–4 (11 deaths) and 0.04 in 1995–7 (1 death). The incidence rate doubled from 1.5 per million (37 cases) in 1971–4 to 3.0 per million (110 cases) in 1985–9, before declining slightly in 1990–2.

Trends by birth cohort

In males, mortality reached a peak in the cohort born in 1900–4, and then decreased substantially, although this decrease ceased for those born in 1950 and later. In females, the greatest rates were in the cohorts born in 1910–14 and 1920–4, with a subsequent decline, largely ceasing for those born since 1940.

For incidence, a peak was reached in males born in 1925–9 and females born in 1920–4, with the subsequent trend in males downward, but in females, after a decrease, a rising trend for those born from 1940 onwards.

Mortality trends by region

Mortality in each sex has tended, but not consistently, to decrease in the south and to increase in the north of England, and there is now a slight north/south gradient which was not apparent in 1960–4.

Comment

The ICD category analysed for bladder cancer includes also cancers of the urethra and other urinary tract

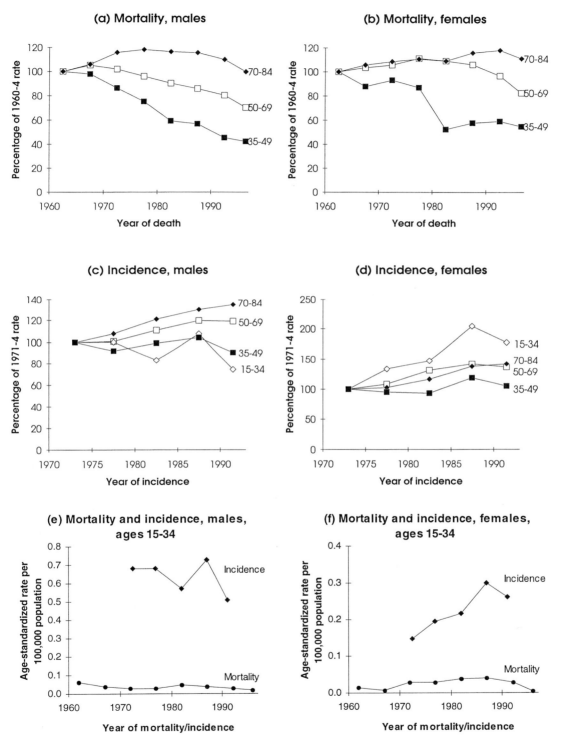

Figure 6.26 Cancer of bladder and urethra (ICD7 181.0, .7, .8; ICD8 188, 189.9; ICD9 188, 189.3–.9), mortality 1960–97, incidence 1971–92.

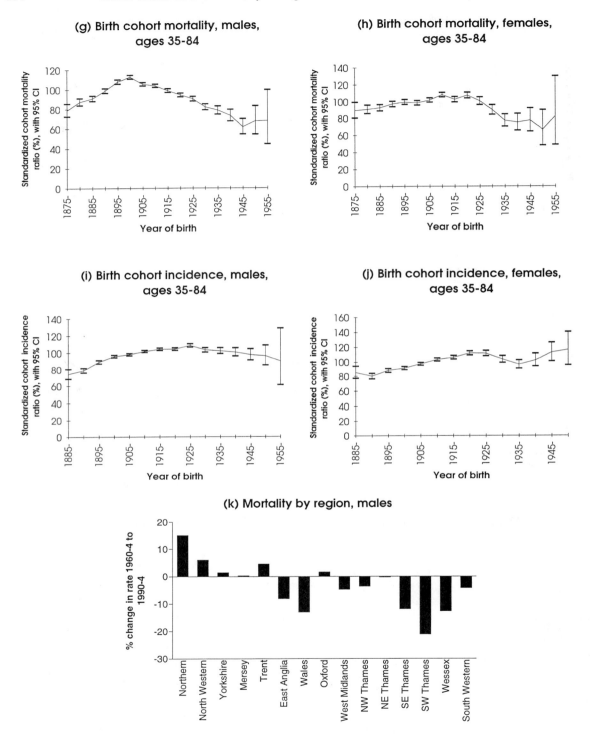

Figure 6.26 Cancer of bladder and urethra (continued).

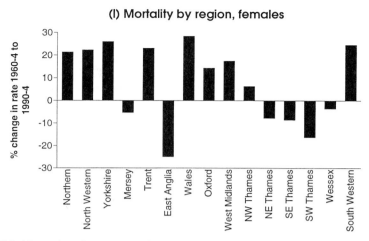

(I) Mortality by region, females

Figure 6.26 Cancer of bladder and urethra (continued).

tumours except the kidney and ureter, but these were under 2% of the total. There is potential for artefact in trends of bladder cancer incidence if there have been changes in clinicopathological terminology or criteria for papillomas of the bladder (Saxén 1982) or in cancer registry coding of invasiveness of bladder tumours (Lynch *et al.* 1991). The approximately unaltered survival[89] in East Anglia over time (Figure A18) would suggest that such changes in criteria have not occurred (as these would be expected to lead to apparent improvements in survival). On the other hand, the increases in survival in England and Wales data (Figure A18) would be compatible with such a diagnostic change (or, of course, with better results of treatment), as would the divergence between national trends for incidence and mortality. It is possible that constant diagnostic and coding criteria for bladder cancer registrations have been maintained over time by the East Anglia registry but not nationally.

Incidence and mortality rates for bladder cancer in women in England and Wales are high by international standards. The main known cause of bladder cancer is smoking. The coincidence of birth cohort peaks of mortality from bladder cancer with those for lung cancer (Figure 6.11) and for tar-adjusted smoking (Figure 5.51)[90] implies that smoking explains much of the trends in this tumour, although the cohort trends

for bladder cancer incidence do not accord so well with those for lung cancer and smoking.

Bladder cancer is also caused by various occupational exposures, which were estimated collectively to account for 3–19% of cases in Yorkshire, England in the period from the 1950s through to 1980 (Vineis and Simonato 1986). Reduction in certain of these exposures will have contributed a downward element to bladder cancer rates. Raised risk has been found in workers in the dyestuffs industry, aromatic amine manufacturing, rubber and electric cable manufacturing, and coal gas and coke production, and associations that are less clearly aetiological have been found for several other occupations including painting and leather working. Certain of these exposures have ceased—exposures to carcinogenic intermediates in the dyestuffs industry decreased from about 1935, and especially after 1945 (Case *et al.* 1954), use of 1- and 2-naphthylamine in the rubber industry stopped in 1949 (Baxter and Werner 1980), the use of 2-naphthylamine was banned in about 1950 and of benzidine in about 1962 (Boyko *et al*, 1985), and the only plant making α-naphthylamine and one making benzidine in Britain were closed in 1965 (Lancet 1965). After a lag period, these measures appear to have had a successful effect: deaths from urinary tract epithelial neoplasms in workers making or handling chemicals such as

---

[89] With fairly narrow confidence intervals.

[90] For men, there is a close correspondence for cumulative smoking at older ages; for women, the same appears to be true as far as can be gauged from the available smoking data, but these do not give as full information on the peak at older ages.

β-naphthylamine for which industrial death benefit was paid in Great Britain reached a peak in 1965–9, and then decreased (Swerdlow 1990). The coal gas manufacturing plants in the mainland UK all closed with the advent of natural gas supplies from the North Sea.

Bladder cancer can also be caused by chronic heavy use of analgesic mixtures that include the drug phenacetin, for which we have no detailed data on trends in use. Phenacetin was first used therapeutically in 1887 (Piper *et al.* 1985). Because prolonged high doses may cause kidney damage, its use in Britain was restricted by law in 1974 and banned completely in March 1980 (IARC 1980). Heavy long-term use occurred particularly in women, and renal cancers in association with analgesic abuse were first reported in the 1960s (IARC 1980).

The doubling of bladder cancer incidence in young women in England and Wales from 1971–4 to 1985–9, and the peak of mortality in this group in the 1980s were at younger ages than cases of phenacetin-induced urinary tract tumours have generally been reported to occur (Bengtsson *et al.* 1968; IARC 1980; McCredie *et al.* 1982) and were not accompanied by increases in bladder cancer at older ages or increases in renal cancer. Furthermore, as the peak occurred many years after use of phenacetin was restricted, and several years after it ceased completely, bladder cancers at young ages in the late 1980s would need to have been related to use at substantially younger ages again[91], if they were related to this drug. Thus overall it seems unlikely that the peak was due to phenacetin. Its cause is unclear, but there is a similarity between the trends for bladder cancer and cervical cancer in young women, and it is possible that the bladder cancer peak is due to occasional misdiagnoses (or misregistrations) of cervical cancers that have spread to the bladder[92] or that the two malignancies have an aetiology in common from sexually transmitted infection (Dolin 1992). Bladder cancer occurs too infrequently as a second cancer after radiotherapy of cervical cancer for such second cancers to explain the shared trends of these tumours in young women (Dolin 1992).

The drugs chlornaphazine and cyclophosphamide, which have been used in cancer chemotherapy, can also cause bladder cancer, but in too few people to have affected national trends. Thirty years ago on the basis of animal experiments of dubious relevance, artificial sweeteners were suggested as possible causes of bladder cancer in man. Epidemiological studies have not supported this, however, and bladder cancer trends in England and Wales did not parallel those for saccharin consumption (Armstrong and Doll 1974).

Cancer of the kidney (Figure 6.27)

Secular trends

Renal cancer mortality has decreased greatly in children, reduced or remained little changed in young adults, and increased substantially at ages 50 years and above. Incidence of renal cancer in children has not appreciably altered since 1971–4, but in adults, especially at older ages, there have been substantial increases.

Trends by birth cohort

Mortality from renal cancer in each sex increased in cohorts born from late in the nineteenth century until the 1920s, and then decreased slightly in men and more greatly, in the most recent cohorts, in women. Trends in incidence were similar to those for mortality, except that the most recent trend has not been downward, and indeed in women, at least, rates have been rising for cohorts born in 1945–54.

Mortality trends by region

Mortality has been unchanged or increasing in all regions, although the degree of increase has varied greatly. Generally, but not uniformly, percentage increases have been greater in the north than the south of England. In men, the absolute extent of increase has been inversely proportional to the original rates in 1960–4 ($p<0.001$ for linear correlation), but this has not been clear in women ($p = 0.07$).

Comment

Renal cancers occur mainly in the renal parenchyma, where almost all are adenocarcinomas, and less often

---

[91] And at younger ages than the main ones for analgesic abuse (Murray 1978).

[92] Cervical cancer is far more common than bladder cancer at these ages, so the percentage misdiagnosed would only need to be small.

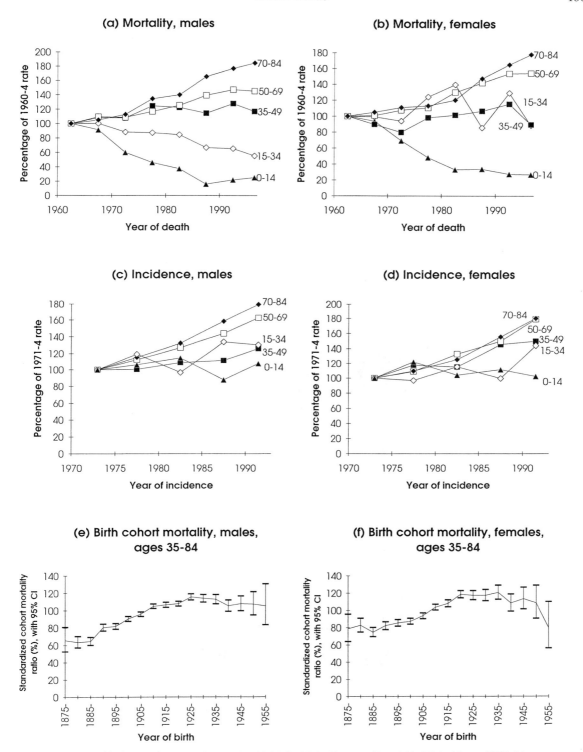

Figure 6.27 Cancer of kidney and ureter (ICD7 180; ICD8&9 189.0–.2), mortality 1960–97, incidence 1971–92.

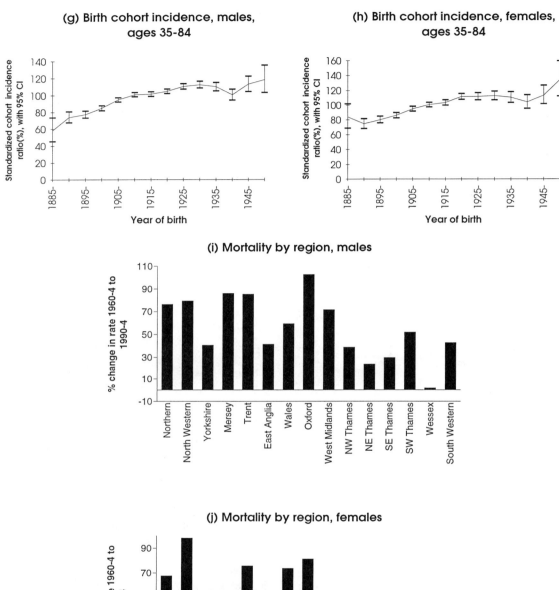

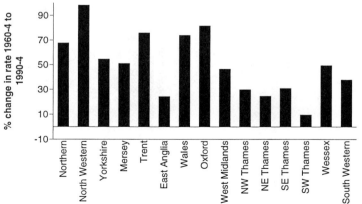

Figure 6.27   Cancer of kidney and ureter (continued).

in the renal pelvis, where the tumours are largely transitional cell. In children, most renal malignancies are nephroblastomas (Wilms' tumours). The ICD codes analysed for renal cancer also include cancer of the ureter, which accounts for about 5% of the total.

As the kidney is a deep abdominal organ, diagnostic factors may have played a part in apparent trends. The regional trends in men, with increases in inverse proportion to the original rates, is a pattern that might be seen if at least part of the increase at older ages was an artefact of improved diagnosis; such a pattern was less clearly present in women, however. Autopsy can reveal substantial numbers of renal cancers not diagnosed clinically (Heasman and Lipworth 1966), so that declining rate of non-coroner's autopsy (Figure 4.1) may have added an artefactual downward component to renal cancer trends. Artefacts from cessation of medical enquiries and changes in interpretation of ICD coding rule 3 (see pp. 11–12), have been small[93].

The increasing incidence of renal cancers, particularly at older ages, parallels increases seen also in the US (Devesa *et al.* 1987, 1995). The main known risk factor for renal cancer—both transitional cell cancers of the pelvis and adenocarcinomas of the body of the kidney (Doll 1996)—is cigarette smoking. The rise in renal cancer in early cohorts showed similarities to the pattern for lung cancer (Figure 6.11), but thereafter there was not the large decrease in rates for cohorts of men born since 1900–4 and women born since 1925–9 seen for lung cancer[94].

Risk of renal cancer is also raised in heavy users of the analgesic phenacetin, and there is weaker evidence that acetaminophen, a more recently introduced over-the-counter analgesic and the main metabolite of phenacetin, may also be causal. Analgesic nephropathy has been comparatively uncommon in England and Wales (Murray 1978). In a case-control study in England in the 1970s, 14% of cancers of the renal body were associated with use of analgesics daily for 6 months or more (Armstrong *et al.* 1976). Use of phenacetin was restricted in 1974 and banned in 1980 (see p. 152). Heavy use of phenacetin-containing analgesics occurred mainly in women, but there is no indication of an epidemic of renal cancer affecting women

specifically, and indeed renal cancer trends have been fairly similar between the sexes.

Risk of renal cell cancer is associated with obesity, particularly in women. In the data available, since 1980, the prevalence of obesity has been increasing in both sexes in England and Wales (Figure 5.6), while renal cancer incidence and mortality rates have risen at older ages and incidence has risen in younger adults too.

The large divergence between incidence and mortality trends for renal cancer in children reflects the great improvement that has taken place in survival from Wilms' tumour (Figure B4). In adults, although recorded incidence has generally risen somewhat more rapidly than mortality, there was only a large divergence in men aged 15–34 years. East Anglia all-age data showed no improvement in survival, while data for England and Wales suggested substantial improvements (Figure A19)[95].

Cancer of the eye (Figure 6.28)

Cancer of the eye is comparatively uncommon, and therefore to give stability of larger numbers, rates for this tumour are shown for only two age groups, under 15 years and older than this. Data for finer age-groups can be found in Appendix C, Table 25.

Secular trends

In children aged 0–14 years mortality from eye cancer decreased, albeit unevenly, through the study period. At older ages rates showed a small rise and fall before 1990, and then decreased sharply. Examining the adult data by age group (not shown), the decrease in the 1990s occurred in all age groups, but the peak around 1970–4 occurred mainly at ages 50 and above.

Incidence of eye cancer in children showed no consistent change. In adults overall, rates were little changed through to 1980–4, and then increased by about a quarter. The pattern was similar to this at each adult age-group (not shown), except that rates were uneven at ages 15–34, based on small numbers.

---

[93] Medical enquiries had an effect of less than 5% (Swerdlow 1989) and the 1984 change in rule 3 interpretation raised rates by 2.5%.
[94] And the decrease in smoking seen in men in recent cohorts in Figure 5.51a; for women the available data in Figure 5.51b did not show cumulative smoking at older ages for cohorts born since 1925–9.
[95] England and Wales data were not available for ages 15–34 separately, and there were few cases in East Anglia at these ages.

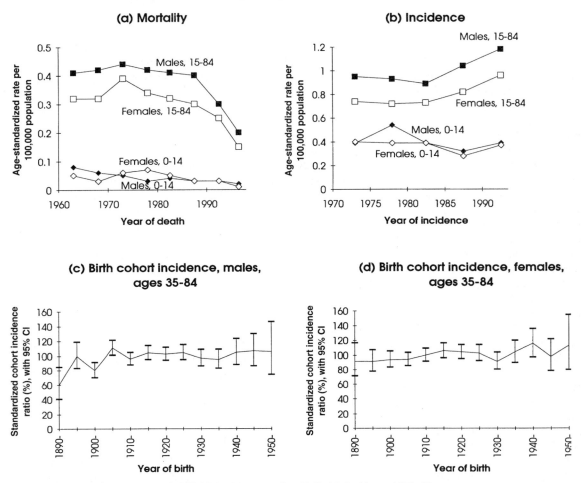

Figure 6.28   Cancer of eye (ICD7 192; ICD8&9 190), mortality 1960–97, incidence 1971–92.

Trends by birth cohort

In each sex, mortality at ages 35–84 (not shown) increased in cohorts born up to about the beginning of the twentieth century and decreased in subsequent cohorts, in both instances inconsistently. Incidence in men has shown no substantial change in cohorts born since early in the twentieth century, while in women there has been a slight and inconsistent increase.

Mortality trends by region

Trends by region (not shown) were erratic, based on small numbers.

Comment

In adults, ocular cancers are mainly melanomas, whereas in children they are almost all retinoblastomas, with a different aetiology (often genetic) and clinical characteristics. The data for ages 15 years and above effectively represent trends in eye melanoma and those for younger ages are effectively for retinoblastoma (Hakulinen *et al.* 1978). The absence of a large secular increase in incidence of eye melanoma in adults contrasts with the more than doubling in cutaneous melanoma incidence over the same period. Changes in exposure to the eye will not, however, have been the same as changes in exposure to the skin of the body, as the former will have been affected by the reduction in agricultural and other open air work by men, which will have had less effect on the latter. Even if UVR causes ocular as well as cutaneous melanoma, therefore, one would not expect the trends for the two tumours to be the same, although eye melanoma might resemble head and neck melanoma, which has more than doubled in incidence in men and increased by two-thirds in women since 1971–4 (Table 6.2) while eye cancer rates increased by far less. In epidemiological data generally, the relation to UVR exposure has been less convincing for eye melanoma than for skin melanoma (NRPB 1995), and there is not the north/south gradient in incidence within England and Wales for eye cancer that is seen for melanoma of the skin (Swerdlow and dos Santos Silva 1993). Eye melanoma in men has been found to be more common in rural than urban areas in several countries (Doll 1991) although this was not the case in data for 1968–81 in England and Wales (Swerdlow and dos Santos Silva 1993). The increase in incidence of eye cancer in adults in England and Wales in the most recent years is not based on large numbers, and further years of data will be needed to determine whether it represents the start of an upward trend, for which a possible effect of UVR cannot be excluded as a potential explanation.

In children, the divergence between incidence and mortality trends somewhat accords with the modestly improved survival from retinoblastoma seen in Figure B5. The declining mortality from eye cancers in adults in recent years, while incidence has increased somewhat, implies improved survival. The available information on survival, from East Anglia, did not show any clear improvement (Figure A20), but with wide confidence intervals for the data on this uncommon tumour. Part of the apparent decrease in mortality may be an artefact. Mortality rates for eye melanoma are more dependent than those for most cancer sites on the precision of specification of cause on the death certificate, because melanomas of unspecified site are coded to the three-digit rubric for cutaneous melanoma. 'Medical enquiries' to certifiers for imprecisely specified cancers in 1986 and 1992 increased eye cancer mortality rates by a third (Swerdlow 1989; OPCS 1995), and we estimate that the discontinuation of medical enquiries in 1993 would have reduced mortality rates by 24%[96] (Table 4.1). (All-age mortality rates actually decreased by 33% in males and 43% in females from 1992 to 1993[97].)

Tumours of the nervous system

(Figure 6.29)

Secular trends

Trends in mortality from tumours of the nervous system[98] have varied greatly by age. At ages 70–84 years, the rate more than quadrupled in each sex over the study period. In contrast, at 50–69 years of age there was a slight increase, and at ages under 50 substantial decreases, greatest at the youngest ages.

Incidence trends also showed a large divergence by age, with rates approximately tripling at ages 70–84, but increasing by around a third or less at younger ages.

Trends for tumours of the nervous system specified as malignant (not shown) (which constituted about 60–80% of deaths and of registered cases of nervous system tumour) were similar to those described above, but slightly less upward.

Trends by birth cohort

We analysed trends by birth cohort in three age-groups: 0–14, 15–44, and 45–84 years. In each sex, mortality in the oldest age-group increased greatly until a peak in the cohort born in 1915–19, but has since decreased. At younger ages there have been decreases in mortality more or less throughout the span of cohorts for which data are available. Incidence rates at ages 45–84 years also increased strongly up to the 1915–19 birth cohort, but have not changed appreciably since except for a rise in the most recent cohorts analysed. At ages 15–44 there have generally been rising incidence rates, and in children no consistent change.

Cohort trends for malignancies of the nervous system (not shown) were generally similar to those above, except that for incidence in men aged 15–44 there was less evidence of an increase than had been present for benign plus malignant tumours.

Figures 6.29i and j show the age distribution of nervous system tumour mortality in different birth cohorts. In men and women born at the beginning of the twentieth century or earlier, rates in the elderly

---

[96] But double-coded data indicate only a 1% reduction from the change in interpretation of ICD coding rule 3 (see p. 12).

[97] This may have reflected an element of chance in addition to the coding changes: eye cancer rates fluctuate considerably from year to year because of small numbers.

[98] The Figures presented include benign tumours and those of unspecified or uncertain behaviour, as well as malignancies of the nervous system—see the Comment for the rationale for this.

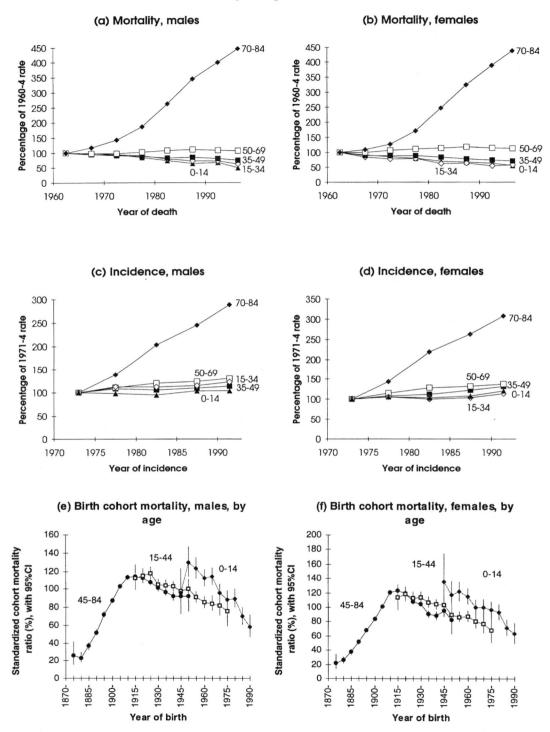

Figure 6.29   Tumours of nervous system (benign and malignant) (ICD7 193.0–.2, .8, .9, 223, 237; ICD8 191, 192.0–.3, 192.9, 225.0–.4, 225.9, 238.1–.5, 238.9; ICD9 191, 192, 225, 237.5–.6, 237.9, 239.6), mortality 1960–97, incidence 1971–92.

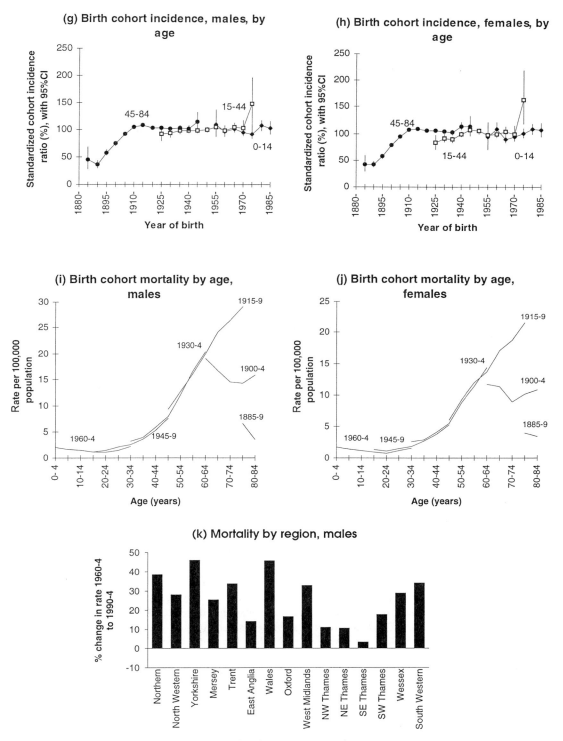

Figure 6.29 Tumours of nervous system (benign and malignant) (continued).

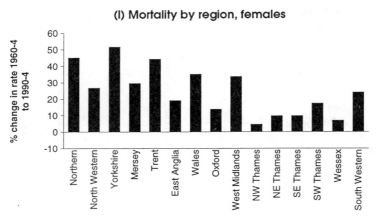

Figure 6.29 Tumours of nervous system (benign and malignant) (continued).

decreased or were approximately unchanged with age, whereas in subsequent cohorts rates have increased steeply with age, as in most other cancers.

Mortality trends by region

Regional trends in nervous system tumours varied from virtually no change to an increase of just over 50%. Rates tended to rise more in absolute terms where they were initially lower (*p*<0.001 in each sex for linear correlation), and there is now only a small variation in rates across the country.

Comment

Nervous system tumours occur mainly in the brain, but the category analysed in Figure 6.29 also includes tumours of the meninges, cranial nerves, and spinal cord (although not tumours of the peripheral, sympathetic, and parasympathetic nerves and ganglia). We have included in the analyses benign tumours of the nervous system and those of unspecified or uncertain behaviour, as well as nervous system tumours specified as malignant, because there is clinical and certification potential for artefact in statistics for these categories separately. The malignant and benign tumours often cannot be distinguished when the diagnosis is made without biopsy; such diagnosis is facilitated by modern imaging techniques. Autopsy leads to re-allocation to the malignant category of many brain and nervous system tumours diagnosed clinically as benign or of unspecified nature (Heasman and Lipworth 1966), so that falling non-coroner's autopsy rates (Figure 4.1) may have diminished apparent rates of malignancy

while having less if any effect on rates of nervous system tumours overall. 'Medical enquiries' by the Registrar General to certifiers have tended to increase the numbers of nervous system tumours recorded as malignant and decrease the numbers recorded as of unspecified nature (Swerdlow 1989), and hence discontinuation of medical enquiries for ages 75 and over in 1984 and for all other ages in 1993 will also have affected apparent rates of nervous system malignancy more than rates of nervous system tumours in total.

Large increases in incidence and mortality rates from nervous system cancers at older ages have been recorded in many countries (Ahlbom 1990; Muir *et al*. 1994). As in England and Wales, it remains uncertain whether these increases are entirely artefactual or in part real. More complete diagnosis, including the introduction of computed tomography (CT) scanning in the 1970s and magnetic resonance imaging (MRI) in the 1980s are likely to account for a substantial part of the increase. This is particularly the case at older ages, because previous diagnostic techniques had high morbidity in the elderly and therefore were likely to be avoided (Greig *et al*. 1990). There is evidence from Norway that the effect of CT was to increase diagnosis rates largely at ages 60 years and above (Helseth *et al*. 1988). An analysis of case notes in Canada, however, suggested that CT and MRI could account for detection of about 20% extra cases both at ages under 65 and at older ages, and would explain only a minority of the rise in rates (Desmeules *et al*. 1992). Furthermore, the beginning of the upward trend in nervous system cancer rates in England and Wales considerably antedated the introduction of these technologies, confirming that they cannot alone explain the full increase.

The brain is a frequent site of metastasis of tumours originating elsewhere in the body. Changing precision of diagnosis therefore has potential to affect nervous system cancer trends artefactually, especially at older ages, by changing the extent to which tumours metastasizing to the brain are counted as if they had originated there. If there has been a reduced propensity to make diagnoses by biopsy, for instance because of greater use of non-invasive diagnostic technologies, this could have increased the numbers of secondary tumours in the brain misdiagnosed as primaries. The proportion of nervous system malignancies for which histological verification was available in cancer registrations at England and Wales registries[99] showed no consistent trend during 1970–90, however, although there were considerable variations within individual registries.

As autopsy can detect appreciable numbers of brain tumours undiagnosed in life (Muir *et al.* 1994), declining rates of non-coroner's autopsy (Figure 4.1) could have reduced detection of nervous system tumours, especially those that are non-fatal. In the large study of the diagnostic effects of autopsy conducted by Heasman and Lipworth (1966) in England and Wales in 1959, however, although autopsy greatly increased the number of diagnoses of malignant and benign nervous system tumours, this was almost exactly counterbalanced by a decrease in the number of diagnoses of nervous system tumours of unspecified nature, such that the number of nervous system tumours overall was virtually unaltered[100]. The changes in 1984 in the Registrar General's interpretation of ICD coding rule 3 (see p. 12) increased recorded nervous system tumour mortality by about 4% (based on data in OPCS (1985)), and the reversal of this change in 1993 presumably caused a decrease of similar magnitude. No direct data are available on the effect of medical enquiries (and hence of their cessation in 1993, see p. 11) on nervous system tumour mortality rates, but the effect was probably mainly on whether or not these tumours were recorded as malignant rather than on the numbers of nervous system tumours overall (Swerdlow 1989)[101].

The very large changes between birth cohorts in the age distribution of nervous system tumours seen in Figures 6.29i and j would be difficult to explain as other than artefactual. In particular, it is likely that the apparently decreasing risk of these tumours with age beyond 65 years in the early cohorts is an artefact of underdiagnosis. In places such as Rochester, Minnesota where diagnostic standards and autopsy rates have been exceptionally high for many years, incidence rates have long been found to increase with age (Percy *et al.* 1972) as they do within recent cohorts in England and Wales. Similarly, the strong inverse correlation between the extent of increase in recorded mortality in different regions of England and Wales and their initial rates, is the pattern that might be expected if increases were due to rising completeness of diagnosis, for which there would be greater scope where rates were initially low.

If there is an element of the increasing rates that is real, the cause is not known, but either it has affected people aged 70 and above far more than those who are younger, or, more plausibly, it ceased to increase for those born since about 1919. Little is understood about the aetiology of nervous system tumours. A small proportion of cases are associated with neurofibromatosis and other phakomatoses, or are due to ionizing radiation exposure, but too few to explain the trends. There has been considerable public concern, although there is no consistent scientific evidence, that use of mobile telephones might cause brain tumours. As can be seen in Figure 5.33, use of mobile telephones has risen enormously in the last few years, while the trend in nervous system tumours in adults of working ages (the main users in those years) has not altered appreciably. If there is an effect of mobile telephone use on the incidence of brain tumours, however, it would have affected trends to date materially only if the induction period for malignancy was unusually short. The absence of any apparent effect at present does not therefore give strong evidence about the plausibility of a hypothesized aetiological relationship.

Several studies have found associations of brain cancer incidence with exposure to electromagnetic radiation fields (EMF). In children these have mainly related to residential exposure to electrical power lines and in adults mainly to occupation, but in neither instance are there well-confirmed relationships, and no relationship was observed in a national study of childhood cancer in the UK (UK Childhood Cancer Study Investigators 1999). Trends in general population

---

[99] Examining data from *Cancer Incidence in Five Continents* (not shown), in a similar fashion to Table 4.2.

[100] No data are available on time trends in the proportion of deaths in England and Wales from nervous system tumours that have been certified after autopsy.

[101] Examination of secular trends around 1993 by single calendar year suggests that the overall effect of the rule 3 and medical enquiry changes in that year was slight, if any.

exposures to power-frequency magnetic fields (Figure 5.35), showed no resemblance to those for brain tumours in children or adults, except to some extent in adults aged 70–84 and above, for whom the artefactual factors discussed above are more likely than EMF exposure to explain the increase.

Mortality rates from nervous system tumours in children and in adults under age 35 years decreased substantially while incidence rates were unchanged or rising, and there were lesser discrepancies between incidence and mortality rates at ages 35–69 although none at older ages. The childhood divergence would accord with the improvement in survival in children shown in Figure B6, but the adult data do not accord with the lack of improvement in survival for all-ages in data for East Anglia in Figure A21. Data for East Anglia by age (not presented) showed an inconsistent picture—there was an improvement in survival in young men, but not in men aged 50 and above or in women of any adult age.

Cancer of the thyroid (Figure 6.30)

Secular trends

Mortality from thyroid cancer has decreased greatly since 1960–4, especially in women and at younger ages. In women at each age group and in men aged under 50 years, rates are now about a half or less of those in 1960–4.

Figures 6.30k and l show mortality rates since 1931–5, the first years for which data are available. With the exception of the period from 1931–5 to 1936–40, when trends were erratic, the data show that the downward trend in young women has occurred virtually throughout the period of data available, but in older women the decrease started later, and indeed at ages 70 and above rates increased to a peak in about 1960 before falling. In men, aside from erratic trends in the 1930s, rates at almost all ages decreased only after about 1960 or later, and as in women the initial trend at ages 70 and above was upward.

By contrast, incidence rates of thyroid cancer have risen considerably since 1971–4 at ages under 50, and to a lesser extent at ages 50–69, while changing little or decreasing at older ages.

Trends by birth cohort

We examined risks by birth cohort separately at ages 15–44 and 45–84. Mortality in the older age-group has decreased almost throughout the span of cohorts studied, and the rates in women at younger ages have also generally decreased; in young men numbers of deaths have been small and rates inconsistent[102].

Incidence in men aged 45–84 has not changed greatly between cohorts. In women aged 45–84, there was somewhat of a diminution in rates in cohorts born until early in the twentieth century, and a marked increase in cohorts born since 1930. In younger adults of each sex, there were considerable increases through the span of cohorts for which data were available.

Examination of incidence trends at young ages since 1940 by single year of birth (Figures 6.30i and j) did not show any major deviations from the general trend in particular birth years, and there were no large peaks consistent between the sexes; the closest to such a peak was in the 1952 cohort, for which the SCIR in males was 147 (95% CI 110–193) and in females 118 (99–139).

Mortality trends by region

For men, there were decreases in all regions, the extent varying considerably based on small numbers. In women, there have been substantial decreases in all regions, with no geographical pattern.

Comment

The best-established cause of thyroid cancer is ionizing radiation; in children the thyroid is a particularly sensitive site. Birth cohort analyses in the US have shown increasing incidence for cohorts born from 1920–50 (and a subsequent decrease) which may have been related to the widespread use of radiation therapy for benign head and neck conditions, including supposedly dangerously large thymus glands at birth, from 1920 up to the late 1950s (Pottern *et al.* 1980). In England and Wales there have been substantial increases in thyroid cancer incidence in cohorts born since the late 1920s (except in older men), which continued in cohorts born after 1950. Radiation therapy for benign conditions of the head and neck had not commonly

---

[102] As a consequence of instability of small numbers, the data for thyroid cancer are displayed for a considerably lesser span of cohorts for men than for women.

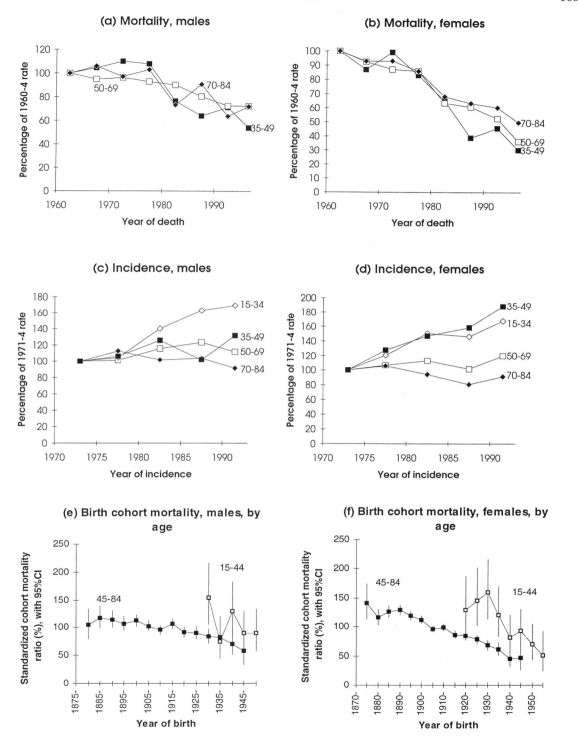

Figure 6.30 Cancer of thyroid (ICD7 194; ICD8&9 193) (a), (b), (e), (f) mortality 1960–97; (c), (d), (g)–(j) incidence 1971–92; (k), (l) mortality 1931–97; (m), (n) mortality 1960–4 to 1990–4.

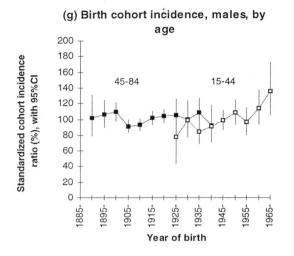

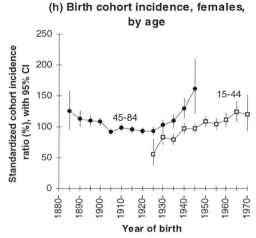

(i) Incidence by single year of birth, males, ages 0-44

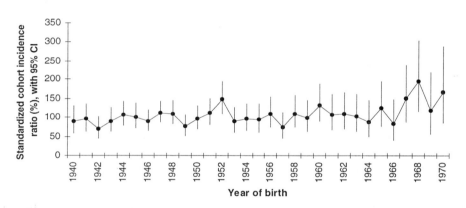

(j) Incidence by single year of birth, females, ages 0-44

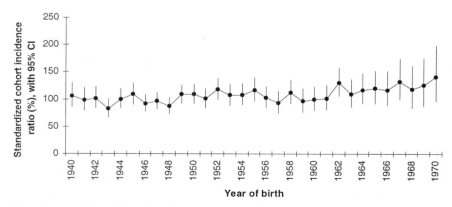

Figure 6.30   Cancer of thyroid (continued).

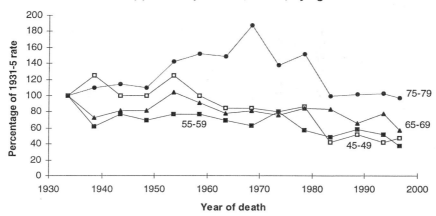

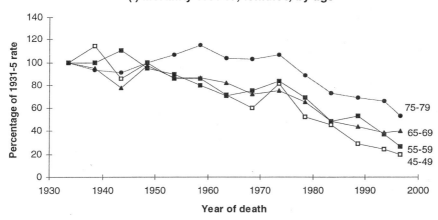

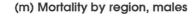

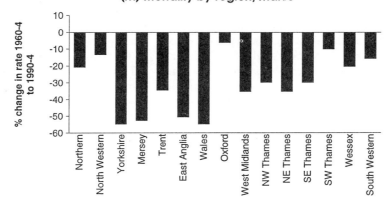

Figure 6.30 Cancer of thyroid (continued).

(n) Mortality by region, females

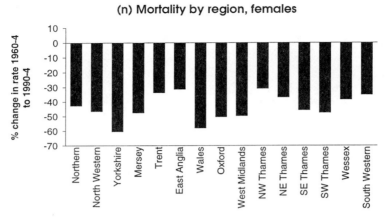

Figure 6.30   Cancer of thyroid (continued).

been used: in 1957, less than 2 children per 10 000 per year received radiation therapy for benign conditions of the head and neck, mainly for skin disorders and rarely (less than 2 per million per year) for glandular enlargements (Ministry of Health and Scottish Home and Health Department 1966). The only radiological procedure to the head and neck whose frequency increased greatly in Britain between surveys in the 1950s and 1970s was dental X-ray[103]; this examination was most often performed on older children and young adults (Kendall *et al.* 1980).

In Norway, raised incidence rates of thyroid cancer occurred in 1965–84, particularly 1975–9, which the authors considered might have been related to fallout radiation with a 15–25 year induction period (Akslen *et al.* 1993). In the data for England and Wales, however, there was no evidence of such a secular pattern, and no raised risk of thyroid cancer in the cohorts exposed to the greatest levels of fallout radiation, and specifically of I^{131} in milk, in infancy (Figure 5.28)[104]. In general, thyroid cancer incidence increased in cohorts born since the Second World War, including those born after 1962 when I^{131} from fallout had declined to relatively low levels. Studies of thyroid cancer incidence after childhood irradiation, however, have found that the relative risk rises for more than 15

(Ron *et al.* 1995) or 20 (Tucker *et al.* 1991) years after first exposure, and remains raised for 40 or more years (Ron *et al.* 1995), so that the years for which thyroid cancer incidence data for England and Wales are currently available are not all of those that could potentially be affected by fallout in the early 1960s.

Associations of thyroid cancer risk have been found with prior benign thyroid disease, although the possible aetiological effects of different specific diseases remain uncertain, and there has been inconsistent evidence for an association with endemic goitre and iodine deficiency. In Zurich, Switzerland, thyroid cancer mortality appears to have decreased as iodine supplementation was introduced (Wynder 1952), but this did not occur in the US (Pendergrast *et al.* 1961). Iodized salt has not been introduced in the UK[105], but average per caput intake of iodine is estimated to have increased from 80 μg per day in the 1940s to about 250 μg per day in the late 1970s (Wenlock *et al.* 1982), while trends in thyroid cancer mortality were complex, and although generally downward, not uniformly so.

There has been some evidence for an association of thyroid cancer in women with high parity, a history of miscarriage and, in some studies, with use of oral contraceptives. The trends in parity by birth cohort in

---

[103] Dental examinations outside NHS hospitals, which are over 95% of all dental X-rays, increased from 40 per thousand population in 1957 to 212 per thousand in 1977 (Kendall *et al.* 1980).

[104] The dose to the thyroid of infants from the tests in 1961 and 1962 is estimated to have been about 0.1 rad (0.001 Gy) (Medical Research Council 1966). Whether such a low dose is carcinogenic is unknown: raised risk has been demonstrated from doses down to 0.1 Gy, a lower dose than has been shown for any other organ (Ron *et al.* 1995), and raised incidence of thyroid cancer has been observed after fallout exposure at Rongelap Island (Conard *et al.* 1970) at much higher radiation levels than occurred in the UK.

[105] Only 2.5% of table salt was iodized in the early 1980s (Wenlock *et al.* 1982).

Figure 5.40, however, were not like those for thyroid cancer in women. We have no data on trends in miscarriage rates. The great increase in use of oral contraceptives between cohorts born in the 1920s and those born in the 1950s (Figure 5.32) was paralleled by an increase in thyroid cancer incidence in women at both ages 15–44 years and older ages. Furthermore, these were cohorts for which cohort trends in men were less upward than in women at ages 15–44, and not upward at all at older ages. There was a further increase in thyroid cancer incidence in subsequent cohorts of women, whose prevalence of ever-use of the pill cannot have been much above that of the generation born in the 1950s although their mean duration of use, on which we have no data, might have increased (see p. 47). Incidence increased also in the contemporary cohorts of men, however, and the sex ratio did not alter substantially.

Clinical diagnosis of thyroid malignancy as the cause of death is usually fairly straightforward, and changes in this are unlikely to have affected trends greatly, even in the early data (Campbell *et al.* 1963). Occult cancers of the thyroid have been detected with high prevalence at autopsy in some but not all studies (Ron 1996), so that there is potential for thyroid cancer registration trends to have been affected by the diminishing frequency of non-coroner's autopsy in recent decades (Figure 4.1)[106]. Use of more sophisticated diagnostic methods, such as fine-needle biopsy and radioisotope scanning, might have led to greater diagnosis of occult cancers ante-mortem. The pattern of increase in incidence, greatest at younger ages, however, is not that which has occurred for other cancers where diagnostic improvements are believed to have resulted in increasing registration rates, and occult carcinomas of the thyroid do not appear to be more common at younger ages (Fukunaga and Yatani 1975; Harach *et al.* 1985; Franssila and Harach 1986).

There is a particularly large divergence between incidence and mortality trends for thyroid cancer at young ages, and a lesser but still substantial divergence at older ages. There is a large variation by age in the ratio of incidence to mortality—at ages 15–34, the incidence rate in males was about 10 times or more the mortality rate, and in females about 30 times or more, whereas at ages 70–84 incidence was less than twice the contemporary mortality rate in each sex. Correspondingly,

the survival data for East Anglia (Figure A.22)[107] showed large improvements in survival from this tumour, and high current survival rates, especially at young ages (not in Figure): at ages 15–49 years, 5-year survival in males improved from 75% for cases incident in 1971–6 to 87% for those incident in 1987–92, and in females there was an improvement from 87% to 97%.

Hodgkin's disease (Figure 6.31)

Secular trends

Mortality from Hodgkin's disease has decreased by over two-thirds in each sex and age group since the late 1960s. The decrease has been particularly great in children, in whom there is now only about 1 death per year nationally compared with an average of 16 per year in the 1960s.

Incidence at ages 50 years and above has decreased by over 40% in each sex, while at younger ages there were modest decreases or increases. As Figures 6.31i and j show, in 1971–4 Hodgkin's disease incidence showed two clear age peaks, one in young adults and one in persons aged in their 60s and 70s, whereas by the early 1990s the peak in young adults remained (indeed in women had become more pronounced), but the peak at older ages had diminished in women and almost disappeared in men. Taking advantage of the entire data set to study the difference between the sexes in more detail, Figure 6.31k shows the distribution of incidence by single year of age. A male excess can be seen in children and in adults aged 20 years and upwards, but the difference between the sexes virtually disappeared at ages 15–19 years. Rates in the two sexes ran approximately in parallel from ages 25 to 70 years.

Trends by birth cohort

We analysed rates by cohort in three age-groups: 0–14, 15–44, and 45–84. Mortality at each age-group in each sex decreased across more or less the entire span of cohorts for whom data were available. (The rates in children are not presented in the Figures because they are based on small numbers, but can be found in Appendix C, Table 28.)

---

[106] No data are available on time trends in the proportion of deaths from thyroid cancer in England and Wales that were certified after autopsy.
[107] Survival data were not published for England and Wales.

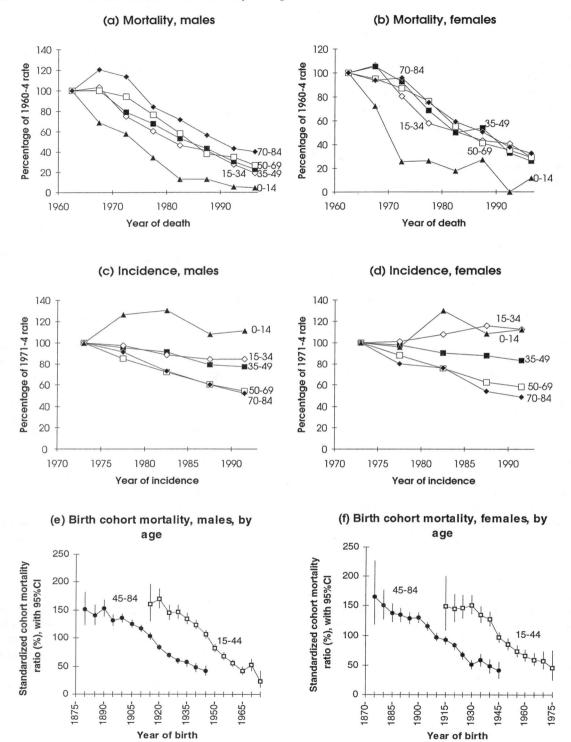

Figure 6.31 Hodgkin's disease (ICD7–9 201), mortality 1960–97, incidence 1971–92.

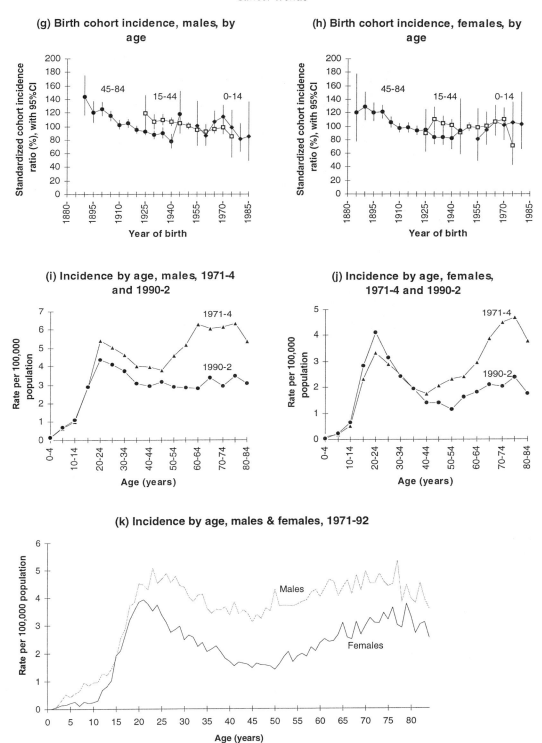

Figure 6.31 Hodgkin's disease (continued).

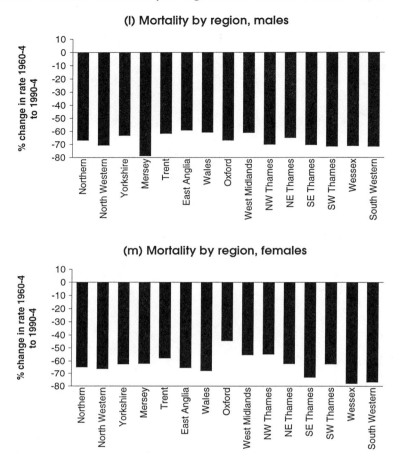

Figure 6.31 Hodgkin's disease (continued).

Incidence at ages 45–84 decreased substantially from cohorts born in 1890–4 to those born in 1940–4, but in each sex increased in the last cohort for whom substantial data were available, namely that born in 1945–9. In young adults, rates in males decreased between successive cohorts, while in females there was no consistent change. In children, based on relatively small numbers, trends were irregular.

Mortality trends by region

There were large, fairly similar, decreases in Hodgkin's disease mortality in all regions in each sex.

Comment

Hodgkin's disease was first described in 1832 by Thomas Hodgkin, the 'Inspector of the Dead' at Guy's Hospital, London. The large decrease in Hodgkin's disease mortality, while incidence has not decreased comparably, has been one of the great successes of modern oncology. Since the late 1960s, intensive radiotherapy and chemotherapy have dramatically improved the prognosis of this tumour (Figures A23, B7), although much more at young than at older ages[108].

The decreasing incidence rates of Hodgkin's disease at most ages may be in part artefactual, but there may also have been real changes in incidence. Pathological

---

[108] 5-year survival in East Anglia (data were not available for England and Wales overall) improved from 67% to 86% in men and 64% to 88% in women aged 15–49, but only from 34% to 44% in men and 28% to 36% in women aged 50–84. This corresponds well with the greater divergence of incidence and mortality trends at young than at older ages.

reclassification of certain histological types of Hodgkin's disease as non-Hodgkin's lymphoma (Banks 1992) may have influenced Hodgkin's disease rates downward, as would any deterioration in specificity of reporting of the histology of lymphomas, because lymphomas not further specified are coded in the ICD to a rubric within non-Hodgkin's lymphoma. Another potential source of artefactual decrease in rates of Hodgkin's disease, primarily at older ages, would have occurred if the frequency of erroneous pathological diagnosis of Hodgkin's disease has diminished over time. This has been shown in the United States (Glaser and Swartz 1990), where the proportion of histological Hodgkin's disease diagnoses in routine practice that were erroneous on expert review was found to diminish from 1969–74 to 1980–4, especially at older ages. Similarly in Uppsala, Sweden (Martinsson *et al.* 1992), a review of the pathology of cases of Hodgkin's disease recorded in the cancer registry found that erroneous diagnoses (mainly of cases of NHL, and mainly at older ages) had diminished during 1969–87. Decreasing rates of non-coroner's autopsy over time (Figure 4.1) could also have led to a reduction in recorded Hodgkin's disease at older ages: in a Danish study, a substantial proportion of cases of Hodgkin's disease at older ages, but not at younger, were diagnosed only at post-mortem (Hasle and Mellemgaard 1993). (There are no data available on trends in the proportion of deaths from Hodgkin's disease in England and Wales certified after post-mortem.)

Recorded mortality from Hodgkin's disease was artefactually increased by 6% in 1984 when the Registrar General's interpretation of ICD coding rule 3 was altered (see p. 12), and presumably decreased by a similar amount in 1993 when there was reversion to the previous coding scheme. The exact effect of medical enquiries to certifiers (see p. 11), and hence presumptively of the cessation of these enquiries in 1993, has not been published, but in 1986 it was less than ±5% (Swerdlow 1989). Examination of mortality rates by single calendar year suggests that a several per cent artefactual decrease occurred in 1993, but with uncertainty about its magnitude because there are appreciable year-to-year variations in rates and there has been a background secular decline.

The epidemiology of Hodgkin's disease in children, young adults, and older adults, differs, and there may

well be differences in aetiology between these ages (MacMahon 1966; Correa and O'Conor 1971). It has been speculated that the young adult peak of the disease relates to late infection with a common (unknown) infectious agent, which rarely causes Hodgkin's disease, but is more likely to do so if infection is delayed to adolescence or young adulthood (Gutensohn and Cole 1977). Delay in this infection, it is suggested, would occur more often in prosperous societies, while childhood infection would be more common in less prosperous societies. This would parallel the epidemiology of paralytic polio in the pre-vaccine era (Gutensohn and Cole 1977), for which incidence in childhood was greater in poorer people, but risk in young adulthood was greater in prosperous circumstances, where infection was more often delayed. On this model, one would expect that with increasing prosperity, rates of Hodgkin's disease would decrease in children and rise in young adults (Correa and O'Conor 1971). Reliable incidence data for young adults are not available before 1971, but since then incidence at the young adult peak has decreased a little in males and increased in females, while rates in children have been inconsistent but not downward. To gain further information on the latter point from a more complete source of childhood cancer data than the national cancer registry files and over a longer period, we have also examined published data from the Childhood Cancer Research Group (see p. 10): these show rates in boys rising from 4.9 per million in 1962–70 to 5.6 in 1971–80 and 6.2 in 1981–90, while rates in girls have risen over the same period from 2.0 to 2.4 to 2.9 per million[109].

The polio analogy would lead one to expect Hodgkin's disease risk in children to be reduced, and in young adults to be increased, by factors that decrease the chance of early infection, such as reductions in overcrowding and in sibship size. Raised risk in young adults has indeed been shown in relation to these factors (Gutensohn and Cole 1981; Mueller and Grufferman 1999). In the more limited data available for children, risk was decreased in those with fewer sibs (Westergaard *et al.* 1997). In England and Wales, household crowding has diminished steadily for at least the last 70 years (Table 5.17). Direct data on sibship size are not available, but mean birth order (i.e. sibship size at the time of birth) (Figure 5.10) dipped for the

---

[109] 1962–70 rates calculated from data in Draper *et al.* (1982); 1971–80 rates from Draper *et al.* (1988); 1981–90 rates from Stiller *et al.* (1998). All rates age-standardized to the 'World Standard' population. 1962–70 data for Britain and subsequent data for England and Wales, but the difference probably had a negligible effect because the population of England and Wales constituted 91% of the British total.

cohorts born during the Second World War and declined between those born in the mid-1960s and mid-1970s, and data on completed family size of mothers (Figure 5.40) imply that sibship size rose to a peak for children born around 1960 and then declined. Neither the over-crowding nor the sibship size trends match the trends in Hodgkin's disease incidence in Figure 6.31 or in the Childhood Cancer Research Group data above—for instance, childhood Hodgkin's disease incidence has risen as overcrowding has decreased and sibship size has been static or declining.

It has been hypothesized that increasing parity may be protective against Hodgkin's disease in young adult women (Glaser 1994), and evidence from a large cohort study supports this (Kravdal and Hansen 1993). The age-incidence distributions in Figure 6.31k, however, unlike those in the US (Glaser 1994; Mueller and Grufferman 1999), do not show different shapes for males and females beyond age 25 years, but instead approximately parallel curves[110]. Additionally, the trend in parity by birth cohort in Figure 5.40 showed little resemblance to that for Hodgkin's disease in women in the corresponding cohorts, and examination of the sex ratio of Hodgkin's disease incidence by birth cohort (not shown) did not indicate proportionately fewer female cases in middle age in the cohorts born in the 1930s who had the greatest mean parity.

The prime candidate for the infection causing Hodgkin's disease has been the Epstein–Barr virus (EBV). Several cohort studies have shown a raised risk, of around three, of Hodgkin's disease in persons who have had infectious mononucleosis, the symptomatic form of EBV infection. Evidence of EBV genome has been found in the malignant cells in about a third to a half of cases of Hodgkin's disease, and in cohort studies there has been serological evidence indicating prior EBV activation (Mueller and Grufferman 1999). EBV infection generally occurs early in childhood in less 'developed' societies (and in lower social classes in 'developed' countries), and is more often delayed to the late teens or older in devel-oped countries and higher social classes (Straus and Fleisher 1990). One might therefore expect, although there do not appear to be direct data to examine this, that late seroconversion has become more common over time in England and Wales. There is evidence, however,

that the incidence of infectious mononucleosis[111] increased in Western countries between about 1940 and 1970 (Straus and Fleisher 1990). The Hodgkin's disease incidence data we examined were for years after 1970, but did not show substantial increases in incidence at young adult ages for the cohorts born from the 1920s to 1950s, who would have reached ages 15–19 years[112] during 1940–70.

The almost identical rates of Hodgkin's disease in the two sexes from ages 15–19 but not surrounding ages is a notable epidemiological feature. A similar pattern is seen at ages 15–19 in 5-year age-group data for Hodgkin's disease in the US, although extending there to a wider childhood and young adult age range (Glaser 1994). Data are not available to test whether this has parallels with sex differences in age-specific rates of EBV seroconversion and infectious mononucleosis.

Non-Hodgkin's lymphoma (NHL)
(Figure 6.32)

Secular trends

Since 1960–4, NHL mortality in each sex has more than tripled at ages 70–84, more than doubled at ages 50–69, and increased by about a half at ages 35–49. At ages 15–34, however, there has been no change in women and a modest decrease in men, and in children of each sex there has been a large decline. At most age groups, including 70–84, there is evidence of a stabilization in recent years.

Incidence data also show rising NHL rates in each sex, with the greatest rises at oldest ages. Unlike the mortality data, however, the increases in incidence extend even to the youngest adult age-group, and in males to children[113], and there has been no stabiliza-tion of rates in recent years, although the data available are for years before those for which mortality has stabilized.

Examining the age distribution of incidence at young ages, using the entire period of data available to give stability of large numbers, shows an unusual pattern compared with other cancers (Figure 6.32e). Rates

---

[110] Of course, this implies greater male to female *ratios* at adult ages when absolute rates are lowest (i.e. in persons aged in their 40s), which could be taken as weak support for a role of female reproductive factors.
[111] Which usually occurs late (in young adulthood).
[112] That is, the ages when late seroconversion usually occurs.
[113] In girls the trend was inconsistent.

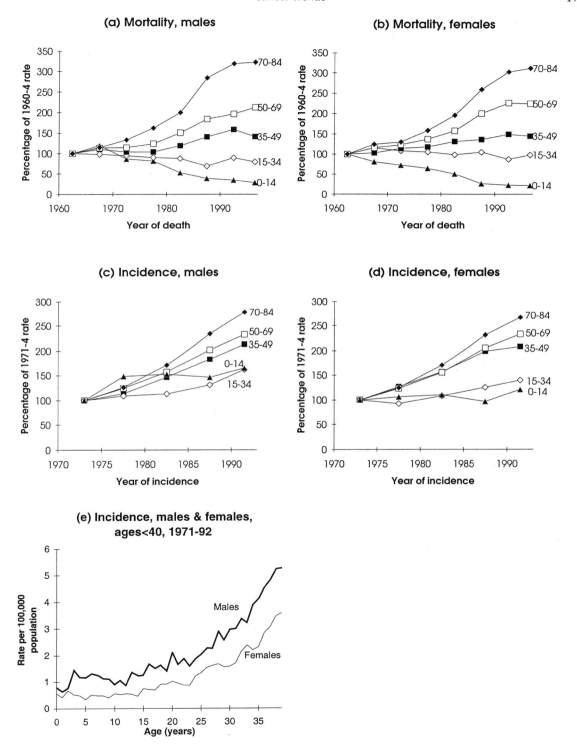

Figure 6.32   Non-Hodgkin's lymphoma (ICD7 200, 202, 205; ICD8&9 200, 202), mortality 1960–97, incidence 1971–92.

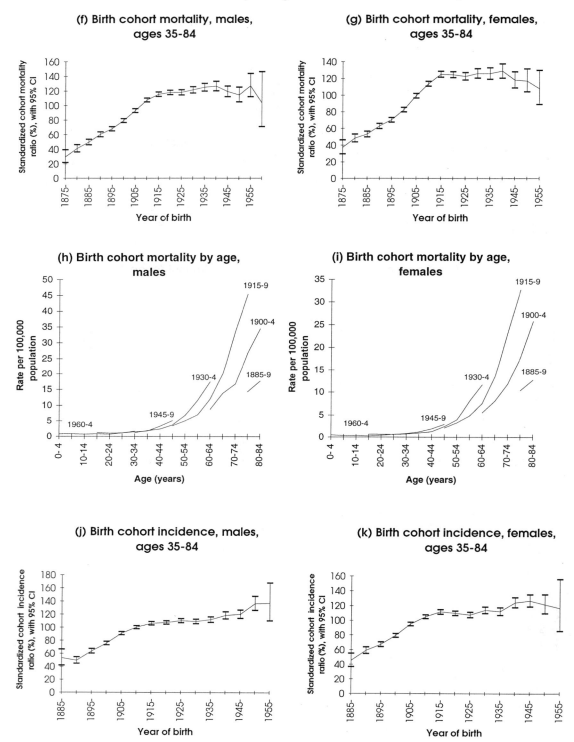

Figure 6.32   Non-Hodgkin's lymphoma (continued).

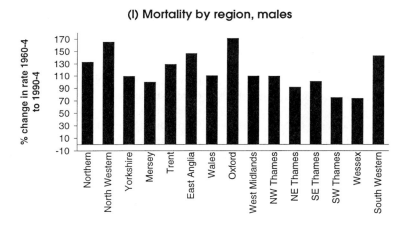

(l) Mortality by region, males

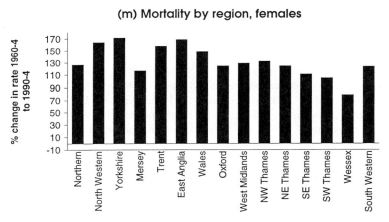

(m) Mortality by region, females

Figure 6.32 Non-Hodgkin's lymphoma (continued).

were fairly constant across childhood ages, and then increased smoothly and about exponentially from approximately age 15 years onwards. Unlike most other tumours, there was neither a peak nor a virtual absence of cases in childhood. (This may be an artefact due to a proportion of cases, decreasing with age, being misdiagnosed cases of acute lymphoblastic leukaemia, which at very young ages are distinguished from NHL only arbitrarily.) At each age there was a male excess, as there is for acute lymphoblastic leukaemia.

Trends by birth cohort

The increasing mortality from NHL occurred almost entirely in cohorts born before 1920. There was then little change until a decline in women, and less con-

sistently in men, beginning with the cohort born in 1945–9. Incidence data showed a similar increase followed by a period of stability, but differed by showing a small increase rather than a decrease in cohorts born after 1939.

Unlike the pattern for nervous system tumours (Figures 6.29i and j), the large secular increase in mortality from NHL has not been accompanied by any substantial change in the age distribution of the tumour within birth cohorts (Figures 6.32h and i).

Mortality trends by region

There were increases of over 70% in NHL mortality in each sex in each region, with no obvious geographical pattern.

Comment

Several subclassifications of NHL have been proposed, on histological, immunological, and clinical grounds, and it is unknown whether the subgroups differ aetiologically; the data available for England and Wales, however, do not allow reliable examination of trends in these groups.

The percentage increase in incidence of NHL over the study period (1971–92) is the second largest (after pleura) for any site analysed in this book for women, and the third largest (after pleura and melanoma) for men. The large increases in NHL rates in England and Wales parallel similar increases in many other countries around the world over several decades (Stalsberg 1973; Devesa and Fears 1992). The main cause of this rising trend in England and Wales, as elsewhere, is unknown, although several factors affecting the rate can be identified.

Risk of NHL is raised in persons with immunodeficiency, whether congenital, acquired, or therapeutic. A small part of the increase in NHL over time arises from the increasing frequency of lymphoid neoplasms (mainly EBV-associated) arising after organ and bone marrow transplantation and of AIDS-associated lymphomas. Organ transplantation in the UK started in the early 1960s, increased until 1990 and then approximately stabilized (see p. 48 and Figure 5.34). The number of deaths from transplant-related lymphoma (Figure 6.37) was less than 25 per year in the earliest data available (1984–6), and has since diminished. Even if incidence was a few times greater than this, the impact on all-age general population rates of NHL will have been slight (there have been over 5000 cases of NHL incident in England and Wales per annum in recent years). In children, however, for whom the risk of post-transplant lymphoid neoplasia is much greater than in adults, and in whom the background incidence of NHL is comparatively low (under 100 cases per year), the impact will have been more noticeable. The number of childhood transplants rose up to 1993 (Figure 5.34b), and there are now about 10 cases of lymphoproliferative disease per annum in childhood transplant patients in England and Wales (A. Thomas, personal communication), i.e. 10% or more of the national total.

Unlike in the US, where AIDS led to a large increase in NHL incidence in men aged 25–44, and to a lesser extent aged 45–54, in the 1980s, and to an obviously different trend for young men than for men of other ages and for women (Devesa and Fears 1992), in England and Wales there was no major deviation from prevailing trends in young men in this period. (The most that can be said is that the increase in incidence in recent years has been somewhat steeper in young men than young women.) The AIDS epidemic in England and Wales reached a peak in men in 1994 (Figure 5.1), when 1502 incident cases were recorded. The number of cases of lymphoma in the country occurring as an initial AIDS-defining illness reached a peak in young men in 1992, when there were 23 cases at ages 15–34 and 33 cases at ages 35–49 (see p. 195). Lymphomas usually occur late in the course of AIDS, however, rather than being present at its diagnosis, and there is no national reporting system for later-presenting lymphomas in AIDS patients. Estimation of the numbers of these later-presenting lymphomas is complex, depending on the pattern of AIDS incidence in previous years, AIDS survival rates, and lymphoma incidence rates in survivors of different durations. Estimates for the US in the early 1990s suggest that total lymphoma incidence in young men with AIDS was about 3 to 5.5 times the number of initial, AIDS-defining cases (Gail *et al.* 1991). If this applied approximately in England and Wales[114] then the total number of AIDS-related lymphomas incident in 1990–2 in men in England and Wales would have been about 55 to 101 per annum at ages 15–34, and 67 to 123 per annum at ages 35–49. This compares with a total NHL incidence of 236 cases per annum at ages 15–34 and 497 cases per annum at ages 35–49 in the country at that time. Thus AIDS might then have been responsible for between a quarter and almost a half of cases in men aged 15–34 and up to a quarter of cases at ages 35–49. It is notable, however, that the rise in NHL incidence in young men in cancer registration data does not appear to have accelerated commensurately with these estimates. It is possible that AIDS-related lymphomas have not been registered as completely as other lymphomas.

Raised risks of NHL are also seen in other patients receiving immunosuppressive drugs, persons with genetic immunodeficiency, and those with various medical conditions in which there is immune dysfunction, for instance patients on renal dialysis and those with

---

[114] Not all of the variables will have had exactly the same values as in the US, of course, but the percentage of AIDS patients presenting initially with lymphoma was not greatly different: 4.2% of men in the data for England and Wales in Figure 5.1 and p. 195 compared with 3.4% in men in the US (Gail *et al.* 1991).

coeliac disease. Again, however, these exposures probably account for a small fraction of cases and would not explain the rising rates in the population overall. Several other factors, including exposures to UV radiation, pesticides and phenoxyherbicides, have been suggested as possible reasons for the rising rates, but there is no strong evidence that they are aetiological.

Part of the increase may be artefactual. There have been changes in the categorization of lesions on the borderline between NHL and certain leukaemias, and a recategorization as malignant of certain uncommon lymphoid tumours previously considered benign (Banks 1992). If US experience is applicable, however, no more than 5% of lymphomas categorized as NHL now are entities that would not formerly have been included under NHL or Hodgkin's disease (Hartge and Devesa 1992). Certain histological subtypes of lymphoma that would previously have been categorized as Hodgkin's disease have been transferred to NHL in recent years (Banks 1992), and there may also have been a reduction over time, as has been found in reviews of US pathological diagnoses (Glaser and Swartz 1990) and Swedish cancer registry data (Martinsson *et al.* 1992), in the frequency with which NHL has been misdiagnosed as Hodgkin's disease. In the US, the percentage of Hodgkin's disease diagnoses that on review were deemed to be NHL diminished from 9.8% in 1969–74 to 4.0% in 1980–4 (Glaser and Swartz 1990). If this applied to the England and Wales data, 7% in males and 5% in females of the rise in NHL from 1971–4 to 1980–4 could be attributed to diminished misdiagnosis of NHL tumours as Hodgkin's disease[115].

Deterioration in specificity of reporting or coding of lymphomas could lead to artefactual increases in NHL because lymphomas not further specified, which could include cases that are actually Hodgkin's disease, are coded in the ICD to NHL. An element of the increase in NHL could be due to better diagnosis of tumours previously misdiagnosed as other types of cancer, or not diagnosed as cancer, or labelled as cancer of unknown primary site, although the increasing secular trend in rates of cancer of unknown primary site argues against the latter.

In the period since the early 1980s, part of the rise in NHL has probably been due to the increasing use of immunohistological techniques to examine specimens from malignancies of uncertain cell type, which can often prove to be lymphoma on such examination (Gatter *et al.* 1985).

There might also have been some artefactual increase from improved coding of lymphomas of extra-nodal sites such as the stomach, brain, and testis. If the histology was stated and the ICD was followed correctly, these tumours should have been coded to NHL, but if the histology was not stated, or if the ICD coding instructions were not adhered to, then they could have been coded to the extra-nodal sites. Whether this has affected trends in NHL materially is unclear, and it would anyway be insufficient to account for the scale of increase, because extra-nodal sites account for only about 20% of NHLs (Stalsberg 1973; Devesa and Fears 1992). A pathology review of cases of NHL in Yorkshire, England over a 20-year period[116] (Barnes *et al.* 1986) concluded that the increasing incidence rate could not be explained by changes in pathological criteria or completeness of registration or coding.

Exact information has not been published on the effect of 'medical enquiries' by the Registrar General to certifiers of death (see p. 11) on rates of NHL - mortality, but in 1986 it was under ±5% (Swerdlow 1989). The effect of changes in the Registrar General's interpretation of ICD coding rule 3 has been small (see p. 12 and Table 4.1) compared with the scale of trends in NHL mortality overall[117]. Changes in the extent to which NHL, when mentioned on death certificates, is deemed to be the underlying cause of death, may have added a few per cent to the NHL death rates, which are based on underlying cause (Grulich *et al.* 1995).

In summary, although diagnostic, certification and coding artefacts may have contributed to the increase in rates of NHL, they seem insufficient to account for the scale of the rise, much of which seems likely to have been real, mainly of unknown causation. The cohort trends imply, however, that the major causes ceased to rise steeply several decades ago.

---

[115] The effect may not have differed greatly by age, as the improvement appears to have been greater at older ages, when Hodgkin's disease is comparatively uncommon compared with NHL, and smaller at young ages, when Hodgkin's disease is more common compared with NHL.
[116] 1978–82 compared with 1963–7.
[117] Examination of mortality rates from NHL by single calendar year (not shown) also suggest that the effect of the rule 3 and medical enquiry changes in 1993 was comparatively slight.

The divergence between incidence and mortality trends in NHL at young ages, greatest in children but large also in adults under age 50, reflects the success of chemotherapy and radiotherapy. The lesser divergence at older ages, especially ages 70–84, is probably because these treatments cannot be used as aggressively (or successfully) at these ages. In accord with the incidence and mortality trends in children, a great improvement in childhood survival is seen in Figure B7. The all-age survival data in Figure A24, however, are less clearly in accord with the all-age divergence of incidence and mortality: in East Anglia there was a small improvement in survival in men and none in women, and in the data for England and Wales there was some improvement in each sex. Furthermore, survival data by adult age (not in Figure) do not clearly show greater improvements at young than at older ages in East Anglia, and generally show greater improvements at old than at younger ages in England and Wales.

Multiple myeloma (Figure 6.33)

Secular trends

At ages 50 and above there have been large increases in recorded mortality from myeloma. From 1960–4 to 1985–9 the death rates at ages 70–84 increased by three times or more, and at ages 50–69 there were increases of a half or more; in each instance, rates then stabilized or even slightly decreased in the 1990s. At ages 35–49, in women there was an increase followed by a decrease, while in men there was no clear trend until a recent decline. At age under 85 years in total, rates of myeloma more than doubled in men and doubled in women up to the late 1980s, but the increase then ceased abruptly, and in men there has been a decline.

Incidence of myeloma also increased greatly at ages 70–84 and to a lesser extent ages 50–69. There was in addition, however, an increase at ages 35–49. Since 1985–9 the all-age increase in incidence has halted in each sex.

Trends by birth cohort

The increase in mortality from myeloma occurred essentially in cohorts born before 1915. Thereafter, rates decreased slightly in cohorts of men born up to 1935–9, and were little changed in women born up to 1930–4, and then in each sex decreased markedly. As Figures 6.33i and j show, the large increase in myeloma mortality in early cohorts, unlike the increase for nervous system tumours (Figures 6.29i and j), occurred without any major change in the age distribution of the tumour within cohorts.

Incidence trends by birth cohort were fairly similar to those for mortality, except that the trend in recent cohorts was only slightly downward, with wide confidence intervals.

Mortality trends by region

Myeloma mortality rates increased substantially in all regions. The extent of increase tended to be greatest where rates were initially lowest[118], and the range of rates across the country has diminished.

Comment

Multiple myeloma is a malignancy of plasma cells, which originate, although perhaps not solely, from the bone marrow. The increase in myeloma rates and subsequent stabilization are not explicable by coding artefact, although for mortality data this did make a minor contribution. About a 5% increase in recent years may be attributable to changes in the position of recording of myeloma on death certificates, so that it was more likely to be coded as the underlying cause of death rather than a mentioned cause (Grulich *et al.* 1995). A 6% increase occurred in 1984 when the Registrar General's interpretation of ICD coding rule 3 altered[119] (see p. 12), and there was presumably a corresponding decrease in 1993 when the previous interpretation was reinstated. The exact effect of the discontinuation of medical enquiries to certifiers in 1993 (see p. 11) has not been published, but was probably less than ±5% (Swerdlow 1989). Inspection of mortality secular trends by single calendar year (not in Figure) did not show a step-change in rates in 1993, even at ages 70–84. Peak all-age rates in each sex were reached in 1989.

The trends in myeloma in England and Wales were similar to those in many Western countries, where large increases have been recorded at older ages, but

---

[118] The sex-specific inverse correlations between the absolute increase and the initial rate were borderline significant: $p = 0.04$ in males, $p = 0.05$ in females.
[119] Eight per cent at ages 75 years and above.

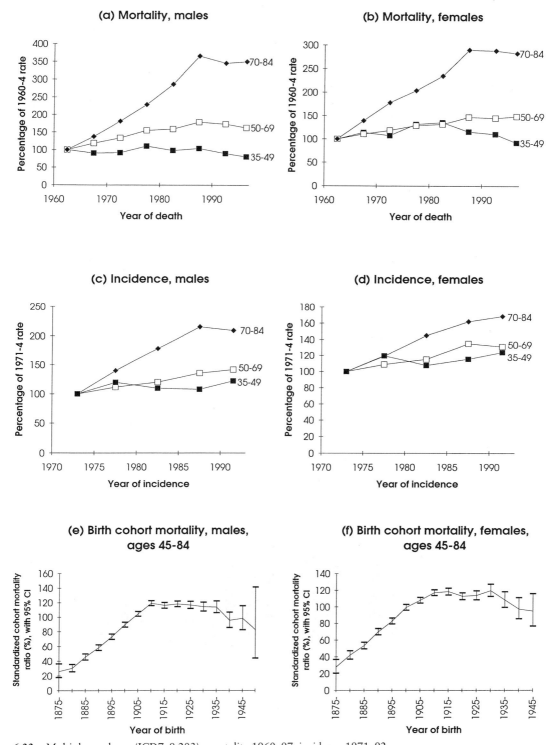

Figure 6.33 Multiple myeloma (ICD7–9 203), mortality 1960–97, incidence 1971–92.

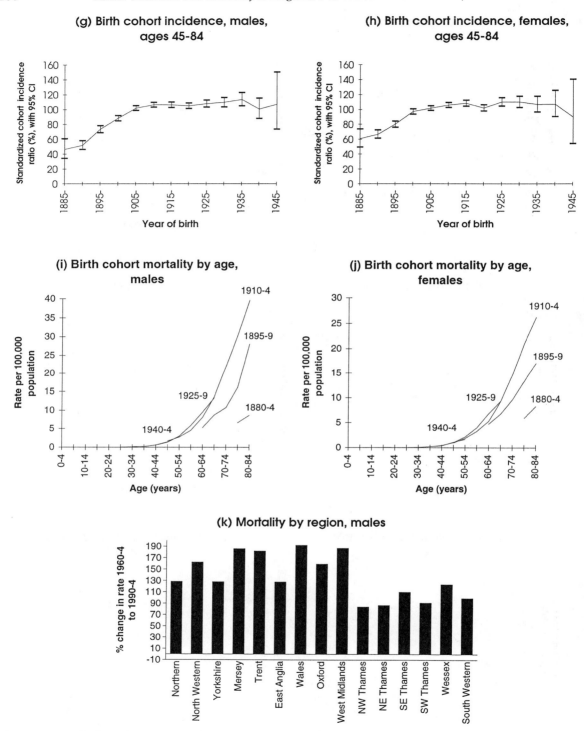

Figure 6.33   Multiple myeloma (continued).

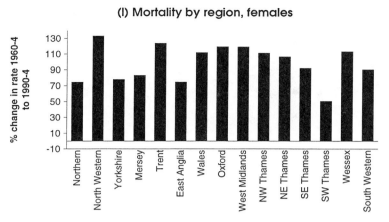

Figure 6.33 Multiple myeloma (continued).

stabilization or a decreasing trend at younger ages (Cuzick 1994). Internationally, the increases have usually been greatest where recorded rates were initially low, and have been less, or there has been no increase, where there was initially particularly good ascertainment (Linos *et al.* 1981; Turesson *et al.* 1984). Diagnosis of myeloma requires sophisticated laboratory tests, so that there is scope for improved diagnosis to have led to apparent increases in rates[120]. If better diagnosis has been the source of the increasing rates of myeloma it is plausible that rises should have been greatest in those places and at those (older) ages where there is likely to have been greatest scope for improvement. Conversely, there is no known cause of myeloma that could have accounted for the rising rates (although little is known of its aetiology). In several studies raised risk has been found in patients with rheumatoid arthritis, and there is an association with ionizing radiation exposure, but these would not explain the secular trends of myeloma. There has been limited support for an association of myeloma incidence with benzene and pesticide exposures.

Overall, therefore, it is likely that at least part, and perhaps almost all, of the increase has been artefactual. If there has been a real element, either the effect has been only in older persons, which seems unlikely, or, more plausibly, the increase has been cohort-based and the cessation of rise in rates for cohorts born since 1915 implies that the aetiological factor ceased to increase several decades ago.

The fairly similar trends for incidence and mortality from myeloma, slightly more upward for the former than the latter, accord well with the continuing poor, but slightly improving, survival from this tumour shown in Figure A25.

Leukaemia (Figure 6.34)

Secular trends

In children, leukaemia mortality has decreased by two-thirds since 1960–4, and at adult ages under 50 there has been a decrease of over a third. At ages 50–69, however, changes have been relatively small, although downward in the most recent years, and at ages 70–84 rates increased until the 1980s and have since decreased slightly.

Incidence rates in children and at adult ages under 70 have increased by 5–20%. At ages 70–84 there were increases of about a third, which levelled off in the most recent years.

Figure 6.34e shows in detail the age distribution of leukaemia incidence in children and young adults of each sex. The childhood peak of the disease was greater and occurred at a slightly older age in boys than in girls. At subsequent ages there was a modest male excess up to about age 50 years, and a widening gap between the sexes at older ages (not in Figure). There was a suggestion of a small peak of incidence, in

---

[120] Although several of these became established before or at the start of the study period—needle biopsy and serum electrophoresis in the 1950s and early 1960s (Velez *et al.* 1982).

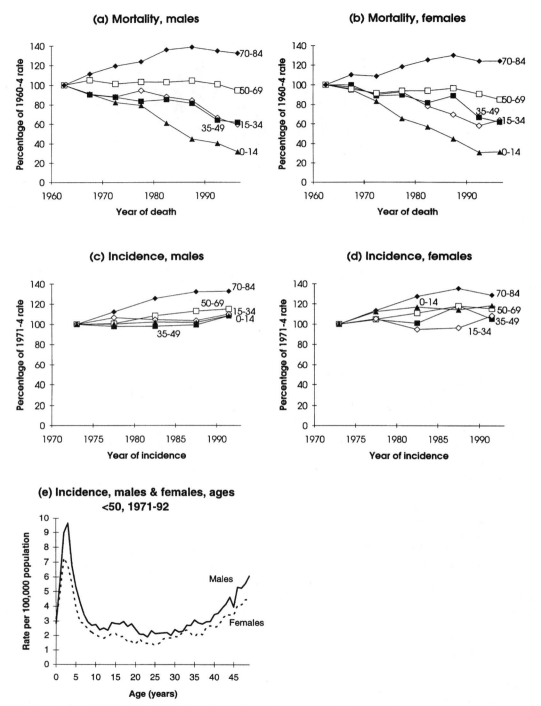

Figure 6.34   Leukaemia (ICD2 53A; ICD3 65a; ICD4 72a (1931-4), 72a, 72b(2) (1935-9); ICD5 74; ICD6&7 204; ICD8 204–7; ICD9 204–8); (a), (b) mortality 1960–97; (c)–(g) incidence 1971–92; (h)–(j) mortality 1911–97; (k), (l) mortality 1911–54, incidence 1971–92; (m)–(t) mortality 1945–57, 1968–97, incidence 1971–92; (u), (v) mortality 1960–4 to 1990–4.

(f) Incidence by single year of birth, males, ages 0-14

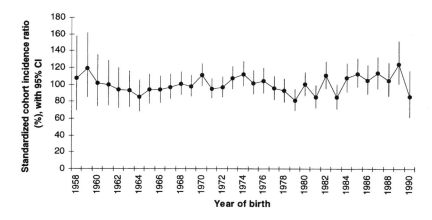

(g) Incidence by single year of birth, females, ages 0-14

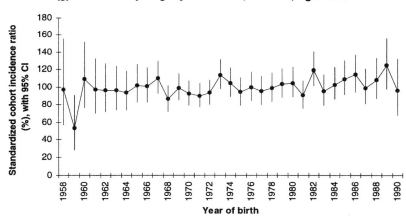

(h) Mortality 1911-97, ages 0-4, by sex

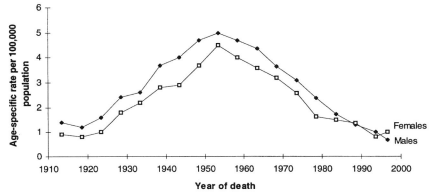

Figure 6.34 Leukaemia (continued).

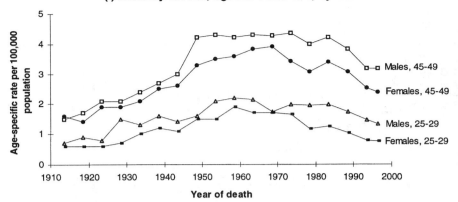

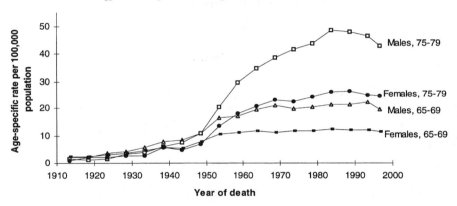

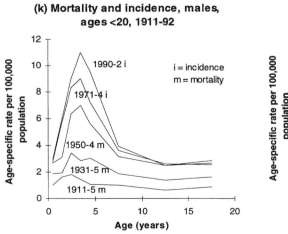

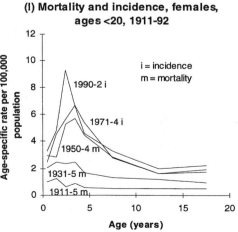

Figure 6.34   Leukaemia (continued).

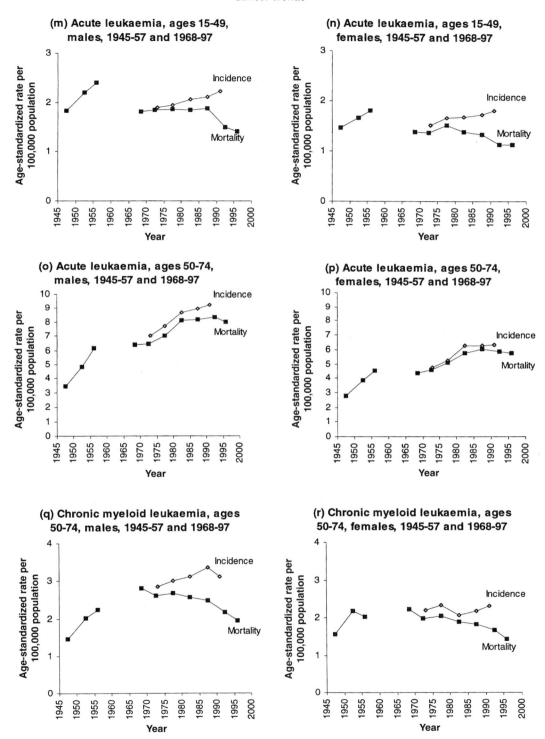

(m) Acute leukaemia, ages 15-49, males, 1945-57 and 1968-97

(n) Acute leukaemia, ages 15-49, females, 1945-57 and 1968-97

(o) Acute leukaemia, ages 50-74, males, 1945-57 and 1968-97

(p) Acute leukaemia, ages 50-74, females, 1945-57 and 1968-97

(q) Chronic myeloid leukaemia, ages 50-74, males, 1945-57 and 1968-97

(r) Chronic myeloid leukaemia, ages 50-74, females, 1945-57 and 1968-97

Figure 6.34 Leukaemia (continued).

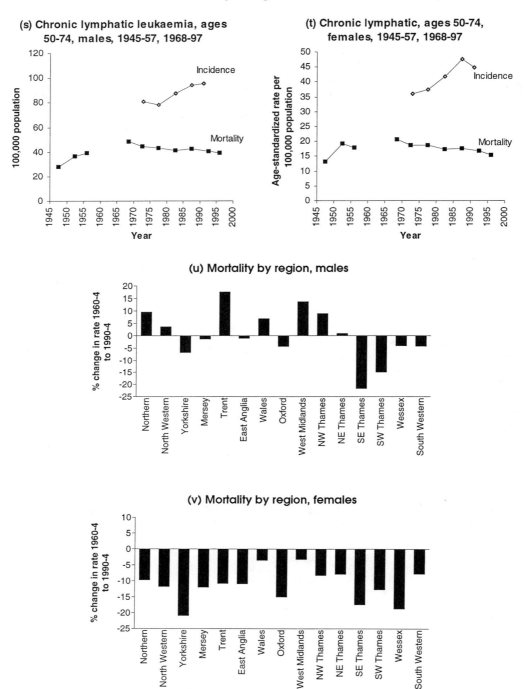

Figure 6.34   Leukaemia (continued).

boys at least, around age 17 years—a feature of leukaemia epidemiology present earlier in the century (see Comment, below). Comparing the age distribution of incidence in children and young adults in 1990–2 with that in 1971–4 (not in Figure), there was no change except that in each sex the childhood peak was greater in the later than the earlier period.

Figures 6.34h to j show secular trends in leukaemia mortality at various ages over a longer period—since 1911. In children aged 0–4 years (Figure 6.34h) rates rose fairly steadily from the 1920s to a peak in 1950–4, and then diminished almost symmetrically. There was a fairly similar pattern of rise and fall in older children (not shown), but at ages 5–9 the peak occurred later, in 1955–9 for boys and 1960–4 for girls, and at ages 10–14 the trends were more inconsistent and the timing of the peak less clear-cut. In adults under age 70 (Figures 6.34i and j) rates rose until the mid-century, with a sharp upward inflexion occurring from 1941–5 to 1946–50 in middle age. There was then little change or a slightly increasing trend from the mid-century through to the 1970s, followed by a decline in the 1980s and 90s. At older ages (Figure 6.34j) there was an increase almost throughout the century, with an upward inflexion in the early 1950s, and a downturn only in the most recent years.

Figures 6.34k and l show the age distribution of leukaemia in children and young adults since 1911. For the early years, only mortality and not incidence data are available, but these should effectively have been a reflection of incidence (as far as it was ascertained) because leukaemia was then almost always rapidly fatal. In recent decades, however, survival has become the rule (see Figure B8), and therefore for these years cancer registration rather than mortality data give the best assessment of the relation of age to incidence, and are shown in the Figures. The data for ages under 5 years are presented by single year of age, using rates published by Court Brown and Doll (1961) for 1911–15 to 1950–4 and using the data we had extracted from the national cancer registry files for 1971 onwards. The rates shown for older ages are by 5-year age group. In each sex, the development of the now-characteristic peak of leukaemia in young children can be seen to have progressed throughout the century.

At older childhood ages and in young adults, however, although increases occurred early in the century, the changes in recent decades have been relatively slight.

Finally, Figures 6.34m to t show secular trends of certain subdivisions of leukaemia: acute, chronic myeloid (CML), and chronic lymphoid (CLL). This classification was employed by Court Brown and Doll (1959) in their publication of mortality data for 1945–57, and is used here in order to maximize the period over which trends can be presented for consistent categories. Court Brown and Doll's data were specially tabulated from death certificates. We added, from our current analyses, mortality data for 1968–97 and incidence data for 1971–92. Data for 1958–67 could not be included because the ICD revision then in use (ICD7) did not provide a sufficiently differentiated classification of leukaemias[121]. In order to assess trends in rates of specific subdivisions of leukaemia, it is necessary to account for cases in which the chronicity and/or cell type of the malignancy are not specified. We included these ill-specified cases in the analysis, as Court Brown and Doll had done for the 1945–57 data, by allocating them to the acute/chronic and cytology-specific categories in the same proportions as these categories constituted within the cases for which the variables were known[122]. For instance, chronic leukaemias of unknown cell type were allocated between chronic myeloid and chronic lymphoid leukaemias in proportion, at each 5-year age group, to the relative proportions of leukaemias of these two cell types known to have occurred at these ages. We have presented the results for acute leukaemia for two broad adult age groups, 15–49 and 50–74 years. For chronic leukaemias we have presented data only for the older age group, because these tumours are comparatively rare in young adults.

Rates of mortality from acute leukaemia at ages 15–49 (Figures 6.34m and n) increased rapidly during 1945–57, but by 1968–9, when data were next available, rates were considerably below those in 1955–7. Subsequently, rates were fairly stable until a decreasing trend after 1985–9 in males and after 1975–9 in females. Incidence increased modestly over the years for which data are available, and diverged considerably from the mortality trend after the latter turned

---

[121] ICD7 divided leukaemias into acute, lymphatic not specified to be acute, and myeloid not specified to be acute, but this categorization aggregated leukaemias that were chronic and of unspecified chronicity, and therefore the latter could not be reallocated between acute and chronic in the same manner as had been employed by Court Brown and Doll and for the ICD8 and 9 data. For the latter (ICD8 and 9) data, we aggregated subacute leukaemias with acute, and we reallocated those uncommon chronic leukaemias that were of specified cell type that was neither lymphoid nor myeloid in the same way as we had reallocated those of unspecified cell type.
[122] See note 121.

downward. At older ages (Figures 6.34o and p) the trend in mortality from acute leukaemia was also sharply upward during 1945–57, and although the rate in 1968–9 was not above that in 1955–7, there was a continuing rise in the 1970s and 1980s, and a downturn only in the most recent years. Trends in incidence since 1971 were similar to those for mortality, diverging only slightly in the most recent data.

Trends in mortality from chronic myeloid leukaemia (Figures 6.34q and r) were generally upward in 1945–57 and downward from 1968–97. Incidence did not change substantially during the period for which data were available, and there was a growing divergence between incidence and mortality rates over time.

Chronic lymphoid leukaemia mortality (Figures 6.34s and t) also generally increased during 1945–57, but since 1968 the trend has been slightly downward. The gap between incidence and mortality rates has been large, and has grown as incidence has increased.

Trends by birth cohort

For the reasons discussed on p. 5, we have not presented birth cohort analyses for leukaemia in adults. We have, however, analysed trends of incidence in children by single year of birth (Figures 6.34f and g). There were peaks of incidence that coincided between the sexes for the cohorts born in 1982 (SCIR = 111 (95% CI 96–128) in males, 120 (102–140) in females) and 1989 (125 (102–153) in males and 125 (99–156) in females).

Mortality trends by region

Leukaemia trends have been slight in all regions, consistently downward in females but not in a consistent direction in males (Figures 6.34u and v).

Comment

Leukaemias are malignancies that arise from the precursor cells of white blood cells and tissue leukocytes. We will discuss leukaemia trends separately for recent decades and earlier in the twentieth century.

Trends in recent decades

Adults

The trend in leukaemia incidence and mortality in old adults in the last few decades, increasing substantially before stabilizing in recent years, is similar to that seen in several other Western countries (Kinlen 1994), although the stabilization appears to have occurred later in England and Wales than in many other countries. Changes in the Registrar General's interpretation of ICD coding rule 3 and in medical enquiry policy (see pp. 11–12) have had relatively little effect on all-age leukaemia mortality rates[123] (Table 4.1), although at ages 75 years and above the change in rule 3 interpretation in 1984 caused a 7% increase, and presumably there was a corresponding decrease in 1993 when the previous interpretation was reinstated. There appears to have been an increasing tendency for leukaemia, when it is mentioned on a death certificate, to be deemed the underlying cause of death (Grulich *et al.* 1995). This had little effect at ages under 75, but at older ages a 10% increase in recent years might be explicable by this mechanism (Grulich *et al.* 1995).

Improved diagnosis may have played a part in the rise in recorded incidence at old ages. In addition there may have been a real increase, but if so, either it was a consequence of factor(s) that affected old far more than younger ages or it was due to factors that mainly increased many decades ago, and therefore largely affected cohorts born early in the twentieth century. Leukaemia in adults can be caused by exposure to ionizing radiation[124], alkylating chemotherapy[125], benzene[126], and probably chloramphenicol; cigarette smoking is a weak cause of myeloid leukaemia. The known effects of these factors, however, would not explain the large increases in leukaemia at older ages, similar between the sexes, and ceasing recently. For instance, an effect of smoking would have led to an earlier peak for men than women (see Figures 5.47, 5.48, 5.50, 5.51, 6.11, 6.12).

The decreasing mortality from leukaemia in young adults, while incidence has not diminished, implies improving survival. All-age survival data (Figure A26) showed slight improvements in East Anglia and greater ones in England and Wales, with the improvements in

---

[123] Medical enquiries had a large (32%) effect in decreasing the numbers of leukaemias of unspecified cell type, but a less than ±5% effect on the numbers of leukaemias overall (Swerdlow 1989).
[124] Acute and non-lymphoid leukaemias, but not chronic lymphoid leukaemia.
[125] Acute and non-lymphoid leukaemias, but not chronic lymphoid leukaemia.
[126] Acute myeloid leukaemia.

East Anglia virtually restricted to ages under 35 years and those in England and Wales greater in young than in older adults (not shown).

Children

Leukaemia, mainly acute lymphocytic leukaemia (ALL), accounts for about one-third of malignancies incident in children in England and Wales. Completeness of registration of childhood cancers by the national registry at ONS was probably over 90% during 1971–84 (Hawkins and Swerdlow 1992), so the registration data are likely to have given a fairly good reflection of actual incidence trends. These data showed evidence of a modest rise in incidence in girls, and a slight rise in boys, at ages 0–14 years overall, and an increase in incidence at the early childhood peak ages in each sex. In high-quality data for Britain from the Childhood Cancer Research Group (Draper *et al.* 1994), there were significant increases of about 1% per annum in incidence of leukaemia from 1953–91 in each sex at ages 1–4 years, while at other childhood ages there were lesser, non-significant changes. In other countries there has been some evidence for an increase in rates of acute lymphocytic leukaemia in children, but not large, not clearly real, and at different times in different places (Draper *et al.* 1994).

Known causes of leukaemia in children are Down's syndrome, certain other rarer chromosome abnormalities, ionizing radiation (both *in utero* and postnatally), alkylating chemotherapy, and perhaps chloramphenicol. Although the number of terminations of Down's syndrome foetuses has increased considerably over recent years, the prevalence of Down's syndrome at birth has only decreased a little over the period for which data are available, since 1989[127] (Mutton *et al.* 1998; Huang *et al.* 1998), because a greater proportion of pregnancies are occurring at older maternal ages when the risk of a Down's syndrome offspring is greater. Prenatal diagnostic irradiation may have caused 5% of all cases of leukaemia in children exposed in the period 1953–67 (Doll 1989), when just over 10% of children born had been irradiated *in utero* (Table 5.12). The frequency of such examinations does not appear to have decreased (Table 5.12) over the subsequent years for which data are available, to 1981,

but the average number of films per examination has diminished somewhat (Table 5.13) and the dose per film has also fallen, perhaps several-fold (see p. 44). About 2–8% of cases may have been due to prenatal exposure to natural radiation (Doll 1989; Doll and Darby 1990), and a further 16% to natural background LET radiation[128] after birth (Doll and Darby 1990), the extent of which will not have changed. The percentage, if any, due to domestic radon exposure (which may have increased—see pp. 37–8) is too small (Doll and Darby 1990) to have affected trends materially.

Although there has not been a clear demonstration that fallout radiation can increase the risk of leukaemia, there has been evidence suggesting raised risk in people in Utah exposed at ages under 20 years to the fallout from nearby US nuclear weapons tests (Stevens *et al.* 1990). In the Nordic countries, where fallout levels from nuclear weapons tests were about twice those in Britain, leukaemia incidence rates were not clearly raised in children born in the years of greatest fallout, nor did rates by birth cohort relate to average estimated foetal dose or paternal testicular dose in the year before birth (Darby *et al.* 1992). Leukaemia rates in the period of highest exposure were, however, slightly and borderline significantly greater than in the immediately surrounding periods. The England and Wales incidence data are from several years after the high fallout levels from nuclear tests in 1962–5 (see Figures 5.26–5.30)[129]. Because the induction period of leukaemia after ionizing radiation exposure tends to be short, with a peak 5–9 years after exposure, leukaemia incidence in the years analysed, from 1971–92, did not have great potential to be affected by fallout from nuclear tests, bone-marrow doses from which reached a peak in the mid-1960s (Figures 5.30)[130]. Although the leukaemia data did include the time of the Chernobyl accident, in 1986, and the years immediately afterwards, fallout levels in Britain from this were far lower than those in earlier decades from nuclear weapons tests (Figures 5.26, 5.28, Table 5.10). Overall, therefore, the absence of a detectable relation between leukaemia incidence in children in England and Wales in 1971–92 and annual fallout is unsurprising, and the modest peaks for children born in 1982 and 1989 might have been due to chance or to a cause other than fallout.

---

[127] There was about a 10% decrease in births of Down's syndrome babies (data are not available to separate livebirths from stillbirths) from 1989 to 1997.

[128] Low linear energy transfer radiation, e.g. gamma-rays.

[129] The peak dose rate will also have occurred around the same time because the biological half-life in bone of radioactive caesium, the main isotope concerned, is under one year.

[130] See note 129.

There has been a great deal of interest in recent years in the possibility that childhood leukaemia might be caused by exposure to low-frequency electromagnetic fields (EMF) produced by power lines and domestic electrical appliances[131]. A large national population-based case-control study has shown that high EMF exposure ($\geq$0.4 µT) occurs in less than 1% of children in Britain, and confirmed that at least for children with lower exposures than this, leukaemia risk is not materially increased by EMF exposure (UK Childhood Cancer Study Investigators 1999). For children with exposures of $\geq$0.4 µT, however, there is evidence that risk may be raised, although whether this is caused by the EMF exposure is unclear (Ahlbom *et al.* 2000). The small rise in leukaemia incidence at ages 1–4 from 1953 to 1991, of about 1% per year[132], and the lesser changes at other ages, were certainly not commensurate with the scale of increase in average power frequency magnetic field exposures from 1949 to the mid 1970s shown in Figure 5.35, but this is not incompatible with EMF exposure as a minor cause of childhood leukaemia.

It has been suggested that childhood infection, with an as yet unknown agent, may be a cause of childhood leukaemia, and that population mixing may facilitate the transmission of this agent and hence lead to increased leukaemia rates (Kinlen 1996). National trends in population mixing are not known and indeed it is uncertain quite what types of mixing would affect relevant infectious disease transmission. It seems plausible that transmission would have been increased by the evacuation of children (sometimes with their mothers) from London and other dangerous areas of the country during the Second World War, which affected the largest numbers of children in 1939, 1941, and 1944 (Kinlen and John 1994). In a different way, the spread of infections may have been increased by National (military) Service in the post-war period, which involved large influxes of young servicemen into military camps around Britain, often in rural areas. National Service existed from 1947 to 1963, but intakes reduced from 1957 onwards (Kinlen and Hudson 1991). Although there was no obvious upsurge in childhood leukaemia (as measured by mortality data) in response to either of these events, they affected only a minority of children and the effect, if any, may have been hidden in national data (Kinlen 1996). In more recent times, a decrease

from 1971 to 1991 in residential movements between localities is apparent from census data on population mobility (Table 5.19), although it is unclear to what extent these data give a good measure of population mixing relevant to infectious diseases.

An alternative hypothesis (Greaves 1997) has been that ALL may be caused by an abnormal immunological response to an infection in childhood. Under this hypothesis, programming of the immune system normally occurs early in life by exposure to infectious diseases around birth and in infancy, in the context of immune protection or dose limitation from the mother deriving from immunoglobulins transferred transplacentally and in breast milk. If this prior programming is absent, it is argued, leukaemia may be the consequence of an immunological response to late infection; i.e. childhood leukaemia may essentially be a consequence of late infection in affluent societies. One specific element of this hypothesis on which we had secular information is breast feeding, which decreased in frequency from 1920 to 1970 (Figure 5.39, Table 5.21), in accord with the recorded rise in childhood leukaemia, but then increased sharply from 1970 onwards, while leukaemia at the childhood peak ages increased. It is possible, however, that pregnant mothers in recent years may themselves not have been exposed appropriately to infections, and therefore may not have been competent to provide protection to their offspring (Greaves 1997).

In the context of a possible infectious aetiology of leukaemia, it is notable that the age-sex distribution of leukaemia in children and young adults in Figure 6.34e shows in several respects a similar pattern, although at a much younger age, to that shown in Figure 6.31k for another malignancy strongly suspected of being caused by a late infection, Hodgkin's disease. In both there was little difference between the sexes in rates as they increased toward a peak (in young childhood for leukaemia, in young adulthood for Hodgkin's disease), there was then a greater and probably slightly later peak in males than females, and there was a male excess thereafter. Although this might be coincidence, it might alternatively indicate a sex-difference in the age distribution of occurrence of relevant infections or in age-specific responses to these infections.

As well as the peak of leukaemia in young children, Lee (1961) noted a lesser peak of leukaemia mortality

---

[131] There has also been interest in a possible association of leukaemia risk in adults with occupational exposures to electromagnetic fields, but there is no strong evidence in favour of this, and there are no data on trends in occupational exposures (Swanson 1996).
[132] Draper *et al.* (1994); see p. 189 above.

in adolescents, especially males, aged around 17 years, in data from several Western countries for the 1950s. This peak had been present in England and Wales data back to 1911 (Court Brown and Doll 1961). Although it was present to some extent also in the England and Wales incidence data for 1971–92 (Figure 6.34e), it was less pronounced there than in the mortality data from the middle of the century.

The large divergence between incidence and mortality trends for leukaemia in children in the data since 1971 reflects the successes of chemotherapy and bone marrow transplantation in treatment (Figure B8).

Trends since 1911

The trends in leukaemia mortality during the first half of the twentieth century, shown in Figures 6.34h–l, are more difficult to interpret than those subsequently. There has long been interest in these trends; in the mid twentieth century, the recorded rates of leukaemia mortality were rising faster than those of any other malignancy except lung cancer (Hewitt 1955). One artefact can be identified, when coding of aleukaemia was transferred from the rubric for Hodgkin's disease to that for leukaemia, and the basis of selection of underlying cause of death was altered, with the change from ICD4 to 5 in 1940. The net result of this, however, was a small *reduction* in recorded leukaemia mortality of 3% overall (Table 4.1), and larger reductions of 18% in men and 9% in women at ages 75 years and above (Case *et al.* 1976). The abrupt increase in rates in middle age from 1941–5 to 1946–50[133] must have been an artefact, perhaps due to cases revealed by the increasing availability and effectiveness of antibiotics and by the advent of the National Health Service. These factors may also have been responsible for the subsequent upturns in rates at ages 65 and above.

The main reason for the great long-term increase in recorded rates of leukaemia could either be improved diagnosis and certification or a real increase in incidence, and there must be uncertainty about the contribution of each. There has been ample scope for increases due to better diagnosis and certification, particularly at old ages, but Court Brown and Doll (1961) considered that at least part of the increase at young ages must have been real, and that in young adults from 1945 to 1959 it had particularly affected acute and chronic myeloid leukaemias. The development of the childhood peak from 1920 onwards in England and Wales is similar to the pattern observed in other populations that now have high rates (Hewitt 1955; Court Brown and Doll 1961; Doll 1989), and could imply that a new leukaemogenic agent was introduced in the UK from about 1920 (Court Brown and Doll 1961).

Stewart and Kneale (1969) suggested that the rise in leukaemia in young children was a consequence of better survival of children with pre-leukaemia, who in the early part of the century would have died of pneumonia before the leukaemia was recognized, but who with the introduction of sulphonamides and then antibiotics survived long enough to be diagnosed with leukaemia, and then to die of it. In support of this they showed that annual leukaemia mortality rates at ages 2–4 years since 1911–15 correlated inversely with pneumonia mortality rates at these ages, but there was not a similar correlation at ages under 2 years. It should be noted, however, that sulphonamides were introduced in 1936 and laboratory preparations of penicillin in 1941, so that an appreciable part of the increase occurred before these drugs were available.

One other aspect of the long-term data deserves comment. In general the downturn in leukaemia mortality in recent decades at young ages, particularly in childhood, reflects the success of treatment, by chemotherapy and bone marrow transplantation. The downturn at ages 0–4, however, started in the mid 1950s, before modern chemotherapy became available, and hence requires some other explanation. A similar change in rates has been noted in data for the US and Australia (Adelstein and White 1976). Although it is possible that there was a downturn in incidence in the 1950s, the most likely reason is that improvements in medical care resulted in a slight lengthening of survival, such that more children with leukaemia incident at the young childhood peak ages of the disease survived to age 5 years and hence were recorded as dying at ages 5–9 years[134].

---

[133] Figure 6.34i shows the increase at ages 45–9 years. There were similar abrupt increases at other age groups from 40–64 years, not shown in the Figure, although it varied whether the major rise occurred over the 5 or the 10 years after 1941–5.

[134] Data from the long-running Manchester Children's Tumour Registry give some support to this, although not strongly: 2-year survival from leukaemia improved from 5% in 1954–8 to 12% in 1959–63 while 3-year survival increased from 2% to 5% (Draper *et al.* 1982); although these data were for all childhood ages, about half of the cases in childhood were at ages 0–4, so that survival at these ages too probably improved. National mortality trends at ages 5–9 years continued to rise until around 1960 (see p. 187), but did not show a compensatory acceleration in this trend as rates declined at ages 0–4.

Trends by histology and chronicity

Assessment of trends in leukaemia by histology and chronicity is difficult because incompleteness of ascertainment of these factors, and potential changes in criteria for their categorization, are added to the problems in interpretation of leukaemia data generally, discussed above. Consideration of the trends must therefore be tentative. Nevertheless, the existence of data on leukaemia rates subdivided by these factors back to 1945, more than 20 years before the ICD provided such a categorization, gave an exceptional opportunity to gain some information on trends over 50 years. Acute leukaemias of different histological types were combined in these analyses because the distinction between them has not always been uniform (Court Brown and Doll 1959), whereas chronic lymphoid and chronic myeloid leukaemias were separated because this distinction has historically been less uncertain. Medical enquiries to certifiers requesting information on cell type of leukaemias when this had not been stated on the death certificate, were made by the Registrar General from 1950 (Court Brown and Doll 1959) to 1992. Such enquiries reduced the numbers of leukaemias of unspecified cell type by a third (Swerdlow 1989). Medical enquiries were also pursued up to 1992 when the certifier had failed to specify whether the leukaemia was acute or chronic (Swerdlow 1989).

The percentage of leukaemia deaths for which chronicity and/or cell type were not specified, and for which one or both of these variables therefore had to be estimated for our analyses, decreased greatly from 46.1% of deaths in men[135] in 1945–9 to 35.7% in 1950–4, 28.2% in 1955–7, and under 8% since 1968. (The percentage for incidence was, surprisingly, initially worse than the contemporary figure for mortality, and decreased from 13.4% in 1971–4 to 6.7% in 1990–2).

Although the factors just discussed and the discontinuity between the two periods of data available give limitations, certain conclusions about the trends can be drawn. It has remained the case, as in the 1940s and 1950s, that the male: female ratio for CLL mortality is around 2:1 (it has increased a little over time), and that the male predominance is less than this for acute leukaemias and less again (or in some years absent) for CML. The incidence data show a similar picture.

The gap between incidence and mortality for CLL has been much greater than that for CML or acute leukaemias. There have been diverging trends between incidence and mortality especially for acute leukaemia in young adults and chronic myeloid leukaemia at older ages, suggesting improved survival for these categories.

The rapid increase in recorded mortality from acute leukaemia during 1945–57 has not continued at the same pace in more recent years. The apparent decline in acute leukaemia mortality at young ages between 1955–7 and 1968–9 might be an artefact of the estimation process used to include leukaemias of unknown chronicity or an artefact of diagnostic categorization: the overall rates of leukaemia in young adults were little changed over this period (Figure 6.34i), and the proportion, after use of the estimation process, that were categorized as acute was considerably greater in 1955–7 than 1968–9. The near-identity of incidence and mortality rates in the early 1970s suggests that better survival did not explain the apparent decline in mortality from 1955–7 to 1968–9. In conclusion, the data show an increase in mortality from acute leukaemia from 1945–57, which occurred at all ages under 65 and which Court Brown and Doll (1959) considered was likely largely to be real, and increases in incidence at all adult ages since 1971, which may also largely have been real. Ionizing radiation exposure and smoking must at least have contributed to this rise. In analyses of long-term trends in acute leukaemia incidence elsewhere, large increases in each sex from 1943 to 1977 were seen in Denmark (Hansen *et al.* 1983), although this reflected increases for older rather than younger adults, and an increase in males but not females was seen from 1935 to 1974 in Olmsted County, Minnesota (Linos *et al.* 1978), particularly for acute myeloid leukaemia at older ages.

For CML, the mortality data for 1945–57 showed an increase in males but not consistently in females, and the incidence data since 1971 did not show a convincing increase in either sex. For CLL the early mortality data showed large increases only at ages 65 and above, when diagnostic artefacts might particularly have pertained, and the more-recent incidence data showed inconsistent evidence of an increase. In Danish data there was little change in either CML or CLL incidence since 1943 (Hansen *et al.* 1983), except for a rise

---

[135] Court Brown and Doll did not present data in this detail for women, but in our data since 1968 the percentages for women were similar to those for men.

in CLL at older ages, whereas in Olmsted County CLL incidence[136] increased in males but not females (Linos *et al.* 1978).

The percentage of leukaemias in England and Wales that were of unspecified histology and/or chronicity has been low enough since 1968 that the assumptions made in reallocating these tumours to more-specific categories are unlikely to have affected the results materially. For the 1945–57 mortality data, the percentage unspecified was much greater, but, as Court Brown and Doll (1959) pointed out, the main unspecified categories were lymphoid and myeloid leukaemias of unspecified chronicity, and the age distribution of these was intermediate between the distributions for leukaemias specified as acute and those specified as chronic, suggesting that they were truly a mixture of the two.

Conclusions

Uncertainty about the extent to which diagnostic factors have contributed to trends, and deficiencies in knowledge of the major aetiological factors for leukaemia, limit the degree to which one can reach firm conclusions on either the trends in leukaemia over the last century or the reasons for them. Nevertheless, in children it seems probable that there was a large increase in rates at young ages in the first half of the twentieth century and that there was a lesser increase (of under 1% per annum) in the second half of the century. The earlier rise might have been due to better hygiene and reduced exposure to infectious agents in early life and effects of this on programming of the immune system to deal with infections encountered later in childhood (Greaves 1997). A small contribution must have come from the introduction of prenatal (and postnatal) diagnostic irradiation. In recent decades a small part of the increase will have been due to leukaemias caused by chemotherapy and radiotherapy. Also, through the century increased population mixing may have contributed by increasing the transmission of a putative infectious agent causing leukaemia (Kinlen 1996). In adults, much of the increase at older ages may well have been artefactual, but there have been increases in acute leukaemia in adults at younger ages which are likely to have been real, at least in part, and for which contributory factors[137] must have been smoking, and

diagnostic and occupational ionizing radiation exposure, as well as a small contribution from alkylating chemotherapy, and some contribution from benzene exposure.

Cancer of unspecified primary site

(Figure 6.35)

Secular trends

Mortality from cancer of unspecified primary site has increased greatly since 1960 in each sex at all adult ages, particularly the elderly: at ages 70–84 there has been an over four-fold increase in rates. Large increases have occurred in all regions (not shown). Malignancies of unspecified primary site constituted 2.6% of all deaths from malignancy at ages under 85 years in 1960–4, but 10.1% in 1995–7, with the greatest increase at the oldest ages: at ages 70–84 there was an increase over this period from 2.8% to 11.0%, whereas at ages 15–34 the increase was from 2.3% to 5.8% and in children from 1.4% to 2.5%.

Incidence of cancer of unspecified primary site has increased by a half or more at ages 50 years and above since 1971, but has increased less or been unchanged at younger ages. Unspecified site malignancies were 4.0% of all cancers except non-melanoma skin cancer registered at ages under 85 years in 1971–4 and 5.7% in 1990–2. This reflected an increase at older ages – from 4.7% to 7.0% at ages 70–84 and 3.9% to 5.2% at ages 50–69 – while at ages under 50 the percentage has been lower and little changed.

Comment

The increasing proportion of cancer deaths and registrations for which no primary site is specified implies that the true trends in cancers of specified primary sites, especially those for which diagnosis is difficult, are more upward than the recorded data for these sites would suggest. Numerically this may have affected particularly lung and liver cancers in men and ovarian and stomach cancers in women, based on analysis of deaths certified to unknown primary site but for which

---

[136] No trend data were presented for CML.
[137] Which will have affected older adults too.

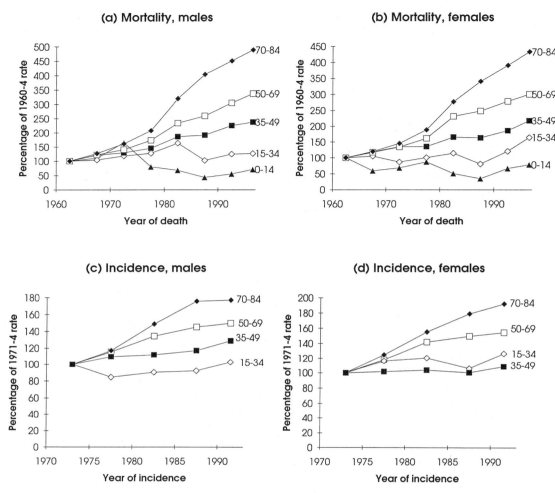

Figure 6.35   Cancer of unspecified primary site (ICD7 156, 165, 198, 199; ICD8 195-199; ICD9 155.2, 195–199), mortality 1960–97, incidence 1971–92.

a site was stated at cancer registration (Grulich *et al.* 1995)[138]. As the data above show, the effect will mainly have been at older ages, especially for mortality.

While to some extent the increase in malignancy of unspecified site might be explicable if there has been a rise in incidence of tumours that metastasize early and aggressively[139], the steepness of the increase is greater than would easily be explained on such a basis, and suggests that much of the increase must have been a consequence of diminished specificity of diagnosis and/or of death certification and cancer registration. The greater increase in unspecified primary site mortality than incidence suggests that at least part of the increase in the former is an artefact of poorer specificity in completion of death certificates. There may also have been a tendency toward less intensive investigation of patients with terminal cancer of unknown primary site. A contribution toward diminished diagnostic precision is likely to have come from the decrease over time in rates of non-coroner's autopsy

---

[138] In a large study in England and Wales in 1959, cancers certified clinically as of unknown primary site were particularly likely to be found at post-mortem to be cancers of the lung, stomach, pancreas, breast, and ovary (Heasman and Lipworth 1966). Those data were, however, from a time before many modern diagnostic aids were available.
[139] We have no evidence on whether there has been a rise in incidence of such tumours.

(Figure 4.1), as autopsy often discloses the primary site of tumours for which it is not known clinically (Heasman and Lipworth 1966). A part of the rise in rates is a consequence of the cessation of the Registrar General's 'medical enquiries' for imprecisely certified cancer deaths at ages 75 and over in 1984, and for all other ages in 1993 (see p. 11, and also note the abrupt increase in rates in 1993 shown in Figure 4.2b). A marked upturn in mortality but not substantially in incidence took place from 1978–82, starting in the year of the introduction of ICD9 but continuing beyond it, and, from examination of data double-coded to ICD8 and 9 (OPCS, 1983a), not due primarily to it[140].

Cancer in people with AIDS

(Figure 6.36)

Data on incidence of Kaposi's sarcoma as an AIDS-defining cancer have been available since the start of the AIDS epidemic, and show similar trends to those for AIDS (Figure 5.1). The peak of the AIDS epidemic in men occurred in 1994, while the peak of Kaposi's sarcoma in male AIDS patients was in 1993–4[141] (Figure 6.36a). The great majority of the Kaposi's cases in males with AIDS were at ages 15–49, and there were few in children (1 case) or over age 69 (3 cases) (not in Figure). In females (not shown), only 68 cases have been recorded since 1979, all but four during the 1990s and most (47) during 1992–6; almost all cases occurred at ages 15–34 (47) and 35–49 (18).

Unlike Kaposi's sarcoma, most lymphomas in AIDS patients do not occur as the AIDS-defining illness. Data are only available, however, on AIDS-defining cases, and these are therefore shown for men in Figure 6.36b. The pattern was similar to that for Kaposi's sarcoma. The peak numbers of cases in men occurred in 1992 (63) and 1995 (62), and most cases (84%) were at ages 15–49. In women (not shown) only 49 cases occurred in the period, mainly at ages 15–49 (82%); all but three cases were in the 1990s, with a peak of nine in 1993[142].

Cancer mortality in people who have received organ transplants

(Figure 6.37)

Figure 6.37a shows mortality from lymphoid and other neoplasms after transplantation in England and Wales, since 1984 when such data were first available. In men

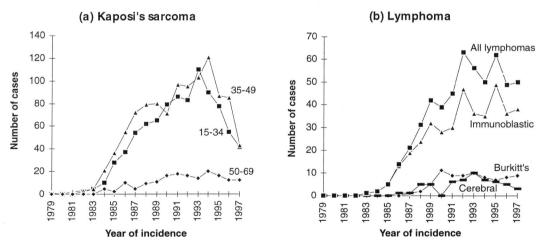

Figure 6.36 Incidence of (a) Kaposi's sarcoma and (b) lymphoma, as AIDS-defining illnesses, England and Wales, males, 1979–97.

---

[140] The double-coded data show a 4% increase in each sex due to the new ICD revision.

[141] 228 cases in 1993; 231 in 1994.

[142] For discussion of the likely total numbers of AIDS-related lymphomas, including cases that were not AIDS-defining, and the effect of AIDS-related lymphomas on trends in lymphoma overall, see p. 176.

(a) Type of neoplasm, by sex

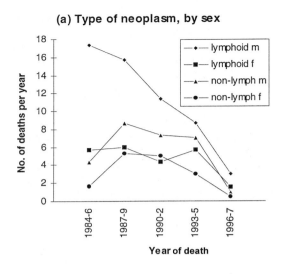

(b) Lymphoid neoplasms, by age

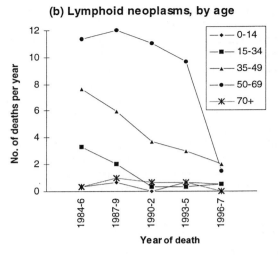

(c) Non-lymphoid neoplasms, by age

Figure 6.37 Mortality from neoplasms in patients who had received organ transplants in England and Wales, 1984–97.

lymphoid neoplasm mortality decreased from 17 deaths per annum in 1984–6 to 3 per annum in 1996–7. In women there were fewer cases, with an inconsistent trend downward in the most recent years. Neoplasms of other sites occurred less often. Again there were more cases in men than women, with trends inconsistent but downward in the most recent years. Most lymphoid and other neoplasms occurred at ages 35–69, with few in children or the elderly (Figures 6.37b,c).

The decreasing trend in cancer deaths in organ transplant recipients is not due to a decrease in numbers of transplants (Figures 5.34a,b), which increased before the 1990s and have since been little changed. The decrease in mortality might reflect improvement in

control of levels of immunosuppression, which may have led to a decrease in incidence of neoplasms caused by immunosuppression (although we have no data on this). The decreased mortality might also reflect more successful treatment of incident cases.

Trends in mortality from and incidence of the most common cancers: summary (Figure 6.38)

Figures 6.38a and b summarize the extent of change since 1960–4 in mortality from the cancers that had the

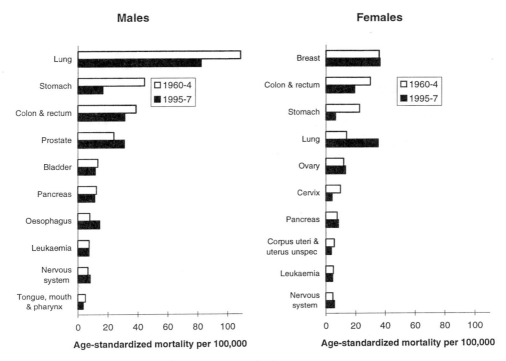

Figure 6.38 (a) Mortality at ages 0–84 from the most common fatal cancers, 1960–4 and 1995–7.

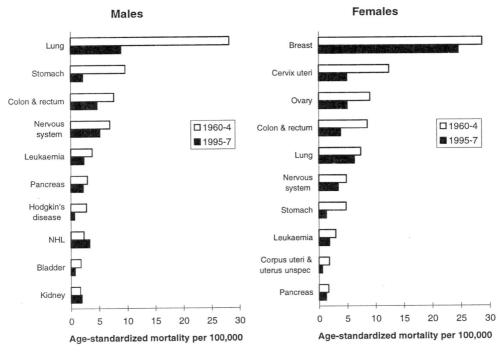

Figure 6.38 (b) Mortality at ages 35–49 from the most common fatal cancers, 1960–4, and 1995–7.

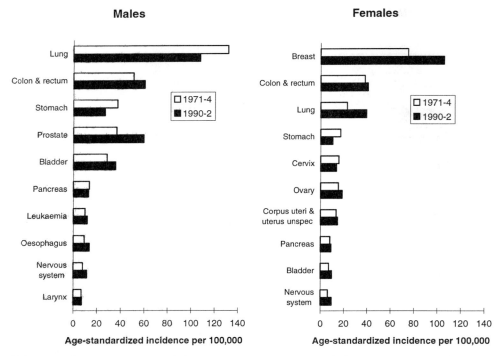

Figure 6.38 (c) Incidence at ages 0–84 of the most common cancers (excluding non-melanoma skin cancer) 1971–4 and 1990–2.

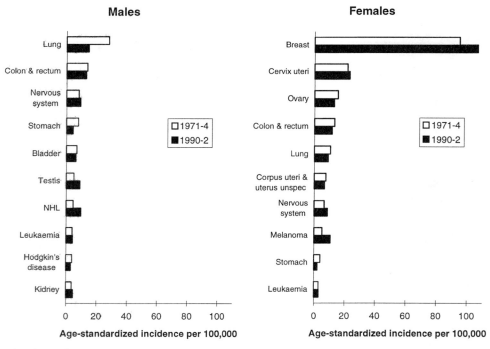

Figure 6.38 (d) Incidence at ages 35–49 of the most common cancers (excluding non-melanoma skin cancer), 1971–4 and 1990–2.

highest rates at that time, for all-ages and for ages 35–49 years. Figures 6.38c and d show the same analyses for incidence since 1971–4. The Figures display rates of mortality and incidence rather than percentage changes, and therefore can be used to compare the absolute magnitude of mortality from and incidence of different specific cancers. In each Figure the same scale is used for both sexes, to facilitate comparison between men and women.

Appendix A

Five year survival from selected cancers[1] incident 1971–92 in East Anglia and 1981 and 1989 in England and Wales. Ages 0–84 years at incidence unless otherwise specified

---

[1] Fewer sites are presented for England and Wales than for East Anglia because of data availability. Confidence intervals were not available for England and Wales results.

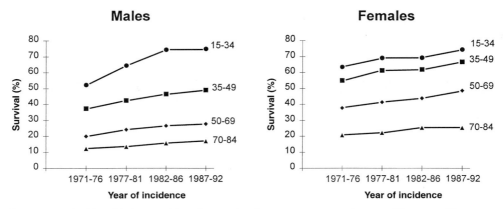

Figure A1 Five-year survival (crude), by age. All malignant neoplasms except non-melanoma skin cancer. Five-year survival by age, East Anglia, cases incident 1971–92.

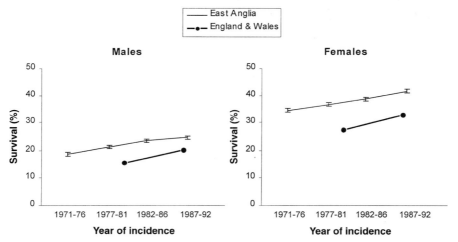

Figure A2 All malignant neoplasms except non-melanoma skin cancer. Five-year survival (crude), ages 0–84 years, East Anglia, cases incident 1971–92, with 95% CI, and England and Wales, cases incident 1981 and 1989.

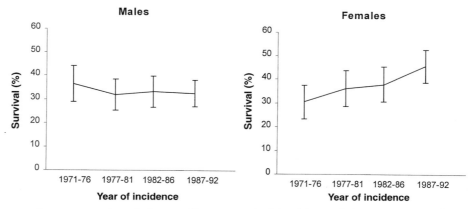

Figure A3 Cancers of tongue, mouth, and pharynx. Five-year survival (crude), ages 0–84 years, East Anglia, cases incident 1971–92, with 95% CI.

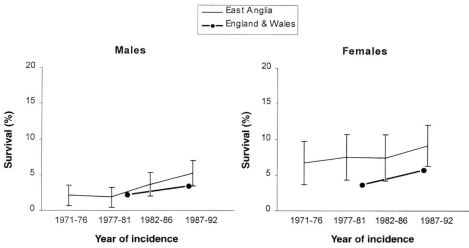

Figure A4   Cancer of oesophagus. Five-year survival (crude), ages 0–84 years, East Anglia, cases incident 1971–92, with 95% CI, and England and Wales, cases incident 1981 and 1989.

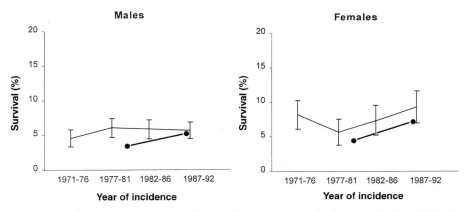

Figure A5   Cancer of stomach. Five-year survival (crude), ages 0–84 years, East Anglia, cases incident 1971–92, with 95% CI, and England and Wales, cases incident 1981 and 1989.

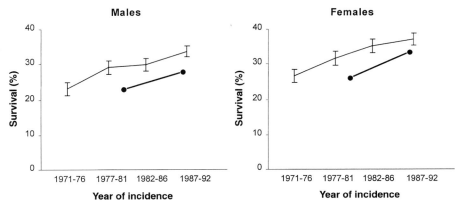

Figure A6   Cancers of colon and rectum. Five-year survival (crude), ages 0–84 years, East Anglia, cases incident 1971–92, with 95% CI, and England and Wales, cases incident 1981 and 1989.

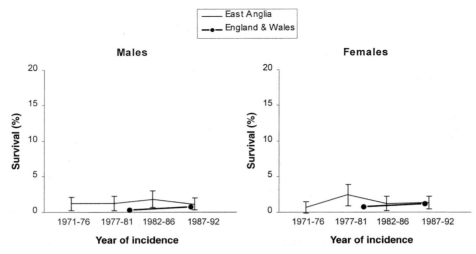

Figure A7 Cancer of pancreas. Five-year survival (crude), ages 0–84 years, East Anglia, cases incident 1971–92, with 95% CI, and England and Wales, cases incident 1981 and 1989.

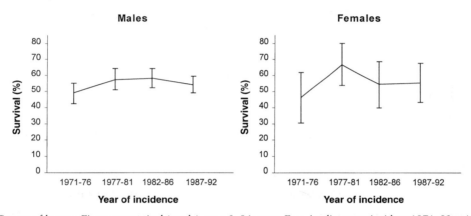

Figure A8 Cancer of larynx. Five-year survival (crude), ages 0–84 years, East Anglia, cases incident 1971–92, with 95% CI.

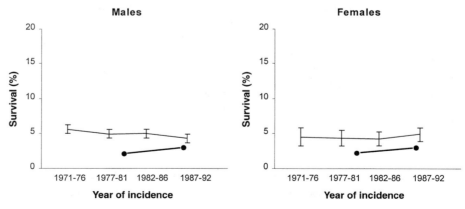

Figure A9 Cancer of lung. Five-year survival (crude), ages 0–84 years, East Anglia, cases incident 1971–92, with 95% CI, and England and Wales, cases incident 1981 and 1989.

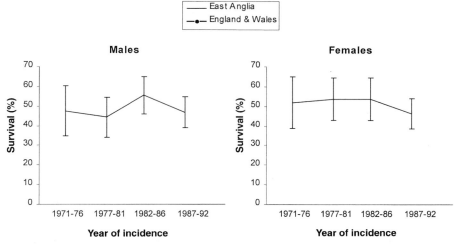

Figure A10 Cancer of soft tissues. Five-year survival (crude), ages 0–84 years, East Anglia, cases incident 1971–92, with 95% CI.

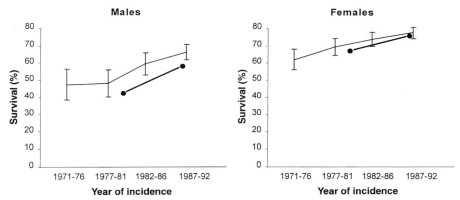

Figure A11 Malignant melanoma of skin. Five-year survival (crude), ages 0–84 years, East Anglia, cases incident 1971–92, with 95% CI, and England and Wales, cases incident 1981 and 1989.

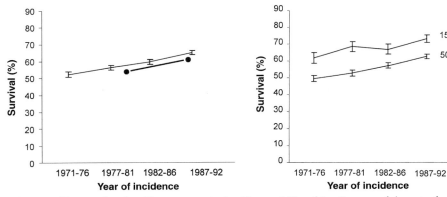

Figure A12 (a) Cancer of breast, females. Five-year survival (crude), ages 0–84 years, East Anglia, cases incident 1971–92, with 95% CI, and England and Wales, cases incident 1981 and 1989.

Figure A12 (b) Cancer of breast, females. Five-year survival (crude) by age, East Anglia, cases incident 1971–92, with 95% CI.

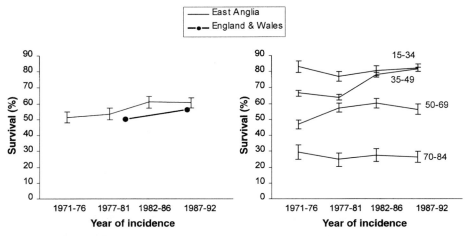

Figure A13 (a) Cancer of cervix. Five-year survival (crude), ages 0–84 years, East Anglia, cases incident 1971–92, with 95% CI, and England and Wales, cases incident 1981 and 1989.

Figure A13 (b) Cancer of cervix. Five-year survival (crude) by age, East Anglia, cases incident 1971–92, with 95% CI.

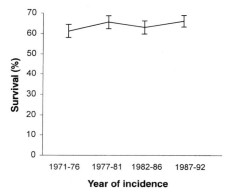

Figure A14 Cancer of corpus uteri and uterus unspecified. Five-year survival (crude), ages 0–84 years, East Anglia, cases incident 1971–92, with 95% CI.

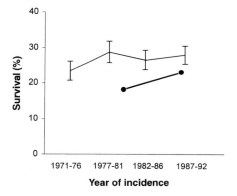

Figure A15 Cancer of ovary. Five-year survival (crude), ages 0–84 years, East Anglia, cases incident 1971–92, with 95% CI, and England and Wales, cases incident 1981 and 1989.

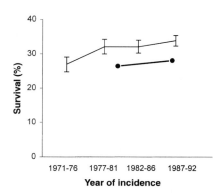

Figure A16 Cancer of prostate. Five-year survival (crude), ages 0–84 years, East Anglia, cases incident 1971–92, with 95% CI, and England and Wales, cases incident 1981 and 1989.

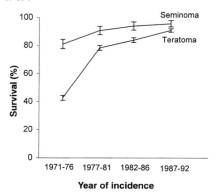

Figure A17 Cancer of testis. Five-year survival (crude) by histological type, ages 0–84 years, East Anglia, cases incident 1971–92, with 95% CI.

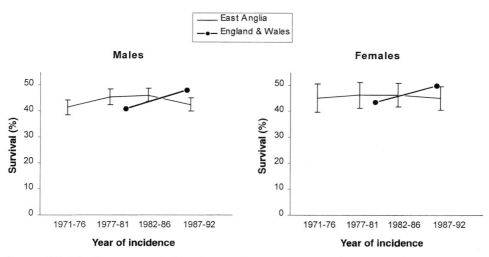

Figure A18   Cancer of bladder. Five-year survival (crude), ages 0–84 years, East Anglia, cases incident 1971–92, with 95% CI, and England and Wales, cases incident 1981 and 1989.

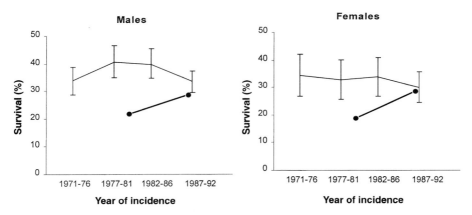

Figure A19   Cancer of kidney. Five-year survival (crude), ages 0–84 years, East Anglia, cases incident 1971–92, with 95% CI, and England and Wales, cases incident 1981 and 1989.

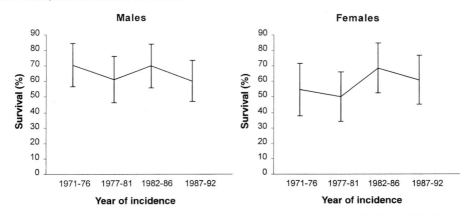

Figure A20   Cancer of eye. Five-year survival (crude), ages 0–84 years, East Anglia, cases incident 1971–92, with 95% CI.

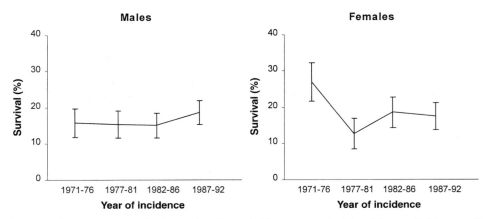

Figure A21 Tumours of nervous system (benign and malignant). Five-year survival (crude), ages 0–84 years, East Anglia, cases incident 1971–92, with 95% CI.

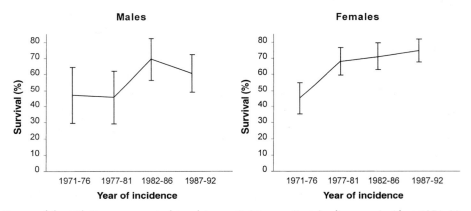

Figure A22 Cancer of thyroid. Five-year survival (crude), ages 0–84 years, East Anglia, cases incident 1971–92, with 95% CI.

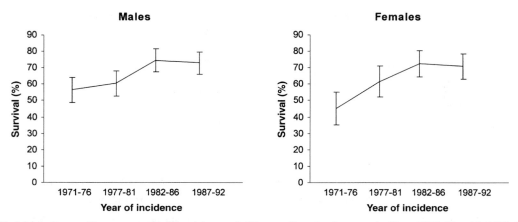

Figure A23 Hodgkin's disease. Five-year survival (crude), ages 0–84 years, East Anglia, cases incident 1971–92, with 95% CI.

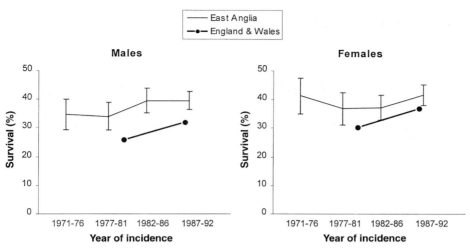

Figure A24 Non-Hodgkin's lymphoma. Five-year survival (crude), ages 0–84 years, East Anglia, cases incident 1971–92, with 95% CI, and England and Wales, cases incident 1981 and 1989.

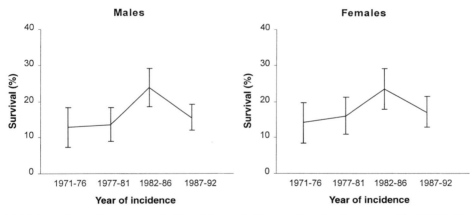

Figure A25 Multiple myeloma. Five-year survival (crude), ages 0–84 years, East Anglia, cases incident 1971–92, with 95% CI.

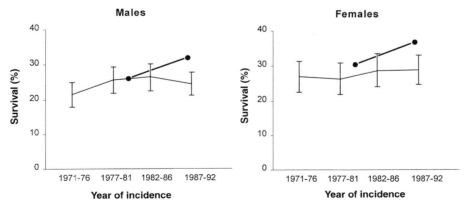

Figure A26 Leukaemia. Five-year survival (crude), ages 0–84 years, East Anglia, cases incident 1971–92, with 95% CI, and England and Wales, cases incident 1981 and 1989.

Appendix B

Five-year survival from selected cancers incident 1962–91 in children in Britain

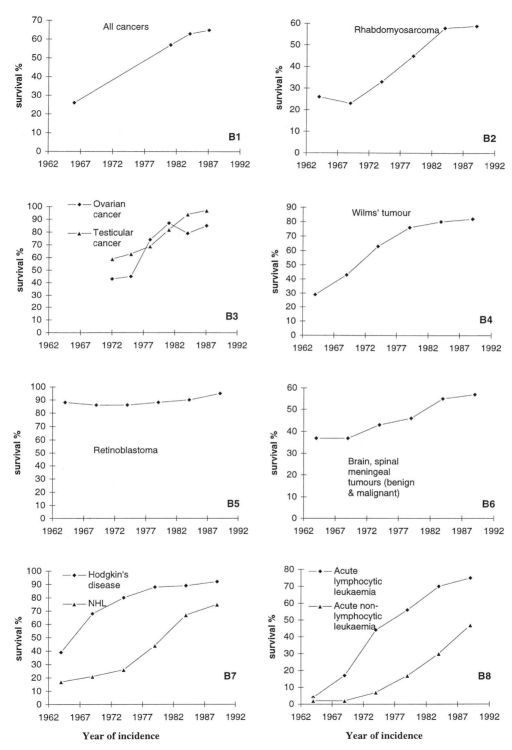

Figures B1–B8 Five-year survival (crude), cancers incident at ages under 15 years, both sexes combined (except for ovarian and testicular cancers), Britain, 1962–91.

Appendix C

Tables of cancer trends, secular and cohort, ages 0–84 years, England and Wales. Mortality 1960–97, incidence 1971–92

For ICD codes see Figures in Chapter 6.

The tables in this appendix cover most of the cancer sites in the Figures, but not quite all for reasons of space.

Rates are per 100,000 per annum, and are directly standardized by single year of age (see pp. 5 and 7). The rates were printed from a computer program that generated more digits after the decimal point than were usually needed, in order that there was sufficient precision for uncommon tumours. Where less than 4 digits are shown to the right of the decimal point, the truncated digits are zeros.

n = number of cases

SCMR = standardized cohort mortality ratio (%)

SCIR = standardized cohort incidence ratio (%)

U 95% CI = upper 95% confidence interval

L 95% CI = lower 95% confidence interval

SCMRs, SCIRs, and confidence intervals are generally shown with one digit after the decimal point; where no decimal point and digit to its right are shown, this is because the truncated digit after the decimal point is a zero.

Table C1 All malignant neoplasms (mortality); all malignant neoplasms except non-melanoma skin cancer (incidence)*

(a) Mortality, males, 1960–97

Age		1960–4	1965–9	1970–4	1975–9	1980–4	1985–9	1990–4	1995–7
0–14	n	2261	2283	2116	1807	1275	998	985	488
	Rate	8.0543	7.6879	6.9993	6.3935	5.0074	4.1174	3.9224	3.1697
15–34	n	4373	4368	4432	4473	3999	3682	3428	1763
	Rate	14.2364	13.5893	13.0991	12.3316	10.6792	9.5935	8.6146	7.324
35–49	n	18695	18247	16902	14786	13800	14014	14357	8164
	Rate	78.3391	76.5508	73.1773	67.0119	61.6755	58.5971	54.3423	48.7853
50–69	n	143113	156923	160919	156852	147743	142962	133427	72368
	Rate	627.5561	637.4293	626.7908	611.6197	589.7823	567.9638	534.9225	485.6044
70–84	n	94904	105719	123074	144388	166260	182088	186301	109927
	Rate	1591.711	1701.2539	1818.1596	1900.1655	1935.8084	1985.0678	1920.4337	1814.505
0–84	n	263346	287540	307443	322306	333077	343744	338498	192710
	Rate	304.5332	316.1882	323.7146	326.4681	323.205	321.8747	307.5595	285.4204

(b) Incidence, males, 1971–92

Age		1971–4	1975–9	1980–4	1985–9	1990–2
0–14	n	2704	3290	3033	2979	1975
	Rate	11.0295	11.7303	11.8254	11.9043	12.6249
15–34	n	6942	9342	9517	11086	7131
	Rate	25.4902	25.8041	25.4691	28.7277	29.5683
35–49	n	20726	24399	24195	26717	17517
	Rate	113.3266	110.8703	108.2084	111.5898	113.672
50–69	n	164601	206629	205184	205891	123968
	Rate	796.4529	803.0926	815.5709	816.9151	819.9957
70–84	n	114768	170962	207164	231015	146463
	Rate	2098.321	2242.6911	2408.3003	2515.3632	2553.3663
0–84	n	309741	414622	449093	477688	297054
	Rate	398.5779	413.1285	430.5601	442.318	447.2673

(c) Mortality, females, 1960–97

Age		1960–4	1965–9	1970–4	1975–9	1980–4	1985–9	1990–4	1995–7
0–14	n	1743	1725	1538	1224	1007	858	704	388
	Rate	6.544	6.0874	5.3288	4.6	4.1674	3.6851	2.9308	2.6755
15–34	n	3656	3704	3613	3906	4027	3717	3437	1989
	Rate	12.1452	12.0525	11.1919	11.1055	11.0843	10.1462	8.8453	8.4499
35–49	n	23276	22819	22013	19547	18689	19765	19579	11040
	Rate	95.2458	94.5598	95.4477	89.8178	84.6562	82.9947	74.5329	66.7237
50–69	n	102541	110187	115689	118717	117470	117048	107903	58728
	Rate	364.97	377.0926	390.2449	405.9497	416.2554	422.2032	401.4243	369.09
70–84	n	88795	96272	107141	120851	135846	150845	155180	92776
	Rate	859.7301	856.5363	877.626	911.2742	944.209	1012.0635	1027.6303	1027.0692
0–84	n	220011	234707	249994	264245	277039	292233	286803	164921
	Rate	181.4168	183.5475	188.123	193.5006	197.7879	204.6614	199.4656	190.7365

(d) Incidence, females, 1971–92

Age		1971–4	1975–9	1980–4	1985–9	1990–2
0–14	n	2002	2457	2335	2353	1475
	Rate	8.6501	9.3395	9.6005	9.8595	9.9586
15–34	n	8207	11662	12857	14639	8904
	Rate	31.8263	33.339	35.4824	39.9866	38.4493
35–49	n	38023	44382	45527	53962	34594
	Rate	209.2807	204.4807	206.3434	225.7895	224.5696
50–69	n	138862	180009	184303	194191	123279
	Rate	584.1338	615.3499	652.6452	702.4635	761.6639
70–84	n	104073	150735	176271	198952	124979
	Rate	1059.5561	1138.677	1229.0067	1343.2886	1395.915
0–84	n	291167	389245	421293	464097	293231
	Rate	274.7316	288.7054	306.1942	332.5565	349.7664

* Cohort data not shown – see text

Table C2 Cancer of lip

(a) Mortality, males, 1960–97

Age		1960–4	1965–9	1970–4	1975–9	1980–4	1985–9	1990–4	1995–7
0–14	n	0	1	0	0	0	0	0	0
	Rate	0	0.0036	0	0	0	0	0	0
15–34	n	1	0	0	1	0	0	0	0
	Rate	0.0038	0	0	0.0027	0	0	0	0
35–49	n	9	6	7	6	3	1	2	0
	Rate	0.0375	0.024	0.03	0.0277	0.0135	0.0033	0.0075	0
50–69	n	86	68	68	63	48	30	22	14
	Rate	0.3984	0.2838	0.2594	0.2439	0.1899	0.1229	0.0874	0.0965
70–84	n	180	120	113	102	90	70	51	37
	Rate	3.1467	1.9804	1.7713	1.4415	1.0876	0.7635	0.5238	0.6007
0–84	n	276	195	188	172	141	101	75	51
	Rate	0.3851	0.2497	0.2254	0.1921	0.1443	0.0979	0.0688	0.0765

(b) Incidence, males, 1971–92

Age		1971–4	1975–9	1980–4	1985–9	1990–2
0–14	n	0	0	1	0	0
	Rate	0	0	0.0038	0	0
15–34	n	20	14	11	14	5
	Rate	0.08	0.0404	0.0298	0.0357	0.0212
35–49	n	147	114	95	68	34
	Rate	0.8055	0.5116	0.426	0.2862	0.2244
50–69	n	752	683	560	437	209
	Rate	3.6225	2.6498	2.2227	1.737	1.3896
70–84	n	554	530	473	461	223
	Rate	10.2943	7.0532	5.5286	5.0153	3.9199
0–84	n	1473	1341	1140	980	471
	Rate	1.9122	1.3355	1.0836	0.9056	0.7129

(c) Mortality, females, 1960–97

Age		1960–4	1965–9	1970–4	1975–9	1980–4	1985–9	1990–4	1995–7
0–14	n	1	0	0	0	0	0	1	0
	Rate	0.0031	0	0	0	0	0	0.0034	0
15–34	n	0	0	0	0	0	0	0	0
	Rate	0	0	0	0	0	0	0	0
35–49	n	1	0	0	1	0	0	1	0
	Rate	0.0049	0	0	0.0045	0	0	0.0036	0
50–69	n	11	14	11	5	6	10	3	0
	Rate	0.0398	0.0501	0.037	0.0167	0.0198	0.0368	0.0104	0
70–84	n	19	25	21	30	20	24	23	6
	Rate	0.1841	0.2129	0.1697	0.2208	0.1339	0.1534	0.1344	0.062
0–84	n	32	39	32	36	26	34	28	6
	Rate	0.0272	0.0306	0.0238	0.0248	0.0167	0.0222	0.016	0.0057

(d) Incidence, females, 1971–92

Age		1971–4	1975–9	1980–4	1985–9	1990–2
0–14	n	2	0	0	0	2
	Rate	0.0076	0	0	0	0.0137
15–34	n	2	1	2	4	4
	Rate	0.008	0.0027	0.0057	0.01	0.0157
35–49	n	19	11	18	10	14
	Rate	0.1034	0.051	0.0822	0.0421	0.0884
50–69	n	102	78	88	87	44
	Rate	0.4198	0.268	0.3066	0.3198	0.2767
70–84	n	117	113	151	144	71
	Rate	1.1778	0.8515	1.0459	0.9589	0.7793
0–84	n	242	203	259	245	135
	Rate	0.2231	0.1472	0.1801	0.1692	0.1559

Table C3   Cancer of tongue and mouth

(a) Mortality, males, 1960–97

Age		1960–4	1965–9	1970–4	1975–9	1980–4	1985–9	1990–4	1995–7
0–14	n	3	2	3	1	1	0	1	1
	Rate	0.0115	0.0058	0.0102	0.0032	0.004	0	0.0049	0.0051
15–34	n	13	9	13	29	20	24	28	13
	Rate	0.0418	0.0291	0.0381	0.0801	0.0538	0.0642	0.0723	0.0502
35–49	n	100	115	107	111	149	235	222	121
	Rate	0.4223	0.4922	0.4636	0.5001	0.6682	0.9911	0.8392	0.7172
50–69	n	903	806	781	922	1162	1152	1194	635
	Rate	4.0824	3.3572	3.0366	3.577	4.5779	4.535	4.7792	4.2296
70–84	n	1268	982	854	848	870	855	831	515
	Rate	21.8345	16.1626	12.9215	11.4859	10.2004	9.3201	8.5441	8.5603
0–84	n	2287	1914	1758	1911	2202	2266	2276	1285
	Rate	2.9981	2.3238	1.9535	1.9582	2.0823	2.0515	2.0104	1.8625

(b) Incidence, males, 1971–92

Age		1971–4	1975–9	1980–4	1985–9	1990–2
0–14	n	8	11	9	5	3
	Rate	0.0364	0.04	0.0358	0.0209	0.0265
15–34	n	50	74	73	87	66
	Rate	0.1914	0.2081	0.1975	0.2279	0.2797
35–49	n	261	329	417	582	426
	Rate	1.4171	1.499	1.8653	2.4476	2.7672
50–69	n	1455	2053	2286	2425	1617
	Rate	6.996	7.9077	9.0015	9.5819	10.7227
70–84	n	1091	1227	1241	1327	890
	Rate	20.3701	16.3866	14.3328	14.4439	15.4944
0–84	n	2865	3694	4026	4426	3002
	Rate	3.732	3.5865	3.6993	3.9468	4.3683

(c) Mortality, females, 1960–97

Age		1960–4	1965–9	1970–4	1975–9	1980–4	1985–9	1990–4	1995–7
0–14	n	1	2	1	1	3	0	4	2
	Rate	0.0032	0.0091	0.0028	0.0037	0.0126	0	0.0148	0.0157
15–34	n	11	13	10	9	17	15	8	12
	Rate	0.0359	0.0449	0.0312	0.0247	0.048	0.0426	0.022	0.0542
35–49	n	59	52	49	56	58	67	94	53
	Rate	0.2412	0.214	0.2142	0.2572	0.2625	0.279	0.3612	0.3176
50–69	n	410	401	412	457	466	486	445	236
	Rate	1.47	1.3774	1.3947	1.5453	1.6404	1.7484	1.6517	1.4859
70–84	n	558	551	567	603	661	695	633	367
	Rate	5.3909	4.8751	4.5811	4.512	4.5489	4.5612	4.1297	3.9631
0–84	n	1039	1019	1039	1126	1205	1263	1184	670
	Rate	0.8741	0.8054	0.7767	0.8093	0.8435	0.8672	0.8175	0.7679

(d) Incidence, females, 1971–92

Age		1971–4	1975–9	1980–4	1985–9	1990–2
0–14	n	7	6	9	5	5
	Rate	0.0334	0.0226	0.0378	0.0216	0.0325
15–34	n	34	54	60	53	44
	Rate	0.1266	0.1494	0.165	0.1455	0.1951
35–49	n	134	181	185	241	175
	Rate	0.7278	0.8229	0.837	1.0034	1.1345
50–69	n	795	1066	1077	1099	722
	Rate	3.3616	3.6364	3.8041	3.9602	4.4412
70–84	n	770	974	1101	1154	697
	Rate	7.838	7.3452	7.7003	7.7822	7.8803
0–84	n	1740	2281	2432	2552	1643
	Rate	1.636	1.6727	1.7527	1.8149	1.9704

(e) Birth cohort mortality, ages 35–84 years, males, 1960–97

Year of birth	1875–79	1880–84	1885–89	1890–94	1895–99	1900–4	1905–9	1910–14	1915–19	1920–24	1925–29	1930–34	1935–39	1940–44	1945–49	1950–54	1955–59	1960–64
n	191	600	864	1087	1260	1496	1653	1709	1563	1714	1208	895	668	454	245	89	39	3
U 95% CI	279.3	223.2	161.6	135.3	113	92.8	83.5	79.2	93	100.4	106.6	118.6	137.4	155.2	137.8	130.3	163.6	164
SCMR	242.4	206	151.2	127.5	106.9	88.2	79.5	75.6	88.5	95.8	100.7	111.1	127.3	141.5	121.6	105.9	119.7	56.1
L 95% CI	209.2	190.2	141.4	120.2	101.2	83.9	75.8	72.1	84.2	91.4	95.2	104.1	118	129.1	107.3	85	85.1	11.6

(f) Birth cohort mortality, ages 35–84 years, females, 1960–97

Year of birth	1875–79	1880–84	1885–89	1890–94	1895–99	1900–4	1905–9	1910–14	1915–19	1920–24	1925–29	1930–34	1935–39	1940–44	1945–49	1950–54	1955–59	1960–64
n	84	266	518	617	775	970	1094	1110	838	828	493	356	192	135	102	33	24	1
U 95% CI	168.6	134.8	133.1	111	104.2	102.8	100.7	98.5	103.1	109.5	106.7	122.3	108.2	126.6	148.6	123.9	244.6	240.9
SCMR	136.2	119.5	122.1	102.6	97.1	96.5	94.9	92.8	96.4	102.3	97.7	110.2	93.9	106.9	122.4	88.2	164.4	43.2
L 95% CI	108.6	106	112	94.8	90.5	90.7	89.4	87.5	90.1	95.6	89.5	99.3	81.1	89.6	99.8	60.7	105.3	1.1

(g) Birth cohort incidence, ages 35–84 years, males, 1971–92

Year of birth	1885–89	1890–94	1895–99	1900–4	1905–9	1910–14	1915–19	1920–24	1925–29	1930–34	1935–39	1940–44	1945–49	1950–54	1955–59
n	102	447	809	1402	2125	2435	2230	2683	1942	1360	998	628	350	102	14
U 95% CI	207.6	154.5	118.3	99.2	95.2	92.7	99	105.5	106.6	107.5	122.2	138.2	142.1	138.7	186.8
SCIR	171	140.8	110.5	94.1	91.2	89.1	95	101.6	101.9	101.9	114.8	127.8	128	114.3	111.3
L 95% CI	139.5	128.4	103.1	89.3	87.4	85.6	91.1	97.8	97.5	96.7	107.9	118.2	115.3	93.2	60.9

(h) Birth cohort incidence, ages 35–84 years, females, 1971–92

Year of birth	1885–89	1890–94	1895–99	1900–4	1905–9	1910–14	1915–19	1920–24	1925–29	1930–34	1935–39	1940–44	1945–49	1950–54	1955–59
n	74	339	727	1143	1574	1561	1309	1320	898	603	348	245	164	58	8
U 95% CI	137.4	115.3	108.9	100.9	101.3	98.9	108.6	108.9	112.4	113.1	101.4	125.9	146.2	161.2	267.1
SCIR	109.4	103.6	101.3	95.3	96.4	94.1	102.9	103.2	105.3	104.4	91.3	111	125.4	124.7	135.6
L 95% CI	85.9	93.2	94.2	89.9	91.8	89.5	97.5	97.8	98.6	96.4	82.2	98	107	94.7	58.5

Table C4 Cancer of pharynx

(a) Mortality, males, 1960–97

Age		1960–4	1965–9	1970–4	1975–9	1980–4	1985–9	1990–4	1995–7
0–14	n	2	3	2	1	2	2	0	0
	Rate	0.0071	0.011	0.0069	0.0037	0.0076	0.0096	0	0
15–34	n	12	16	6	8	8	5	9	1
	Rate	0.0383	0.0486	0.0178	0.0232	0.0214	0.0138	0.0224	0.0049
35–49	n	62	75	80	92	95	134	152	106
	Rate	0.2579	0.3182	0.3413	0.4108	0.4296	0.568	0.5754	0.6224
50–69	n	694	771	853	821	886	917	1039	633
	Rate	3.1196	3.1569	3.3216	3.1806	3.4864	3.6531	4.133	4.1886
70–84	n	708	699	720	634	623	599	652	396
	Rate	12.042	11.3272	10.7784	8.5358	7.2403	6.5235	6.7445	6.5963
0–84	n	1478	1564	1661	1556	1614	1657	1852	1136
	Rate	1.8538	1.8109	1.7905	1.5664	1.5181	1.5115	1.6395	1.641

(b) Incidence, males, 1971–92

Age		1971–4	1975–9	1980–4	1985–9	1990–2
0–14	n	5	9	0	6	1
	Rate	0.0221	0.0301	0	0.0257	0.0059
15–34	n	26	24	23	18	12
	Rate	0.0997	0.067	0.0634	0.0512	0.0495
35–49	n	140	194	211	282	223
	Rate	0.757	0.8735	0.9456	1.1863	1.4369
50–69	n	999	1307	1548	1590	1067
	Rate	4.8135	5.0626	6.1105	6.2838	7.0554
70–84	n	741	818	884	835	605
	Rate	13.6912	10.7811	10.236	9.1047	10.534
0–84	n	1911	2352	2666	2731	1908
	Rate	2.4889	2.2883	2.4743	2.4527	2.7939

(c) Mortality, females, 1960–97

Age		1960–4	1965–9	1970–4	1975–9	1980–4	1985–9	1990–4	1995–7
0–14	n	2	2	3	0	0	0	0	0
	Rate	0.0066	0.0098	0.0104	0	0	0	0	0
15–34	n	22	12	11	5	6	4	0	2
	Rate	0.0743	0.0412	0.0346	0.0168	0.0163	0.012	0	0.0085
35–49	n	171	132	104	69	48	53	45	25
	Rate	0.6993	0.5533	0.4401	0.3144	0.22	0.2305	0.1706	0.1484
50–69	n	685	693	619	606	519	480	358	196
	Rate	2.4104	2.3652	2.0868	2.0825	1.8256	1.7093	1.3217	1.2342
70–84	n	483	492	482	487	477	470	429	255
	Rate	4.6863	4.3889	3.9511	3.6828	3.3445	3.2217	2.8535	2.8343
0–84	n	1363	1331	1219	1167	1050	1007	832	478
	Rate	1.1101	1.0374	0.9138	0.8583	0.7537	0.7173	0.5838	0.5615

(d) Incidence, females, 1971–92

Age		1971–4	1975–9	1980–4	1985–9	1990–2
0–14	n	3	1	5	1	0
	Rate	0.0135	0.0033	0.021	0.0036	0
15–34	n	21	17	13	14	6
	Rate	0.0807	0.0522	0.0358	0.0396	0.0252
35–49	n	134	127	119	121	84
	Rate	0.7264	0.5801	0.5416	0.5179	0.5378
50–69	n	758	956	825	736	437
	Rate	3.1922	3.2908	2.9107	2.6539	2.7042
70–84	n	472	630	653	603	358
	Rate	4.8229	4.7664	4.591	4.193	4.054
0–84	n	1388	1731	1615	1475	885
	Rate	1.3029	1.2826	1.1746	1.0748	1.0715

(e) Birth cohort mortality, ages 35–84 years, males, 1960–97

Year of birth	1875–79	1880–84	1885–89	1890–94	1895–99	1900–4	1905–9	1910–14	1915–19	1920–24	1925–29	1930–34	1935–39	1940–44	1945–49	1950–54	1955–59	1960–64
n	96	300	534	810	1032	1257	1351	1435	1283	1363	1077	751	537	335	193	66	18	3
U 95% CI	242.1	175.9	145.6	137.9	121.2	99.8	86.7	84.6	94.8	96.7	112.7	118.6	134.6	150.6	156.3	158.4	178.5	395.7
SCMR	198.2	157.1	133.8	128.7	114	94.4	82.2	80.3	89.7	91.7	106.2	110.4	123.6	135.3	135.7	124.5	112.9	135.4
L 95% CI	160.6	140.3	122.9	120.1	107.3	89.3	77.9	76.3	85	87	100	102.8	113.6	121.5	117.3	96.3	66.9	27.9

(f) Birth cohort mortality, ages 35–84 years, females, 1960–97

Year of birth	1875–79	1880–84	1885–89	1890–94	1895–99	1900–4	1905–9	1910–14	1915–19	1920–24	1925–29	1930–34	1935–39	1940–44	1945–49	1950–54	1955–59	1960–64
n	49	188	405	596	777	1006	1116	1218	914	901	518	310	193	104	48	28	7	0
U 95% CI	176.6	146.8	142.2	132.1	120	116.7	108.6	111.1	106.8	103.8	90.2	81.5	78	71.4	56.9	87.9	82.3	
SCMR	133.6	127.3	129	121.9	111.9	109.7	102.5	105.1	100.1	97.2	82.7	72.9	67.7	58.9	42.9	60.8	40	
L 95% CI	98.8	109.7	117	112.5	104.3	103.2	96.6	99.3	93.8	91.1	75.9	65.3	58.5	48.1	31.7	40.4	16.1	

(g) Birth cohort incidence, ages 35–84 years, males, 1971–92

Year of birth	1885–89	1890–94	1895–99	1900–4	1905–9	1910–14	1915–19	1920–24	1925–29	1930–34	1935–39	1940–44	1945–49	1950–54	1955–59
n	59	270	569	990	1422	1632	1554	1719	1295	860	522	348	162	36	6
U 95% CI	192.7	150.2	128.6	104.9	94.6	92	102.6	103.4	113.3	114	115.9	149	142.3	138.5	321.2
SCIR	149.4	133.3	118.4	98.6	89.8	87.6	97.7	98.6	107.3	106.6	106.4	134.1	122	100	147.6
L 95% CI	113.7	118.3	109.1	92.6	85.3	83.5	92.9	94.1	101.6	99.7	97.6	120.7	103.9	70.1	54.2

(h) Birth cohort incidence, ages 35–84 years, females, 1971–92

Year of birth	1885–89	1890–94	1895–99	1900–4	1905–9	1910–14	1915–19	1920–24	1925–29	1930–34	1935–39	1940–44	1945–49	1950–54	1955–59
n	31	206	421	741	1034	1084	998	1008	629	395	234	134	70	27	1
U 95% CI	127.9	139	117.1	111.2	106.7	101.2	113.4	108.8	103.4	100.4	99.9	109.9	112.4	165.2	220.4
SCIR	90.1	121.2	106.4	103.5	100.4	95.3	106.6	102.2	95.6	91	87.9	92.8	89	113.5	39.5
L 95% CI	61.2	105.8	96.8	96.3	94.4	89.8	100.2	96.1	88.4	82.4	77.3	77.8	69.4	74.8	1

Table C5 Cancer of oesophagus

(a) Mortality, males, 1960–97

Age		1960–4	1965–9	1970–4	1975–9	1980–4	1985–9	1990–4	1995–7
0–14	n	0	0	0	1	0	0	0	0
	Rate	0	0	0	0.0039	0	0	0	0
15–34	n	26	14	26	35	38	50	35	33
	Rate	0.0866	0.0449	0.0815	0.1013	0.1032	0.1357	0.0835	0.1281
35–49	n	320	390	474	446	475	596	738	516
	Rate	1.3209	1.6287	2.0166	2.0073	2.1346	2.5151	2.7963	3.0572
50–69	n	3075	3786	4425	4984	5571	6453	7089	4271
	Rate	13.6618	15.3637	17.2404	19.3909	22.1285	25.5451	28.2711	28.5136
70–84	n	2953	3094	3489	4028	4986	6266	7533	5025
	Rate	50.1425	50.4238	52.1693	53.4609	58.149	68.2381	77.8612	83.4925
0–84	n	6374	7284	8414	9494	11070	13365	15395	9845
	Rate	7.8827	8.3251	8.9789	9.5763	10.6327	12.3908	13.9104	14.5419

(b) Incidence, males, 1971–92

Age		1971–4	1975–9	1980–4	1985–9	1990–2
0–14	n	0	1	1	4	1
	Rate	0	0.0039	0.0039	0.0157	0.0081
15–34	n	25	38	48	54	25
	Rate	0.0963	0.107	0.1316	0.1478	0.108
35–49	n	401	501	532	646	495
	Rate	2.1496	2.2531	2.3945	2.7295	3.1944
50–69	n	3779	5366	5626	6539	4294
	Rate	18.2806	20.8494	22.3616	25.953	28.4062
70–84	n	2849	4104	4988	6212	4248
	Rate	52.4692	54.2246	58.1495	67.6659	74.2137
0–84	n	7054	10010	11195	13455	9063
	Rate	9.2636	10.013	10.7397	12.4729	13.6843

(c) Mortality, females, 1960–97

Age		1960–4	1965–9	1970–4	1975–9	1980–4	1985–9	1990–4	1995–7
0–14	n	0	0	0	0	0	0	0	0
	Rate	0	0	0	0	0	0	0	0
15–34	n	20	18	14	12	10	7	15	13
	Rate	0.0684	0.0621	0.048	0.0329	0.0288	0.0186	0.0384	0.053
35–49	n	272	251	266	225	201	223	225	120
	Rate	1.0999	1.0255	1.1363	1.0245	0.9164	0.954	0.8571	0.7037
50–69	n	2004	2200	2372	2593	2549	2568	2609	1565
	Rate	7.2327	7.5732	7.9572	8.8242	8.975	9.171	9.5824	9.848
70–84	n	2574	2991	3392	3972	4506	5187	5736	3580
	Rate	24.8454	26.4469	27.6515	29.7688	30.9247	34.0534	37.1882	38.9787
0–84	n	4870	5460	6044	6802	7266	7985	8585	5278
	Rate	4.0946	4.3019	4.5126	4.8739	4.993	5.3276	5.6955	5.8959

(d) Incidence, females, 1971–92

Age		1971–4	1975–9	1980–4	1985–9	1990–2
0–14	n	1	0	0	5	0
	Rate	0.0057	0	0	0.0217	0
15–34	n	17	23	17	25	9
	Rate	0.074	0.0666	0.0479	0.0693	0.0356
35–49	n	248	257	266	239	156
	Rate	1.338	1.1669	1.2106	1.019	1.0185
50–69	n	2211	2996	3054	3050	1876
	Rate	9.2375	10.1591	10.7523	10.9195	11.3985
70–84	n	2822	4171	4686	5378	3600
	Rate	28.5725	31.318	32.2549	35.5161	39.3469
0–84	n	5299	7447	8023	8697	5641
	Rate	4.9241	5.3458	5.5647	5.8786	6.3217

(e) Birth cohort mortality, ages 35–84 years, males, 1960–97

Year of birth	1875–79	1880–84	1885–89	1890–94	1895–99	1900–4	1905–9	1910–14	1915–19	1920–24	1925–29	1930–34	1935–39	1940–44	1945–49	1950–54	1955–59	1960–64
n	331	1279	2414	3630	4919	7738	9580	11696	10403	11032	7516	4599	2863	1646	866	369	96	5
U 95% CI	97.3	92	82.7	80.8	78.1	85.9	88.2	100.2	114.1	121	128.1	125.7	133.6	142.2	136	167.6	155.3	135.7
SCMR	87.4	87.1	79.5	78.2	76	84	86.4	98.4	111.9	118.8	125.2	122.1	128.8	135.5	127.2	151.3	127.1	58.2
L 95% CI	78.4	82.4	76.4	75.7	73.9	82.2	84.7	96.6	109.8	116.6	122.4	118.6	124.2	129.1	119	136.6	103	18.9

(f) Birth cohort mortality, ages 35–84 years, females, 1960–97

Year of birth	1875–79	1880–84	1885–89	1890–94	1895–99	1900–4	1905–9	1910–14	1915–19	1920–24	1925–29	1930–34	1935–39	1940–44	1945–49	1950–54	1955–59	1960–64
n	349	1326	2390	3551	4726	6115	7381	8279	6142	5212	3096	1745	957	531	272	88	19	2
U 95% CI	87.2	88.1	83.3	89.1	91.5	95.5	101.8	111.6	118.3	115.4	119.2	114	108.7	111	101.1	99.3	86.3	175.2
SCMR	78.5	83.5	80	86.2	88.9	93.1	99.5	109.2	115.4	112.3	115.1	108.8	102	102	89.8	80.6	55.3	48.5
L 95% CI	70.7	79.1	76.9	83.4	86.4	90.8	97.2	106.9	112.6	109.3	111.1	103.8	95.8	93.7	79.7	64.7	33.3	5.9

(g) Birth cohort incidence, ages 35–84 years, males, 1971–92

Year of birth	1885–89	1890–94	1895–99	1900–4	1905–9	1910–14	1915–19	1920–24	1925–29	1930–34	1935–39	1940–44	1945–49	1950–54	1955–59
n	199	1095	2511	5217	7842	8880	7470	7413	4656	2588	1469	771	346	116	7
U 95% CI	94.3	92.3	90.2	94.3	95.2	99.1	109	110.6	114.2	108.8	114.8	127.4	124.8	161.5	161.2
SCIR	82	87	86.8	91.8	93.1	97.1	106.6	108.1	111	104.7	109	118.7	112.3	134.6	78.2
L 95% CI	71	82	83.4	89.3	91.1	95.1	104.2	105.7	107.9	100.8	103.6	110.6	101.1	111.2	31.4

(h) Birth cohort incidence, ages 35–84 years, females, 1971–92

Year of birth	1885–89	1890–94	1895–99	1900–4	1905–9	1910–14	1915–19	1920–24	1925–29	1930–34	1935–39	1940–44	1945–49	1950–54	1955–59
n	302	1482	3008	4928	6500	6332	4402	3640	2204	1157	594	286	134	34	7
U 95% CI	94.1	94	94	97.5	100.5	107.6	112	106.6	114.2	107.8	105.4	109.5	110.2	109.5	255.8
SCIR	84	89.4	90.7	94.8	98.1	105	108.8	103.2	109.6	101.8	97.2	97.5	93	78.3	124.2
L 95% CI	75.1	84.9	87.5	92.2	95.8	102.4	105.6	99.9	105.1	96.1	89.7	86.8	77.9	54.2	49.9

Table C6 Cancer of stomach

(a) Mortality, males, 1960-97

Age		1960-4	1965-9	1970-4	1975-9	1980-4	1985-9	1990-4	1995-7
0-14	n	1	2	1	1	0	1	1	0
	Rate	0.0041	0.0076	0.0034	0.0037	0	0.0047	0.0046	0
15-34	n	163	145	113	100	56	84	63	45
	Rate	0.541	0.4713	0.3534	0.289	0.1534	0.2274	0.1556	0.1774
35-49	n	2318	1836	1604	1206	981	847	745	364
	Rate	9.6407	7.6886	6.8782	5.4392	4.4102	3.5829	2.8248	2.1562
50-69	n	19877	19233	18037	15455	12716	10754	8603	3967
	Rate	87.5715	78.3507	70.3771	60.1925	50.7621	42.772	34.3139	26.6008
70-84	n	14962	14337	14589	15458	15829	14995	12790	6748
	Rate	251.463	231.5355	216.7878	203.8101	184.2383	163.2689	131.9291	111.7399
0-84	n	37321	35553	34344	32220	29582	26681	22202	11124
	Rate	44.2954	40.0646	36.7715	33.0603	28.9585	25.1465	20.2441	16.5753

(b) Incidence, males, 1971-92

Age		1971-4	1975-9	1980-4	1985-9	1990-2
0-14	n	2	1	2	8	3
	Rate	0.0088	0.0031	0.0079	0.034	0.0188
15-34	n	111	131	115	133	68
	Rate	0.4329	0.372	0.3141	0.3605	0.2812
35-49	n	1443	1514	1396	1235	654
	Rate	7.8145	6.8458	6.2783	5.2139	4.237
50-69	n	15118	17163	15649	13812	7381
	Rate	73.4752	66.8375	62.3546	54.9043	48.7599
70-84	n	11640	15971	17595	17329	9397
	Rate	213.4906	209.8077	204.4188	188.6117	163.7222
0-84	n	28314	34780	34757	32517	17503
	Rate	37.3417	35.3499	33.7498	30.4856	26.6418

(c) Mortality, females, 1960-97

Age		1960-4	1965-9	1970-4	1975-9	1980-4	1985-9	1990-4	1995-7
0-14	n	0	0	0	1	1	0	0	0
	Rate	0	0	0	0.0039	0.0041	0	0	0
15-34	n	155	114	98	70	74	63	65	35
	Rate	0.5181	0.3847	0.312	0.2004	0.2062	0.1706	0.1673	0.1426
35-49	n	1175	954	843	609	480	396	385	212
	Rate	4.7674	3.9544	3.6526	2.781	2.18	1.6694	1.4816	1.3031
50-69	n	10212	9112	7850	6687	5151	4203	3251	1542
	Rate	36.9	31.2867	26.2524	22.6018	18.0451	14.9994	11.8945	9.7005
70-84	n	15191	14371	13823	13269	12056	10521	8439	4048
	Rate	146.7211	127.2568	112.729	99.3674	82.5381	68.2841	53.8208	43.4445
0-84	n	26733	24551	22614	20636	17762	15183	12140	5837
	Rate	22.6291	19.4173	16.8964	14.6752	12.0185	9.934	7.8852	6.4082

(d) Incidence, females, 1971-92

Age		1971-4	1975-9	1980-4	1985-9	1990-2
0-14	n	0	3	0	5	1
	Rate	0	0.0119	0	0.0238	0.0062
15-34	n	91	99	114	113	59
	Rate	0.3523	0.2849	0.3159	0.3023	0.2487
35-49	n	742	726	585	596	343
	Rate	4.053	3.325	2.6602	2.5083	2.2183
50-69	n	6617	7485	6262	5315	2677
	Rate	27.6569	25.2621	21.9546	18.9866	16.1733
70-84	n	10821	13792	13336	12155	6302
	Rate	109.6128	103.5864	91.594	79.3717	67.6367
0-84	n	18271	22105	20297	18184	9382
	Rate	17.0022	15.7731	13.8304	12.026	10.2554

(e) Birth cohort mortality, ages 35–84 years, males, 1960–97

Year of birth	1875–79	1880–84	1885–89	1890–94	1895–99	1900–4	1905–9	1910–14	1915–19	1920–24	1925–29	1930–34	1935–39	1940–44	1945–49	1950–54	1955–59	1960–64
n	1438	5503	11430	17683	23361	32569	36087	33546	22580	19989	11823	6274	3129	1603	834	291	95	16
U 95% CI	142.3	133.3	131.6	132	126	124.4	115.5	100.7	87.1	77.9	73.2	64.4	56.8	55.9	52.5	50.5	53	93.3
SCMR	135.2	129.9	129.2	130.1	124.4	123.1	114.3	99.6	86	76.9	71.9	62.8	54.8	53.2	49.1	45	43.4	57.4
L 95% CI	128.4	126.5	126.8	128.2	122.8	121.8	113.1	98.5	84.9	75.8	70.6	61.2	52.9	50.7	45.9	40.1	35.1	32.8

(f) Birth cohort mortality, ages 35–84 years, females, 1960–97

Year of birth	1875–79	1880–84	1885–89	1890–94	1895–99	1900–4	1905–9	1910–14	1915–19	1920–24	1925–29	1930–34	1935–39	1940–44	1945–49	1950–54	1955–59	1960–64
n	2067	7197	12346	16655	18897	20741	20230	17453	10554	8516	4937	2435	1369	664	409	209	89	12
U 95% CI	173	162.5	146.3	143.6	127.4	114.3	99.4	84.3	73.3	69.1	71.7	61.7	60.8	53.2	53.4	65.4	77.3	109.6
SCMR	165.7	158.7	143.8	141.4	125.6	112.8	98	83.1	71.9	67.6	69.7	59.3	57.6	49.3	48.5	57.1	62.8	62.7
L 95% CI	158.7	155.1	141.3	139.3	123.9	111.3	96.7	81.8	70.5	66.2	67.8	57	54.7	45.7	44	49.8	50.4	32.4

(g) Birth cohort incidence, ages 35–84 years, males, 1971–92

Year of birth	1885–89	1890–94	1895–99	1900–4	1905–9	1910–14	1915–19	1920–24	1925–29	1930–34	1935–39	1940–44	1945–49	1950–54	1955–59
n	788	4219	9797	19773	27935	27968	19231	17175	10195	5353	2761	1302	601	181	17
U 95% CI	112.1	108.3	107.4	110.7	107.8	102.6	96.3	93.7	97.5	92	90.4	88	82.2	86.1	106.3
SCIR	104.5	105.1	105.3	109.2	106.6	101.4	94.9	92.3	95.6	89.6	87.1	83.4	75.9	74.4	66.4
L 95% CI	97.5	102	103.2	107.7	105.3	100.2	93.6	90.9	93.7	87.2	83.9	79	70	64	38.7

(h) Birth cohort incidence, ages 35–84 years, females, 1971–92

Year of birth	1885–89	1890–94	1895–99	1900–4	1905–9	1910–14	1915–19	1920–24	1925–29	1930–34	1935–39	1940–44	1945–49	1950–54	1955–59
n	1183	5511	10354	15347	17576	14260	8517	6867	3950	2021	1133	557	342	126	10
U 95% CI	125.2	122.5	115.3	110.9	102.4	95.7	91.5	91.4	98.2	89.7	89.8	83.3	91.1	106.6	110.1
SCIR	118.2	119.3	113.1	109.1	100.9	94.1	89.5	89.2	95.2	85.9	84.7	76.7	82	89.5	59.9
L 95% CI	111.7	116.2	110.9	107.4	99.4	92.6	87.6	87.2	92.3	82.2	79.9	70.6	73.7	74.6	28.7

Table C7 Cancers of colon and rectum

(a) Mortality, males, 1960–97

Age		1960–4	1965–9	1970–4	1975–9	1980–4	1985–9	1990–4	1995–7
0-14	n	4	1	5	4	1	2	1	0
	Rate	0.0152	0.0048	0.0194	0.0148	0.004	0.0096	0.0052	0
15-34	n	247	197	232	218	186	162	126	68
	Rate	0.8168	0.6305	0.7144	0.6078	0.5148	0.4281	0.3087	0.2705
35-49	n	1830	1904	1892	1747	1665	1579	1464	792
	Rate	7.6499	8.0164	8.1833	7.9017	7.4631	6.6394	5.5613	4.6918
50-69	n	14074	15205	15960	15913	15302	15768	15384	8364
	Rate	63.0211	62.3545	62.3432	61.9164	60.9152	62.5971	61.4389	56.033
70-84	n	14809	14826	15952	17556	19182	20513	20544	11729
	Rate	251.9503	241.7687	240.0463	235.907	226.0947	223.6078	211.6495	194.3435
0-84	n	30964	32133	34041	35438	36336	38024	37519	20953
	Rate	38.6688	37.5913	37.4885	36.9302	35.6984	35.6682	34.084	31.1344

(b) Incidence, males, 1971–92

Age		1971–4	1975–9	1980–4	1985–9	1990–2
0-14	n	12	13	6	14	6
	Rate	0.0562	0.0478	0.0238	0.0607	0.0477
15-34	n	369	463	415	375	224
	Rate	1.4107	1.2953	1.1349	1.0027	0.9347
35-49	n	2518	3097	3057	3205	2010
	Rate	13.7213	14.0153	13.7101	13.4646	12.9824
50-69	n	19153	25019	26064	27430	17583
	Rate	92.8298	97.1513	103.642	108.834	116.4021
70-84	n	16221	23528	28143	31197	19995
	Rate	300.0969	312.1437	329.0022	339.7442	348.6621
0-84	n	38273	52120	57685	62221	39818
	Rate	50.9288	53.004	55.8762	57.9313	60.3088

(c) Mortality, females, 1960–97

Age		1960–4	1965–9	1970–4	1975–9	1980–4	1985–9	1990–4	1995–7
0-14	n	5	2	1	1	0	1	0	1
	Rate	0.0208	0.0098	0.0044	0.0039	0	0.005	0	0.0086
15-34	n	206	209	165	147	141	96	102	43
	Rate	0.6923	0.7043	0.5283	0.425	0.3924	0.2735	0.2593	0.1833
35-49	n	2110	1951	1776	1487	1313	1364	1244	649
	Rate	8.574	8.1148	7.6459	6.8183	5.9741	5.7649	4.7229	3.8471
50-69	n	14450	14963	14811	14143	12694	12184	10805	5264
	Rate	51.8848	51.2686	49.7506	48.0736	44.6131	43.7021	39.9044	33.107
70-84	n	18926	19722	20954	22245	22174	21874	20330	11219
	Rate	182.7313	174.4326	170.702	166.3607	152.0919	143.3224	131.5277	122.0049
0-84	n	35697	36847	37707	38023	36322	35519	32481	17176
	Rate	29.9749	28.9954	28.1799	27.2327	24.9972	23.9173	21.8055	19.256

(d) Incidence, females, 1971–92

Age		1971–4	1975–9	1980–4	1985–9	1990–2
0-14	n	26	14	14	16	3
	Rate	0.1271	0.0538	0.0575	0.0706	0.0229
15-34	n	365	443	348	372	193
	Rate	1.4373	1.279	0.9667	1.0216	0.8328
35-49	n	2428	2780	2709	2836	1783
	Rate	13.2444	12.7507	12.3188	11.9739	11.5551
50-69	n	17636	22262	21933	21635	12966
	Rate	73.875	75.7588	77.2381	77.7002	79.254
70-84	n	20301	28975	32060	33658	20714
	Rate	205.8472	217.7178	221.3906	223.2085	226.8864
0-84	n	40756	54474	57064	58517	35659
	Rate	38.0211	39.3771	39.8697	40.0968	40.6356

(e) Birth cohort mortality, ages 35–84 years, males, 1960–97

Year of birth	1875–79	1880–84	1885–89	1890–94	1895–99	1900–4	1905–9	1910–14	1915–19	1920–24	1925–29	1930–34	1935–39	1940–44	1945–49	1950–54	1955–59	1960–64
n	1797	6487	11790	17525	22959	31563	36229	37557	28454	28173	18089	11053	6276	3361	1795	624	198	24
U 95% CI	121.7	116.7	107.1	108.4	105.7	104.1	100	97.1	96.8	99.4	102.7	103	99.6	96.2	86.2	75.2	69.7	79.3
SCMR	116.2	113.9	105.2	106.8	104.3	102.9	99	96.1	95.7	98.2	101.3	101.1	97.2	93	82.3	69.5	60.7	53.3
L 95% CI	110.9	111.1	103.3	105.2	103	101.8	98	95.2	94.6	97.1	99.8	99.2	94.8	89.9	78.6	64.3	52.5	34.2

(f) Birth cohort mortality, ages 35–84 years, females, 1960–97

Year of birth	1875–79	1880–84	1885–89	1890–94	1895–99	1900–4	1905–9	1910–14	1915–19	1920–24	1925–29	1930–34	1935–39	1940–44	1945–49	1950–54	1955–59	1960–64
n	2651	9148	16417	23271	29226	34284	37105	36789	25435	23198	13624	7853	4559	2540	1489	486	161	21
U 95% CI	125.4	120.1	113.7	115.5	111.4	104.9	99.8	96.4	94	95.8	94.5	89.1	85	82.3	78.7	64.5	61.8	83.4
SCMR	120.7	117.7	112	114	110.1	103.8	98.7	95.4	92.8	94.6	92.9	87.2	82.6	79.2	74.8	59	53	54.6
L 95% CI	116.2	115.3	110.3	112.6	108.8	102.7	97.7	94.4	91.7	93.4	91.4	85.3	80.2	76.2	71.1	54	45.1	33.8

(g) Birth cohort incidence, ages 35–84 years, males, 1971–92

Year of birth	1885–89	1890–94	1895–99	1900–4	1905–9	1910–14	1915–19	1920–24	1925–29	1930–34	1935–39	1940–44	1945–49	1950–54	1955–59
n	1250	6227	15031	29182	41919	44604	33323	31878	19923	12172	6820	3458	1835	536	61
U 95% CI	97.2	91.2	97.2	98.8	98.7	100.6	102.1	103.7	107.5	109.5	107.1	104.8	103.8	98.4	103.6
SCIR	91.9	89	95.6	97.7	97.8	99.6	101	102.5	106	107.6	104.5	101.3	99.1	90.4	80.7
L 95% CI	87	86.8	94.1	96.6	96.9	98.7	99.9	101.4	104.6	105.7	102.1	98	94.7	83	61.7

(h) Birth cohort incidence, ages 35–84 years, females, 1971–92

Year of birth	1885–89	1890–94	1895–99	1900–4	1905–9	1910–14	1915–19	1920–24	1925–29	1930–34	1935–39	1940–44	1945–49	1950–54	1955–59
n	2087	10319	21273	33676	43971	41560	28771	26767	15881	9618	5524	3073	1645	454	56
U 95% CI	95.5	98.7	99.8	99.3	100.3	101.8	102.2	104.7	103.9	103.1	100.7	104.3	101.4	89	109.1
SCIR	91.5	96.8	98.5	98.2	99.4	100.9	101	103.4	102.3	101	98.1	100.7	96.6	81.2	84
L 95% CI	87.7	95	97.2	97.2	98.5	99.9	99.8	102.2	100.8	99	95.6	97.2	92	74.1	63.5

Table C8 Cancer of pancreas

(a) Mortality, males, 1960–97

Age		1960–4	1965–9	1970–4	1975–9	1980–4	1985–9	1990–4	1995–7
0–14	n	6	1	0	1	0	1	2	1
	Rate	0.0216	0.0036	0	0.0031	0	0.0037	0.0086	0.0081
15–34	n	41	44	58	66	45	47	32	17
	Rate	0.1342	0.1486	0.186	0.1871	0.1234	0.1248	0.0765	0.0663
35–49	n	707	759	757	657	690	647	626	369
	Rate	2.9437	3.1826	3.2328	2.9649	3.1001	2.7184	2.3695	2.1868
50–69	n	5550	6555	7129	7202	6753	6300	5672	3296
	Rate	24.4612	26.6503	27.7495	28.0273	26.8074	25.0545	22.6135	22.0192
70–84	n	4115	4677	5227	6192	6791	6997	6998	3945
	Rate	69.2179	75.5955	77.8098	81.4681	79.0868	76.2171	72.312	65.3501
0–84	n	10419	12036	13171	14118	14279	13992	13330	7628
	Rate	12.3224	13.4343	13.8996	14.2508	13.7671	13.0505	12.0782	11.271

(b) Incidence, males, 1971–92

Age		1971–4	1975–9	1980–4	1985–9	1990–2
0–14	n	1	4	4	2	1
	Rate	0.0042	0.0145	0.0159	0.0086	0.0059
15–34	n	58	58	57	66	32
	Rate	0.2301	0.1567	0.1556	0.1771	0.1314
35–49	n	622	718	719	668	417
	Rate	3.354	3.2483	3.2311	2.7993	2.6936
50–69	n	5638	7110	6814	6304	3638
	Rate	27.3259	27.6895	27.0601	25.0518	24.0747
70–84	n	4088	6154	6873	7166	4375
	Rate	75.1102	80.7981	80.0331	78.0483	76.3977
0–84	n	10407	14044	14467	14206	8463
	Rate	13.5938	14.1582	13.9462	13.2498	12.8496

(c) Mortality, females, 1960–97

Age		1960–4	1965–9	1970–4	1975–9	1980–4	1985–9	1990–4	1995–7
0–14	n	1	0	0	4	0	3	0	0
	Rate	0.0034	0	0	0.0149	0	0.0133	0	0
15–34	n	27	33	33	38	44	35	31	18
	Rate	0.091	0.1114	0.1035	0.1085	0.1229	0.0993	0.0825	0.075
35–49	n	406	455	433	395	345	412	411	209
	Rate	1.642	1.8733	1.835	1.7929	1.5775	1.7493	1.5713	1.2341
50–69	n	3898	4378	4715	4844	4649	4738	4366	2423
	Rate	14.0492	15.0154	15.8444	16.3883	16.3365	16.8891	16.0129	15.2491
70–84	n	4659	5364	6060	6894	7448	7996	7919	4723
	Rate	45.0855	47.6419	49.5538	51.8544	51.5752	53.1886	51.9207	51.9762
0–84	n	8991	10230	11241	12175	12486	13184	12727	7373
	Rate	7.5616	8.0561	8.4054	8.7339	8.6599	8.956	8.607	8.3818

(d) Incidence, females, 1971–92

Age		1971–4	1975–9	1980–4	1985–9	1990–2
0–14	n	1	3	1	7	0
	Rate	0.0057	0.011	0.0043	0.0327	0
15–34	n	31	39	50	57	27
	Rate	0.1203	0.1092	0.138	0.158	0.116
35–49	n	350	439	369	432	281
	Rate	1.8835	1.9935	1.6843	1.8311	1.8454
50–69	n	3691	4819	4723	4809	2780
	Rate	15.4632	16.3555	16.6024	17.1313	16.8313
70–84	n	4643	6743	7567	8253	5032
	Rate	47.167	50.7938	52.3846	54.831	55.1852
0–84	n	8716	12043	12710	13558	8120
	Rate	8.1167	8.6641	8.8173	9.1969	9.1465

(e) Birth cohort mortality, ages 35–84 years, males, 1960–97

Year of birth	1875–79	1880–84	1885–89	1890–94	1895–99	1900–4	1905–9	1910–14	1915–19	1920–24	1925–29	1930–34	1935–39	1940–44	1945–49	1950–54	1955–59	1960–64
n	392	1651	3348	5645	8001	11696	14067	14753	11757	10984	6949	4264	2532	1458	781	251	80	2
U 95% CI	98.5	100.8	95.8	103.7	104.8	107	106.6	104.1	105.6	98	96.2	94.1	94.4	99.6	94.1	84.9	93.6	55.4
SCMR	89.2	96.1	92.6	101	102.5	105.1	104.8	102.4	103.7	96.2	94	91.4	90.8	94.6	87.7	75	75.2	15.3
L 95% CI	80.8	91.6	89.5	98.4	100.3	103.2	103.1	100.8	101.8	94.4	91.8	88.7	87.4	89.9	81.7	66.3	59.6	1.9

(f) Birth cohort mortality, ages 35–84 years, females, 1960–97

Year of birth	1875–79	1880–84	1885–89	1890–94	1895–99	1900–4	1905–9	1910–14	1915–19	1920–24	1925–29	1930–34	1935–39	1940–44	1945–49	1950–54	1955–59	1960–64
n	559	2149	4277	6414	8507	10894	12503	13037	9743	8778	5166	2908	1640	879	465	167	48	6
U 95% CI	95.3	94.8	94.3	98.1	98.4	101.2	102.4	104.1	107.8	107.3	108	103.4	102.4	101.5	97	99.2	98.9	170.2
SCMR	87.7	90.9	91.5	95.8	96.4	99.3	100.6	102.3	105.6	105.1	105.1	99.7	97.6	95	88.5	85.2	74.6	78.2
L 95% CI	80.8	87.1	88.8	93.5	94.3	97.5	98.9	100.6	103.6	102.9	102.2	96.2	93	88.9	80.8	72.8	55	28.7

(g) Birth cohort incidence, ages 35–84 years, males, 1971–92

Year of birth	1885–89	1890–94	1895–99	1900–4	1905–9	1910–14	1915–19	1920–24	1925–29	1930–34	1935–39	1940–44	1945–49	1950–54	1955–59
n	281	1521	3699	7461	10742	11216	8687	7709	4607	2699	1440	794	363	74	11
U 95% CI	101.8	99.4	103	105.7	104.2	102.1	105.7	99.3	99.2	100	98	109.2	101.6	81.8	154.6
SCIR	90.6	94.5	99.7	103.3	102.3	100.3	103.5	97.1	96.4	96.3	93.1	101.9	91.6	65.2	86.4
L 95% CI	80.6	89.9	96.6	101	100.4	98.4	101.3	95	93.7	92.7	88.4	95	82.7	51.2	43.1

(h) Birth cohort incidence, ages 35–84 years, females, 1971–92

Year of birth	1885–89	1890–94	1895–99	1900–4	1905–9	1910–14	1915–19	1920–24	1925–29	1930–34	1935–39	1940–44	1945–49	1950–54	1955–59
n	457	2226	4784	8147	10408	9711	6773	5797	3230	1742	897	450	225	77	7
U 95% CI	95.2	94.2	96.7	102.4	101.7	103	106.8	106.4	107.3	104.4	101.3	106.7	112	140.1	164.1
SCIR	86.9	90.4	94	100.2	99.8	101	104.2	103.7	103.6	99.7	94.9	97.3	98.3	112.1	79.7
L 95% CI	79.3	86.7	91.4	98	97.9	99	101.8	101	100.1	95.1	88.9	88.7	86.2	88.4	32

Table C9 Cancer of larynx

(a) Mortality, males, 1960–97

Age		1960–4	1965–9	1970–4	1975–9	1980–4	1985–9	1990–4	1995–7
0–14	n	0	0	0	0	0	0	0	0
	Rate	0	0	0	0	0	0	0	0
15–34	n	10	7	6	9	3	3	2	3
	Rate	0.0334	0.023	0.0199	0.0261	0.0083	0.0087	0.0052	0.0132
35–49	n	147	130	146	129	131	126	150	103
	Rate	0.6042	0.545	0.6196	0.5836	0.5891	0.5343	0.5665	0.6028
50–69	n	1613	1515	1471	1461	1494	1598	1458	761
	Rate	7.212	6.2597	5.7165	5.6549	5.9088	6.3547	5.8151	5.0753
70–84	n	1273	1183	1318	1331	1353	1451	1459	875
	Rate	21.438	19.1118	19.4759	17.7134	15.8574	15.8319	15.0697	14.4426
0–84	n	3043	2835	2941	2930	2981	3178	3069	1742
	Rate	3.6778	3.2405	3.1667	2.9865	2.8671	2.9533	2.769	2.5574

(b) Incidence, males, 1971–92

Age		1971–4	1975–9	1980–4	1985–9	1990–2
0–14	n	2	1	1	6	0
	Rate	0.0083	0.0031	0.0039	0.0242	0
15–34	n	20	30	33	28	8
	Rate	0.0718	0.0875	0.0921	0.0765	0.034
35–49	n	440	540	532	542	365
	Rate	2.3808	2.4287	2.3951	2.2893	2.3801
50–69	n	3447	4316	4373	4615	2615
	Rate	16.5291	16.6745	17.2447	18.216	17.28
70–84	n	1649	2206	2476	2708	1809
	Rate	29.5496	28.3367	28.3627	29.4831	31.6789
0–84	n	5558	7093	7415	7899	4797
	Rate	6.8042	6.7368	6.8603	7.1579	7.1521

(c) Mortality, females, 1960–97

Age		1960–4	1965–9	1970–4	1975–9	1980–4	1985–9	1990–4	1995–7
0–14	n	0	0	0	0	0	0	0	0
	Rate	0	0	0	0	0	0	0	0
15–34	n	3	5	3	4	4	2	1	0
	Rate	0.0096	0.0172	0.0094	0.012	0.0111	0.006	0.0028	0
35–49	n	68	44	39	38	25	30	28	15
	Rate	0.2739	0.1834	0.1632	0.1737	0.114	0.1271	0.1072	0.0878
50–69	n	372	359	342	399	404	396	339	173
	Rate	1.321	1.2327	1.1497	1.3639	1.4236	1.3968	1.247	1.0892
70–84	n	275	251	233	317	386	357	436	256
	Rate	2.6649	2.2261	1.921	2.4039	2.7098	2.43	2.938	2.9711
0–84	n	718	659	617	758	819	785	804	444
	Rate	0.5876	0.514	0.4617	0.5559	0.5864	0.5555	0.5648	0.5288

(d) Incidence, females, 1971–92

Age		1971–4	1975–9	1980–4	1985–9	1990–2
0–14	n	0	1	3	2	0
	Rate	0	0.0039	0.0124	0.0089	0
15–34	n	20	27	19	11	10
	Rate	0.0817	0.0759	0.0536	0.032	0.0438
35–49	n	123	112	110	125	78
	Rate	0.6679	0.5082	0.5001	0.5287	0.5158
50–69	n	600	935	836	949	533
	Rate	2.5129	3.1997	2.9469	3.424	3.2616
70–84	n	278	459	511	617	424
	Rate	2.8492	3.4909	3.6303	4.3426	4.934
0–84	n	1021	1534	1479	1704	1045
	Rate	0.9589	1.1398	1.0905	1.2588	1.277

(e) Birth cohort mortality, ages 35–84 years, males, 1960–97

Year of birth	1875–79	1880–84	1885–89	1890–94	1895–99	1900–4	1905–9	1910–14	1915–19	1920–24	1925–29	1930–34	1935–39	1940–44	1945–49	1950–54	1955–59	1960–64
n	121	488	955	1486	2106	2748	2879	2942	2447	2592	1674	1010	602	378	173	59	13	2
U 95% CI	145.3	137.7	125	122.3	122.4	111	96.3	91.7	97.3	101.7	102.1	99.6	102.4	123	109.3	124.9	124.6	372
SCMR	121.6	126	117.3	116.3	117.3	107	92.8	88.5	93.5	97.9	97.3	93.7	94.5	111.2	94.2	96.8	72.9	103
L 95% CI	100.9	115.3	110.1	110.5	112.4	103	89.5	85.3	89.9	94.2	92.8	88.1	87.3	100.6	80.7	73.7	38.8	12.5

(f) Birth cohort mortality, ages 35–84 years, females, 1960–97

Year of birth	1875–79	1880–84	1885–89	1890–94	1895–99	1900–4	1905–9	1910–14	1915–19	1920–24	1925–29	1930–34	1935–39	1940–44	1945–49	1950–54	1955–59	1960–64
n	33	130	197	282	452	559	782	797	711	742	444	205	128	75	34	6	5	0
U 95% CI	181	150.8	102.4	92.4	101.1	94.4	111.2	108.1	124.7	130.5	121.5	89.4	94.5	105.3	96.6	74.1	220.3	
SCMR	128.9	127	89.1	82.2	92.2	86.9	103.6	100.9	115.8	121.5	110.7	78	79.5	84	69.1	34.1	94.4	
L 95% CI	88.7	106.1	77.1	73.2	84.1	80	96.6	94.1	107.6	113	100.9	68	66.3	66.1	47.9	12.5	30.6	

(g) Birth cohort incidence, ages 35–84 years, males, 1971–92

Year of birth	1885–89	1890–94	1895–99	1900–4	1905–9	1910–14	1915–19	1920–24	1925–29	1930–34	1935–39	1940–44	1945–49	1950–54	1955–59
n	72	479	1308	2791	4340	5358	4965	5468	3547	2102	1213	640	270	78	2
U 95% CI	103.1	107.1	108.7	102.5	97.6	98.9	106.2	108.7	106.1	100.9	104.6	114.1	103.8	122.2	77
SCIR	81.9	97.9	102.9	98.8	94.8	96.3	103.3	105.8	102.7	96.7	98.8	105.6	92.1	97.9	21.3
L 95% CI	64.1	89.5	97.5	95.2	92	93.8	100.4	103.1	99.4	92.7	93.4	97.7	81.8	77.4	2.6

(h) Birth cohort incidence, ages 35–84 years, females, 1971–92

Year of birth	1885–89	1890–94	1895–99	1900–4	1905–9	1910–14	1915–19	1920–24	1925–29	1930–34	1935–39	1940–44	1945–49	1950–54	1955–59
n	18	117	246	519	890	1086	1016	1171	734	443	230	138	66	15	1
U 95% CI	115.8	109	88.2	93.2	101.7	105.4	114.1	121.2	114.5	110.5	101.2	122.3	120	113.5	204.4
SCIR	73.3	91	77.8	85.5	95.2	99.3	107.3	114.4	106.5	100.7	88.9	103.6	94.4	68.8	36.7
L 95% CI	43.4	75.2	68.7	78.5	89.2	93.6	100.9	108	99.1	91.7	78.1	87	73	38.5	1

Table C10 Cancer of lung

(a) Mortality, males, 1960–97

Age		1960–4	1965–9	1970–4	1975–9	1980–4	1985–9	1990–4	1995–7
0–14	n	5	9	3	6	4	1	1	1
	Rate	0.0189	0.026	0.0097	0.0214	0.0157	0.0049	0.0035	0.0074
15–34	n	390	318	310	221	158	105	105	52
	Rate	1.306	1.0385	0.9644	0.631	0.4373	0.2952	0.2711	0.205
35–49	n	6771	6416	5640	4342	3451	3134	2972	1520
	Rate	28.1027	26.72	23.909	19.4493	15.5582	13.3022	11.2717	8.9174
50–69	n	66341	73769	74534	69778	61382	53769	44598	21794
	Rate	288.5953	298.8985	289.7356	271.6088	244.4886	213.2946	178.088	146.2576
70–84	n	26276	34813	45482	55532	62294	61715	57392	31651
	Rate	431.8096	551.7807	660.2884	719.4733	719.0825	671.5812	593.0575	525.3651
0–84	n	99783	115325	125969	129879	127289	118724	105068	55018
	Rate	108.6574	121.6401	129.0833	129.6483	122.8912	111.2071	95.8628	82.1893

(b) Incidence, males, 1971–92

Age		1971–4	1975–9	1980–4	1985–9	1990–2
0–14	n	10	7	10	13	5
	Rate	0.0396	0.0255	0.0388	0.0505	0.0315
15–34	n	309	326	225	180	108
	Rate	1.1871	0.9225	0.6201	0.4939	0.4651
35–49	n	5187	5366	4222	3855	2245
	Rate	27.7918	24.0522	19.0065	16.3593	14.5828
50–69	n	63567	75629	67870	59525	31877
	Rate	307.3723	294.1722	269.9704	236.0248	210.7434
70–84	n	35366	53881	62690	63375	36434
	Rate	632.4302	694.0258	722.1084	689.7621	635.694
0–84	n	104439	135209	135017	126948	70669
	Rate	131.1655	133.1804	129.4518	118.4965	107.6277

(c) Mortality, females, 1960–97

Age		1960–4	1965–9	1970–4	1975–9	1980–4	1985–9	1990–4	1995–7
0–14	n	7	5	3	2	0	2	6	3
	Rate	0.0276	0.0212	0.0116	0.008	0	0.0097	0.0219	0.0229
15–34	n	125	131	99	104	91	76	58	31
	Rate	0.4211	0.4393	0.3207	0.3043	0.2554	0.218	0.152	0.1308
35–49	n	1808	2038	2058	1770	1573	1665	1834	1057
	Rate	7.3575	8.3851	8.7262	8.0067	7.181	7.0855	6.9537	6.2555
50–69	n	9456	12811	15929	19213	21455	22595	21058	11136
	Rate	33.6019	43.6698	53.6103	65.4386	75.4846	80.2734	77.0604	69.701
70–84	n	5515	7460	10330	13816	18984	23813	27082	17776
	Rate	53.5916	67.0007	85.2886	105.0919	133.9913	164.695	185.6988	203.0967
0–84	n	16911	22445	28419	34905	42103	48151	50038	30003
	Rate	13.769	17.406	21.2995	25.5921	30.2998	34.1531	35.3377	35.1884

(d) Incidence, females, 1971–92

Age		1971–4	1975–9	1980–4	1985–9	1990–2
0–14	n	6	6	6	13	3
	Rate	0.0303	0.0227	0.0245	0.0557	0.0185
15–34	n	132	151	152	197	83
	Rate	0.5276	0.4416	0.4245	0.5462	0.3742
35–49	n	1966	2081	1969	2141	1401
	Rate	10.5306	9.4172	8.976	9.0878	9.0846
50–69	n	14038	21014	24067	25606	14777
	Rate	58.9473	71.6842	84.7864	91.2195	89.3317
70–84	n	8066	13700	19724	25039	16912
	Rate	82.6382	104.3304	139.5562	173.4925	194.2707
0–84	n	24208	36952	45918	52996	33176
	Rate	22.6178	27.1941	33.2349	37.8373	39.2732

(e) Birth cohort mortality, ages 35–84 years, males, 1960–97

Year of birth	1875–79	1880–84	1885–89	1890–94	1895–99	1900–4	1905–9	1910–14	1915–19	1920–24	1925–29	1930–34	1935–39	1940–44	1945–49	1950–54	1955–59	1960–64
n	1200	7397	21438	45308	79443	120817	140853	140943	105388	98675	58311	28778	14729	7301	3411	1101	245	23
U 95% CI	44.1	59.7	74.7	95.3	115.1	121.3	117.8	110.5	103	93.6	85.1	68.5	63.1	63.2	58.8	59.1	49.1	53.7
SCMR	41.7	58.4	73.7	94.4	114.3	120.6	117.2	109.9	102.4	93	84.4	67.7	62.1	61.7	56.9	55.7	43.3	35.8
L 95% CI	39.4	57.1	72.7	93.6	113.5	120	116.6	109.4	101.8	92.5	83.8	66.9	61.1	60.3	55	52.5	38.2	22.7

(f) Birth cohort mortality, ages 35–84 years, females, 1960–97

Year of birth	1875–79	1880–84	1885–89	1890–94	1895–99	1900–4	1905–9	1910–14	1915–19	1920–24	1925–29	1930–34	1935–39	1940–44	1945–49	1950–54	1955–59	1960–64
n	464	2079	5097	9443	16092	24980	34852	44475	39788	41526	26601	13016	6765	3872	2207	755	203	17
U 95% CI	45.2	45.5	48.6	55.7	66.3	79.4	95.6	116.6	133.2	139.2	139.5	109.4	96.2	98.5	97.7	93.2	88.1	87.9
SCMR	41.3	43.6	47.3	54.6	65.3	78.4	94.6	115.6	131.9	137.9	137.8	107.5	94	95.4	93.7	86.7	76.8	54.9
L 95% CI	37.7	41.8	46	53.5	64.3	77.5	93.7	114.5	130.6	136.6	136.2	105.7	91.7	92.5	89.9	80.8	66.9	32

(g) Birth cohort incidence, ages 35–84 years, males, 1971–92

Year of birth	1885–89	1890–94	1895–99	1900–4	1905–9	1910–14	1915–19	1920–24	1925–29	1930–34	1935–39	1940–44	1945–49	1950–54	1955–59
n	1417	9994	30633	69137	103456	112116	85850	78198	43948	20201	9614	4289	1757	452	27
U 95% CI	69.5	82.8	99.9	108.6	107.3	104.1	103.1	98.7	95.3	81.2	79.1	82.8	80.6	83.4	62.2
SCIR	66	81.2	98.8	107.8	106.6	103.5	102.4	98	94.4	80.1	77.5	80.4	76.9	76	42.8
L 95% CI	62.6	79.6	97.7	107	106	102.9	101.7	97.3	93.5	79	76	78	73.4	69.3	28.2

(h) Birth cohort incidence, ages 35–84 years, females, 1971–92

Year of birth	1885–89	1890–94	1895–99	1900–4	1905–9	1910–14	1915–19	1920–24	1925–29	1930–34	1935–39	1940–44	1945–49	1950–54	1955–59
n	507	2948	8370	17758	29414	36082	30693	30729	19001	8783	4414	2271	1220	284	27
U 95% CI	60	61.3	71.4	82.6	94.5	106.6	115.5	118.2	120.6	97.9	92.4	99.2	112.3	99.3	113.1
SCIR	55	59.1	69.9	81.4	93.4	105.5	114.3	116.9	118.9	95.8	89.7	95.2	106.2	88.4	77.8
L 95% CI	50.4	57	68.4	80.2	92.4	104.4	113	115.6	117.2	93.8	87.1	91.3	100.4	78.7	51.2

Table C11 Cancer of pleura

(a) Mortality, males, 1960–97

Age		1960–4	1965–9	1970–4	1975–9	1980–4	1985–9	1990–4	1995–7
0–14	n	1	0	0	2	1	0	0	0
	Rate	0.0044	0	0	0.0068	0.0036	0	0	0
15–34	n	4	6	8	9	2	5	3	1
	Rate	0.0129	0.0181	0.0242	0.0245	0.0057	0.0144	0.0076	0.0036
35–49	n	25	43	66	100	108	153	153	54
	Rate	0.1078	0.1783	0.2816	0.4515	0.4863	0.6422	0.5896	0.3121
50–69	n	108	213	340	557	754	1101	1191	641
	Rate	0.4501	0.8478	1.3086	2.1533	2.9664	4.3642	4.7438	4.2695
70–84	n	33	58	135	242	362	578	783	560
	Rate	0.5532	0.926	1.9513	3.0868	4.1174	6.2935	8.1132	9.2901
0–84	n	171	320	549	910	1227	1837	2130	1256
	Rate	0.174	0.309	0.525	0.8471	1.1208	1.6583	1.8979	1.8513

(b) Incidence, males, 1971–92

Age		1971–4	1975–9	1980–4	1985–9	1990–2
0–14	n	1	0	1	1	2
	Rate	0.0047	0	0.004	0.0043	0.014
15–34	n	7	14	7	9	7
	Rate	0.0258	0.0397	0.02	0.0239	0.0291
35–49	n	62	118	151	264	208
	Rate	0.3353	0.5344	0.6786	1.1124	1.3478
50–69	n	357	681	1047	1673	1368
	Rate	1.7227	2.6189	4.1341	6.617	9.026
70–84	n	123	289	557	982	944
	Rate	2.177	3.646	6.3433	10.6866	16.4537
0–84	n	550	1102	1763	2929	2529
	Rate	0.6479	1.019	1.6212	2.6457	3.7521

(c) Mortality, females, 1960–97

Age		1960–4	1965–9	1970–4	1975–9	1980–4	1985–9	1990–4	1995–7
0–14	n	0	0	0	0	0	0	0	0
	Rate	0	0	0	0	0	0	0	0
15–34	n	2	5	8	8	4	3	0	0
	Rate	0.0064	0.0152	0.0245	0.0213	0.0111	0.009	0	0
35–49	n	16	27	23	25	29	15	30	12
	Rate	0.0639	0.1108	0.1002	0.1177	0.1315	0.0625	0.1145	0.0725
50–69	n	58	85	117	142	148	167	191	73
	Rate	0.2045	0.2878	0.3984	0.4771	0.5216	0.6016	0.7034	0.4546
70–84	n	39	51	55	64	114	134	175	103
	Rate	0.3789	0.4603	0.4599	0.4893	0.8072	0.9832	1.2525	1.1598
0–84	n	115	168	203	239	295	319	396	188
	Rate	0.0932	0.13	0.1553	0.1774	0.2158	0.2367	0.2904	0.2197

(d) Incidence, females, 1971–92

Age		1971–4	1975–9	1980–4	1985–9	1990–2
0–14	n	0	1	1	0	0
	Rate	0	0.0033	0.0041	0	0
15–34	n	8	8	7	5	4
	Rate	0.0305	0.0249	0.0194	0.0157	0.0151
35–49	n	19	33	33	47	51
	Rate	0.1025	0.1563	0.1499	0.194	0.3268
50–69	n	116	212	246	311	268
	Rate	0.4915	0.7177	0.8625	1.1068	1.642
70–84	n	59	121	183	246	260
	Rate	0.6062	0.9232	1.3034	1.7151	3.0894
0–84	n	202	375	470	609	583
	Rate	0.1915	0.279	0.3432	0.4407	0.7084

(e) Birth cohort mortality, ages 35–84 years, males, 1960–97

Year of birth	1875–79	1880–84	1885–89	1890–94	1895–99	1900–4	1905–9	1910–14	1915–19	1920–24	1925–29	1930–34	1935–39	1940–44	1945–49	1950–54	1955–59	1960–64
n	2	14	33	89	166	451	634	1108	1150	1545	1225	821	567	349	150	49	5	0
U 95% CI	37.3	28.2	22.5	30.3	34.9	58.2	64.4	100.8	124.8	151.1	170.7	167.3	180.8	196.5	148.4	140.7	85.6	
SCMR	10.3	16.8	16	24.6	30	53	59.6	95.1	117.8	143.8	161.4	156.2	166.5	176.9	126.4	106.4	36.7	
L 95% CI	1.3	9.2	11	19.7	25.6	48.4	55.1	89.6	111.2	136.8	152.6	145.9	153.4	159.3	107	78.7	11.9	

(f) Birth cohort mortality, ages 35–84 years, females, 1960–97

Year of birth	1875–79	1880–84	1885–89	1890–94	1895–99	1900–4	1905–9	1910–14	1915–19	1920–24	1925–29	1930–34	1935–39	1940–44	1945–49	1950–54	1955–59	1960–64
n	3	17	28	53	88	138	201	278	307	304	209	108	64	57	26	6	5	1
U 95% CI	161.6	114.7	67.8	65.3	69.3	79.3	95.4	122	163.2	150.7	158.5	132.5	128.7	181.5	134.6	92.6	224.8	1005.6
SCMR	55.3	71.7	46.9	50	56.3	67.1	83.1	108.5	146	134.6	138.4	109.8	100.8	140.1	91.8	42.5	96.3	180.5
L 95% CI	11.4	41.8	31.2	37.4	45.1	56.4	72.4	96.5	130.5	120.3	120.8	90	77.6	106.1	60	15.6	31.3	4.7

(g) Birth cohort incidence, ages 35–84 years, males, 1971–92

Year of birth	1885–89	1890–94	1895–99	1900–4	1905–9	1910–14	1915–19	1920–24	1925–29	1930–34	1935–39	1940–44	1945–49	1950–54	1955–59
n	6	35	108	480	875	1332	1306	1613	1229	772	564	331	142	30	1
U 95% CI	56.4	35.8	37.3	69.8	77.9	96.4	109.8	123.5	136.8	131.8	164.2	186.7	167.9	154.9	219.3
SCIR	25.9	25.7	30.9	63.8	72.9	91.4	104	117.6	129.4	122.8	151.2	167.6	142.5	108.5	39.4
L 95% CI	9.5	17.9	25.4	58.4	68.3	86.6	98.5	112	122.4	114.4	139.2	150.5	120	73.2	1

(h) Birth cohort incidence, ages 35–84 years, females, 1971–92

Year of birth	1885–89	1890–94	1895–99	1900–4	1905–9	1910–14	1915–19	1920–24	1925–29	1930–34	1935–39	1940–44	1945–49	1950–54	1955–59
n	6	19	64	158	262	354	386	386	236	124	87	70	44	8	1
U 95% CI	137.6	63.5	68.7	80.5	87.1	104.8	140	139.2	140.5	120.5	138.5	198.7	199.2	160.9	1171.5
SCIR	63.2	40.7	53.8	68.9	77.2	94.4	126.7	126	123.7	101.1	112.3	157.3	148.4	81.7	210.3
L 95% CI	23.2	24.5	41.5	58.6	68.4	85.1	114.7	114.1	108.8	84.1	90	122.6	107.8	35.3	5.5

Table C12   Cancer of bone

(a) Mortality, males, 1960–97

Age		1960–4	1965–9	1970–4	1975–9	1980–4	1985–9	1990–4	1995–7
0–14	n	64	84	92	94	78	49	37	23
	Rate	0.2555	0.3504	0.3462	0.3402	0.3095	0.2262	0.175	0.1695
15–34	n	241	257	235	219	238	215	199	112
	Rate	0.786	0.7808	0.6992	0.6125	0.6231	0.5565	0.5412	0.5346
35–49	n	153	168	109	95	70	73	71	47
	Rate	0.6473	0.7149	0.4844	0.4334	0.308	0.2999	0.2718	0.2885
50–69	n	601	571	536	443	219	198	184	95
	Rate	2.5923	2.3184	2.0776	1.7072	0.8661	0.786	0.7381	0.6139
70–84	n	432	407	384	317	195	149	145	86
	Rate	7.2841	6.5516	5.7619	4.201	2.2539	1.6215	1.4924	1.3925
0–84	n	1491	1487	1356	1168	800	684	636	363
	Rate	1.6479	1.5501	1.3578	1.0959	0.7063	0.5915	0.549	0.5123

(b) Incidence, males, 1971–92

Age		1971–4	1975–9	1980–4	1985–9	1990–2
0–14	n	158	184	181	144	78
	Rate	0.7356	0.6653	0.7208	0.6428	0.5975
15–34	n	238	339	370	375	213
	Rate	0.8879	0.9468	0.9712	0.9787	0.9578
35–49	n	108	138	143	143	108
	Rate	0.6133	0.6348	0.633	0.5807	0.6981
50–69	n	303	332	358	334	184
	Rate	1.478	1.2931	1.4006	1.3123	1.2189
70–84	n	187	238	276	213	115
	Rate	3.373	3.1574	3.1576	2.3159	2.017
0–84	n	994	1231	1328	1209	698
	Rate	1.1664	1.1132	1.1554	1.0355	0.9926

(c) Mortality, females, 1960–97

Age		1960–4	1965–9	1970–4	1975–9	1980–4	1985–9	1990–4	1995–7
0–14	n	101	85	80	77	83	63	35	21
	Rate	0.425	0.3606	0.3143	0.297	0.3483	0.3034	0.1719	0.1667
15–34	n	137	158	140	138	159	114	112	58
	Rate	0.453	0.5005	0.4296	0.4005	0.4349	0.3134	0.3303	0.308
35–49	n	87	84	71	62	47	44	43	25
	Rate	0.3575	0.357	0.3106	0.2878	0.2117	0.1791	0.1693	0.1558
50–69	n	438	373	348	246	131	118	79	47
	Rate	1.5604	1.2811	1.1777	0.8404	0.4616	0.4198	0.2906	0.2927
70–84	n	443	363	385	318	204	169	163	77
	Rate	4.2778	3.23	3.1389	2.3936	1.4193	1.1421	1.0807	0.8509
0–84	n	1206	1063	1024	841	624	508	432	228
	Rate	1.026	0.8692	0.7988	0.6395	0.4739	0.3872	0.3295	0.2985

(d) Incidence, females, 1971–92

Age		1971–4	1975–9	1980–4	1985–9	1990–2
0–14	n	116	160	191	147	65
	Rate	0.5564	0.6102	0.8028	0.708	0.5308
15–34	n	156	230	223	236	131
	Rate	0.5964	0.668	0.6095	0.6496	0.6268
35–49	n	70	83	90	107	65
	Rate	0.3954	0.3932	0.4067	0.4406	0.4281
50–69	n	228	260	254	240	107
	Rate	0.9601	0.876	0.8932	0.8669	0.6502
70–84	n	190	228	279	236	129
	Rate	1.9312	1.7183	1.9449	1.5504	1.4527
0–84	n	760	961	1037	966	497
	Rate	0.7554	0.7498	0.7986	0.7552	0.6529

(e) Birth cohort mortality, ages 0–29, 30–84 years, males, 1960–97

Ages 0–29 years

Year of birth	1875–79	1880–84	1885–89	1890–94	1895–99	1900–04	1905–09	1910–14	1915–19	1920–24	1925–29	1930–34	1935–39	1940–44	1945–49	1950–54	1955–59	1960–64	1965–69	1970–74	1975–79	1980–84	1985–89
n	–	–	–	–	–	–	–	–	–	–	–	18	59	147	274	235	265	348	287	226	114	40	14
U 95% CI												218	150	130.4	130.6	110.4	113.3	126.1	106.7	109.2	94	75.8	101.4
SCMR												137.9	116.3	111	116	97.1	100.5	113.5	95	95.8	78.2	55.6	60.4
L 95% CI												81.7	88.5	93.8	103	85.5	89.1	102.2	84.7	84.1	64.5	39.8	33

Ages 30–84 years

Year of birth	1875–79	1880–84	1885–89	1890–94	1895–99	1900–04	1905–09	1910–14	1915–19	1920–24	1925–29	1930–34	1935–39	1940–44	1945–49	1950–54	1955–59	1960–64	1965–69	1970–74	1975–79	1980–84	1985–89
n	57	156	328	495	569	756	754	669	502	503	344	283	161	111	117	72	40	30	9	–	–	–	–
U 95% CI	351.1	230.5	218.6	201.6	160.3	144	115.9	93.7	86.6	79.7	76	86.9	71	70.1	89.4	95.2	87.8	117.1	253.2				
SCMR	271	197.1	196.2	184.6	147.7	134.1	107.9	86.8	79.4	73.1	68.4	77.4	60.8	58.2	74.6	75.6	64.5	82.1	133.4				
L 95% CI	205.2	167.4	176	169	136	124.9	100.5	80.5	72.7	66.9	61.5	68.9	51.8	47.9	61.7	59.2	46.1	55.4	61				

(f) Birth cohort mortality, ages 0–29, 30–84 years, females, 1960–97

Ages 0–29 years

Year of birth	1875–79	1880–84	1885–89	1890–94	1895–99	1900–04	1905–09	1910–14	1915–19	1920–24	1925–29	1930–34	1935–39	1940–44	1945–49	1950–54	1955–59	1960–64	1965–69	1970–74	1975–79	1980–84	1985–89
n	–	–	–	–	–	–	–	–	–	–	–	10	30	79	183	185	189	230	187	175	94	38	18
U 95% CI												287.6	157	135.4	139.4	130.5	120.1	122.2	102.7	120.1	99.9	73.2	110.8
SCMR												156.4	110	108.7	120.6	113	104.2	107.4	89	103.5	81.6	53.3	70.1
L 95% CI												75	74.2	86	103.7	97.3	89.9	94.4	76.7	88.8	66	37.7	41.5

Ages 30–84 years

Year of birth	1875–79	1880–84	1885–89	1890–94	1895–99	1900–04	1905–09	1910–14	1915–19	1920–24	1925–29	1930–34	1935–39	1940–44	1945–49	1950–54	1955–59	1960–64	1965–69	1970–74	1975–79	1980–84	1985–89
n	63	185	313	501	538	535	587	485	326	304	207	126	103	68	67	50	26	23	1	–	–	–	–
U 95% CI	314	226	182	193.1	153.4	120.3	113.8	90.1	80.7	76.3	78.8	71	82.6	76.8	88.2	109.3	94.2	139.1	123.5				
SCMR	245.4	195.7	162.9	176.9	140.9	110.5	104.9	82.4	72.4	68.2	68.7	59.6	68.1	60.6	69.4	82.9	64.3	92.7	22.2				
L 95% CI	188.6	168.5	145.8	162	129.5	101.5	96.8	75.4	64.9	61	60	49.7	55.6	47	53.8	61.6	42	58.8	0.6				

(g) Birth cohort incidence, ages 0–29, 30–84 years, males, 1971–92

Ages 0–29 years

Year of birth	1885–89	1890–94	1895–99	1900–4	1905–9	1910–14	1915–19	1920–24	1925–29	1930–34	1935–39	1940–44	1945–49	1950–54	1955–59	1960–64	1965–69	1970–74	1975–79	1980–84	1985–89
n	–	–	–	–	–	–	–	–	–	–	–	11	90	163	304	515	456	334	146	68	13
U 95% CI												115.5	128.3	104.3	102.9	117.7	110.5	116	112.2	138.2	127.4
SCIR												64.5	104.4	89.5	92	108	100.8	104.2	95.4	109.1	74.5
L 95% CI												32.2	83.9	76.3	82.2	99	92	93.6	80.6	84.7	39.7

Ages 30–84 years

Year of birth	1885–89	1890–94	1895–99	1900–4	1905–9	1910–14	1915–19	1920–24	1925–29	1930–34	1935–39	1940–44	1945–49	1950–54	1955–59	1960–64	1965–69	1970–74	1975–79	1980–84	1985–89
n	8	78	146	280	414	440	337	385	318	273	186	174	162	111	37	10	–				
U 95% CI	151.3	185.5	136.7	120.2	115.2	106	97.8	103.1	115.1	123.8	102.2	109.5	117.7	144.3	107.1	198.5					
SCIR	76.8	148.6	116.3	106.9	104.6	96.6	87.9	93.3	103.1	109.9	88.5	94.4	100.9	119.8	77.7	107.9					
L 95% CI	33.1	117.5	98.2	95.1	95	88	79	84.4	92.4	97.6	76.3	80.9	85.9	98.5	54.7	51.7					

(h) Birth cohort incidence, ages 0–29, 30–84 years, females, 1971–92

Ages 0–29 years

Year of birth	1885–89	1890–94	1895–99	1900–4	1905–9	1910–14	1915–19	1920–24	1925–29	1930–34	1935–39	1940–44	1945–49	1950–54	1955–59	1960–64	1965–69	1970–74	1975–79	1980–84	1985–89
n	–	–	–	–	–	–	–	–	–	–	–	13	51	119	209	329	310	281	153	44	11
U 95% CI												183.2	120.7	130.7	110	108.8	105.6	127.5	132.2	101.7	115.2
SCIR												107.1	91.8	109.2	96	97.7	94.4	113.4	112.8	75.8	64.4
L 95% CI												57.1	68.4	90.5	83.9	87.7	84.5	100.9	95.6	55.1	32.1

Ages 30–84 years

Year of birth	1885–89	1890–94	1895–99	1900–4	1905–9	1910–14	1915–19	1920–24	1925–29	1930–34	1935–39	1940–44	1945–49	1950–54	1955–59	1960–64	1965–69	1970–74	1975–79	1980–84	1985–89
n	17	82	164	292	393	358	280	292	207	133	139	115	109	73	37	9	–				
U 95% CI	162	128.2	117.5	120.7	118.4	107.2	110.2	111.2	112.5	96.8	117.8	112.5	119	140.3	145.9	275.3					
SCIR	101.2	103.3	100.9	107.6	107.2	96.7	98	99.1	98.1	81.7	99.8	93.7	98.6	111.5	105.9	145					
L 95% CI	58.9	82.1	86	96	97.1	87.2	87.2	88.4	85.6	68.4	83.9	77.4	81	87.4	74.5	66.3					

Table C13 Cancer of soft tissues

(a) Mortality, males, 1960-97

Age		1960-4	1965-9	1970-4	1975-9	1980-4	1985-9	1990-4	1995-7
0-14	n	162	198	209	154	45	45	42	30
	Rate	0.5516	0.6306	0.6685	0.5556	0.1773	0.1821	0.1667	0.1908
15-34	n	98	107	103	129	146	164	184	102
	Rate	0.3163	0.3287	0.2914	0.3601	0.3866	0.4271	0.4677	0.4444
35-49	n	109	103	105	114	143	152	201	117
	Rate	0.4641	0.4411	0.4705	0.5258	0.6333	0.6256	0.7698	0.711
50-69	n	311	269	245	298	473	544	553	313
	Rate	1.3662	1.0476	0.95	1.1586	1.8662	2.17	2.1899	2.0971
70-84	n	142	137	125	216	377	400	472	325
	Rate	2.4066	2.2329	1.8399	2.8381	4.3668	4.3506	4.8567	5.3449
0-84	n	822	814	787	911	1184	1305	1452	887
	Rate	0.8144	0.7442	0.6882	0.8335	1.0794	1.1567	1.2425	1.2544

(b) Incidence, males, 1971-92

Age		1971-4	1975-9	1980-4	1985-9	1990-2
0-14	n	224	220	142	146	103
	Rate	0.9178	0.8065	0.5546	0.5841	0.6704
15-34	n	189	263	296	345	245
	Rate	0.6816	0.7239	0.7874	0.8982	1.0561
35-49	n	200	300	314	399	323
	Rate	1.1138	1.3971	1.3891	1.6286	2.0958
50-69	n	410	666	917	907	662
	Rate	1.9512	2.5535	3.6156	3.5773	4.413
70-84	n	196	421	571	653	475
	Rate	3.5924	5.5323	6.5879	7.0993	8.2967
0-84	n	1219	1870	2240	2450	1808
	Rate	1.3542	1.7057	2.0027	2.1238	2.5667

(c) Mortality, females, 1960-97

Age		1960-4	1965-9	1970-4	1975-9	1980-4	1985-9	1990-4	1995-7
0-14	n	126	164	160	104	42	38	34	27
	Rate	0.4541	0.5387	0.5286	0.3876	0.1716	0.1595	0.1424	0.1767
15-34	n	92	87	93	81	110	124	116	73
	Rate	0.3018	0.2729	0.2882	0.2294	0.3001	0.3323	0.314	0.3169
35-49	n	83	92	78	81	129	143	157	107
	Rate	0.345	0.3978	0.3499	0.3748	0.5864	0.5931	0.603	0.6587
50-69	n	235	240	239	237	382	408	469	339
	Rate	0.8203	0.8227	0.8061	0.8134	1.3479	1.4737	1.7783	2.121
70-84	n	190	199	184	250	376	435	518	291
	Rate	1.8371	1.7728	1.508	1.8948	2.6142	2.9206	3.4646	3.281
0-84	n	726	782	754	753	1039	1148	1294	837
	Rate	0.5962	0.6088	0.5748	0.5695	0.7681	0.8325	0.9423	1.0187

(d) Incidence, females, 1971-92

Age		1971-4	1975-9	1980-4	1985-9	1990-2
0-14	n	159	177	122	148	81
	Rate	0.684	0.6822	0.5014	0.6322	0.5643
15-34	n	151	219	284	294	191
	Rate	0.5679	0.6208	0.7772	0.7842	0.8429
35-49	n	178	194	269	328	271
	Rate	1.017	0.908	1.2131	1.3593	1.7733
50-69	n	377	523	726	748	519
	Rate	1.5907	1.8016	2.5726	2.7216	3.2027
70-84	n	280	472	582	656	494
	Rate	2.8628	3.5781	4.0735	4.4452	5.4821
0-84	n	1145	1585	1983	2174	1556
	Rate	1.1079	1.2165	1.4965	1.6185	1.8972

(e) Birth cohort mortality, ages 35–84 years, males, 1960–97

Year of birth	1875–79	1880–84	1885–89	1890–94	1895–99	1900–4	1905–9	1910–14	1915–19	1920–24	1925–29	1930–34	1935–39	1940–44	1945–49	1950–54	1955–59	1960–64
n	17	54	105	183	287	461	643	828	732	820	644	455	376	256	202	113	53	15
U 95% CI	124.7	83.3	72.4	75.6	80.7	86.2	95.3	109.4	116.7	117.9	128.6	128.5	146.9	140.3	137.6	141.9	145.9	305.9
SCMR	77.9	63.8	59.8	65.4	71.8	78.7	88.2	102.2	108.6	110.1	119	117.2	132.8	124.1	119.8	118	111.5	185.5
L 95% CI	45.4	47.9	48.9	56.2	64	71.8	81.6	95.5	101	102.9	110.2	106.9	120	109.8	104.4	97.3	83.5	103.8

(f) Birth cohort mortality, ages 35–84 years, females, 1960–97

Year of birth	1875–79	1880–84	1885–89	1890–94	1895–99	1900–4	1905–9	1910–14	1915–19	1920–24	1925–29	1930–34	1935–39	1940–44	1945–49	1950–54	1955–59	1960–64
n	30	76	149	239	328	451	668	748	633	707	532	411	315	231	190	101	40	13
U 95% CI	150.6	88.7	81.2	83.2	81.1	83.5	102.1	105.8	112.9	119.7	129.9	141	148.2	152.3	157.1	159.9	154	434.1
SCMR	105.5	70.8	69.2	73.3	72.7	76.1	94.6	98.4	104.4	111.2	119.3	128	132.7	133.9	136.3	131.6	113.1	253.9
L 95% CI	71.2	55.8	58.5	64.5	65.3	69.4	87.7	91.6	96.6	103.3	109.6	116.2	118.9	117.7	117.6	107.2	80.8	135.2

(g) Birth cohort incidence, ages 35–84 years, males, 1971–92

Year of birth	1885–89	1890–94	1895–99	1900–4	1905–9	1910–14	1915–19	1920–24	1925–29	1930–34	1935–39	1940–44	1945–49	1950–54	1955–59
n	14	95	200	504	803	1040	895	1044	801	612	521	378	325	152	34
U 95% CI	94.7	87.4	77.5	92.6	94.7	107.1	110.6	115.3	117	110.8	115.6	116.2	130.1	143	248.1
SCIR	56.6	71.3	67.5	84.9	88.4	100.7	103.6	108.5	109.1	102.4	106.1	105.1	116.7	122	177.5
L 95% CI	30.9	57.4	58.5	77.8	82.5	94.8	97	102.1	101.8	94.6	97.3	95	104.7	103.4	123

(h) Birth cohort incidence, ages 35–84 years, females, 1971–92

Year of birth	1885–89	1890–94	1895–99	1900–4	1905–9	1910–14	1915–19	1920–24	1925–29	1930–34	1935–39	1940–44	1945–49	1950–54	1955–59
n	22	127	303	560	843	914	739	848	628	496	411	344	252	111	19
U 95% CI	97.7	87.4	89.8	95.7	103.2	106.5	109.2	115.1	113.3	111.7	114.7	132.8	130	144.2	228.4
SCIR	64.5	73.4	80.2	88.1	96.5	99.8	101.6	107.6	104.7	102.3	104.1	119.5	114.9	119.7	146.2
L 95% CI	40.4	61.2	71.7	81.1	90.2	93.5	94.6	100.6	96.9	93.7	94.5	107.5	101.6	98.5	88

Table C14 Malignant melanoma of skin

(a) Mortality, males, 1960–97

Age		1960–4	1965–9	1970–4	1975–9	1980–4	1985–9	1990–4	1995–7
0–14	n	4	3	2	1	4	2	0	3
	Rate	0.0138	0.0115	0.0071	0.0037	0.0158	0.0096	0	0.0191
15–34	n	108	116	140	158	178	172	194	89
	Rate	0.3488	0.369	0.412	0.4318	0.4837	0.4517	0.4742	0.3463
35–49	n	205	298	284	350	447	505	578	346
	Rate	0.8599	1.2993	1.2632	1.6093	1.9831	2.0779	2.2081	2.0942
50–69	n	369	496	587	774	898	987	1233	851
	Rate	1.5129	1.9373	2.2294	2.9684	3.5261	3.9127	4.9107	5.5945
70–84	n	160	171	253	306	473	582	885	630
	Rate	2.7118	2.7703	3.7662	4.0026	5.4442	6.3279	9.0757	10.4565
0–84	n	846	1084	1266	1589	2000	2248	2890	1919
	Rate	0.8444	1.0269	1.1887	1.4399	1.78	1.9523	2.4528	2.6751

(b) Incidence, males, 1971–92

Age		1971–4	1975–9	1980–4	1985–9	1990–2
0–14	n	13	21	24	34	11
	Rate	0.0533	0.0763	0.0946	0.1506	0.0841
15–34	n	254	383	484	784	499
	Rate	0.9207	1.0515	1.3067	2.0424	2.0477
35–49	n	451	698	893	1601	1016
	Rate	2.5348	3.2273	3.9623	6.5756	6.5967
50–69	n	754	1273	1703	2660	1908
	Rate	3.5707	4.8681	6.6658	10.5029	12.6512
70–84	n	320	523	799	1325	1058
	Rate	5.8598	6.885	9.2051	14.4182	18.4384
0–84	n	1792	2898	3903	6404	4492
	Rate	2.0669	2.6144	3.4357	5.4599	6.2945

(c) Mortality, females, 1960–97

Age		1960–4	1965–9	1970–4	1975–9	1980–4	1985–9	1990–4	1995–7
0–14	n	4	1	2	3	6	1	3	1
	Rate	0.0157	0.0048	0.0073	0.0119	0.0248	0.0036	0.0162	0.0073
15–34	n	111	127	137	196	186	144	154	85
	Rate	0.3711	0.4133	0.4142	0.5627	0.5123	0.3902	0.3884	0.3503
35–49	n	308	365	385	364	408	488	500	276
	Rate	1.284	1.5542	1.7097	1.7019	1.8399	2.0344	1.916	1.6914
50–69	n	446	542	748	879	971	1049	1051	698
	Rate	1.568	1.8458	2.5297	3.0117	3.44	3.8173	3.9463	4.3437
70–84	n	292	352	390	555	700	954	1148	757
	Rate	2.8325	3.1334	3.1949	4.1994	4.8755	6.4214	7.6125	8.3772
0–84	n	1161	1387	1662	1997	2271	2636	2856	1817
	Rate	0.9501	1.0976	1.2822	1.5256	1.6939	1.9122	2.0312	2.1357

(d) Incidence, females, 1971–92

Age		1971–4	1975–9	1980–4	1985–9	1990–2
0–14	n	11	37	28	31	17
	Rate	0.0517	0.1381	0.1156	0.1419	0.1376
15–34	n	498	876	1026	1532	992
	Rate	1.8418	2.4596	2.8132	4.0985	4.2208
35–49	n	927	1289	1859	2891	1623
	Rate	5.2406	6.0493	8.3665	11.9279	10.5968
50–69	n	1490	2189	2809	4056	2261
	Rate	6.3109	7.5763	10.0427	14.8456	14.0761
70–84	n	687	1099	1656	2367	1643
	Rate	6.9923	8.3075	11.6748	16.4312	18.6005
0–84	n	3613	5490	7378	10877	6536
	Rate	3.3352	4.2844	5.6519	8.1764	8.0066

239

(e) Birth cohort mortality, ages 25–84 years, males, 1960–97

Year of birth	1875–79	1880–84	1885–89	1890–94	1895–99	1900–4	1905–9	1910–14	1915–19	1920–24	1925–29	1930–34	1935–39	1940–44	1945–49	1950–54	1955–59	1960–64	1965–69	1970–74
n	18	67	130	227	376	627	1056	1434	1435	1689	1489	1305	1021	925	824	444	275	161	64	6
U 95% CI	80.8	62.8	55.9	58.8	64.1	67.7	85.3	99	113.5	113.9	125.7	133.1	126.8	142.9	144.5	127	123	117.3	124.1	162.8
SCMR	51.1	49.4	47.1	51.6	57.9	62.6	80.3	94	107.8	108.6	119.4	126.1	119.2	134	135	115.7	109.3	100.5	97.2	74.8
L 95% CI	30.3	38.3	39.4	45.3	52.3	57.9	75.6	89.2	102.3	103.6	113.5	119.4	112.1	125.6	126.1	105.4	97.1	85.6	74.8	27.4

(f) Birth cohort mortality, ages 25–84 years, females, 1960–97

Year of birth	1875–79	1880–84	1885–89	1890–94	1895–99	1900–4	1905–9	1910–14	1915–19	1920–24	1925–29	1930–34	1935–39	1940–44	1945–49	1950–54	1955–59	1960–64	1965–69	1970–74
n	31	131	260	420	644	966	1379	1914	1733	1996	1496	1204	920	817	753	411	259	119	56	4
U 95% CI	71	68.8	63.5	66.6	71.3	79.2	91.2	112	122.2	127.1	125.5	125.8	116.9	125.8	129.9	117.1	116.9	92.9	117.3	123.2
SCMR	50	58	56.2	60.5	66	74.4	86.5	107.1	116.5	121.6	119.3	118.9	109.6	117.5	120.9	106.3	103.5	77.6	90.3	48.1
L 95% CI	34	48.5	49.8	55	61.1	69.8	82.1	102.4	111.2	116.4	113.4	112.4	102.7	109.7	112.6	96.5	91.6	64.3	68.2	13.1

(g) Birth cohort incidence, ages 25–84 years, males, 1971–92

Year of birth	1885–89	1890–94	1895–99	1900–4	1905–9	1910–14	1915–19	1920–24	1925–29	1930–34	1935–39	1940–44	1945–49	1950–54	1955–59	1960–64	1965–69
n	20	115	301	661	1379	1850	1870	2310	2050	1817	1624	1520	1480	819	581	310	54
U 95% CI	77.3	63.3	66	68.7	87.8	95.7	106.5	105.8	110.6	112	112.2	119.8	125.2	118.6	143.6	156	212.6
SCIR	50.1	52.8	58.9	63.6	83.3	91.4	101.8	101.6	105.9	107	106.9	113.9	119	110.8	132.4	139.6	162.9
L 95% CI	30.6	43.6	52.6	58.9	79	87.4	97.3	97.5	101.4	102.2	101.8	108.4	113.1	103.4	122.1	124.9	122.4

(h) Birth cohort incidence, ages 25–84 years, females, 1971–92

Year of birth	1885–89	1890–94	1895–99	1900–4	1905–9	1910–14	1915–19	1920–24	1925–29	1930–34	1935–39	1940–44	1945–49	1950–54	1955–59	1960–64	1965–69
n	66	299	720	1448	2466	3170	2956	3740	3203	2827	2657	2699	2776	1681	1173	568	83
U 95% CI	88.6	69.3	70.9	78.2	90.5	101.6	106.9	109.1	108.2	103.9	103.2	111.5	118.1	118.2	136.5	134.1	157.3
SCIR	69.6	61.9	65.9	74.3	87	98.2	103.1	105.7	104.5	100.2	99.3	107.4	113.8	112.6	128.9	123.5	126.9
L 95% CI	53.8	55.3	61.3	70.6	83.6	94.8	99.5	102.3	100.9	96.6	95.6	103.4	109.7	107.4	121.7	113.7	101.1

Table C15 Cancer of breast, female

(a) Mortality, females, 1960–97

Age		1960–4	1965–9	1970–4	1975–9	1980–4	1985–9	1990–4	1995–7
0–14	n	0	1	0	1	0	0	0	0
	Rate	0	0.005	0	0.0039	0	0	0	0
15–34	n	547	573	637	706	725	712	706	403
	Rate	1.8552	1.9985	2.1129	2.0587	2.0396	2.0468	1.8231	1.6278
35–49	n	7050	7268	7679	7184	7140	7416	7262	4079
	Rate	28.7323	30.0802	33.2665	32.9905	32.4476	31.2036	27.6685	24.5793
50–69	n	23255	25023	27088	27729	27731	27590	24691	12999
	Rate	81.7141	85.1801	91.4685	94.9757	98.7339	100.6504	92.6147	81.3344
70–84	n	13637	14651	16546	19195	21675	24728	24493	13405
	Rate	132.0623	130.4335	135.6518	144.8796	151.0544	165.8071	161.5304	148.4374
0–84	n	44489	47516	51950	54815	57271	60446	57152	30886
	Rate	35.8084	36.7056	39.1698	40.7262	42.0187	43.5795	40.721	36.4249

(b) Incidence, females, 1971–92

Age		1971–4	1975–9	1980–4	1985–9	1990–2
0–14	n	6	8	8	9	3
	Rate	0.0289	0.0305	0.0327	0.0401	0.0199
15–34	n	1876	2553	2563	2908	1949
	Rate	7.6315	7.4613	7.196	8.2563	8.4777
35–49	n	17222	20652	20576	24582	16514
	Rate	95.0477	95.3101	93.4196	102.7993	106.8275
50–69	n	39078	49409	50218	56890	42536
	Rate	164.6313	169.5033	178.8494	207.8808	266.6876
70–84	n	20655	29718	33666	39205	24407
	Rate	210.7522	225.0947	236.2147	267.8411	275.9847
0–84	n	78837	102340	107031	123594	85409
	Rate	74.8454	77.2328	79.8973	91.1888	105.6619

(c) Birth cohort mortality, ages 30–49, 50–84, females, 1960–97

Year of birth	1875–79	1880–84	1885–89	1890–94	1895–99	1900–4	1905–9	1910–14	1915–19	1920–24	1925–29	1930–34	1935–39	1940–44	1945–49	1950–54	1955–59	1960–64	1965–69
									Ages 30–49 years										
n	–	–	–	–	–	–	–	2100	4577	7461	7636	7516	7255	7460	8098	4152	1863	696	63
U 95% CI								97.4	101.3	103.2	108.8	111.6	106.6	103.2	95.4	93.3	94.5	99.6	101.9
SCMR								93.3	98.4	100.9	106.4	109.1	104.2	100.9	93.4	90.5	90.3	92.5	79.6
L 95% CI								89.4	95.6	98.6	104.1	106.6	101.8	98.6	91.3	87.8	86.3	85.8	61.2
									Ages 50–84 years										
n	1580	5929	11544	18163	26530	37264	48549	53305	39921	40157	27305	17632	10677	5055	824	–	–	–	–
U 95% CI	93.7	92.8	88.5	91.2	93.1	96.5	102.3	106.6	106.2	107.5	108.5	102.4	96.9	92.4	94.1				
SCMR	89.2	90.4	86.9	89.9	92	95.5	101.4	105.7	105.2	106.4	107.2	100.9	95	89.9	87.9				
L 95% CI	84.9	88.2	85.3	88.6	90.9	94.5	100.5	104.8	104.2	105.4	105.9	99.4	93.3	87.5	82.1				

(d) Birth cohort incidence, ages 30–49, 50–84 years, females, 1971–92

Year of birth	1885–89	1890–94	1895–99	1900–4	1905–9	1910–14	1915–19	1920–24	1925–29	1930–34	1935–39	1940–44	1945–49	1950–54	1955–59	1960–64
								Ages 30–49 years								
n	–	–	–	–	–	–	–	3560	13042	17958	21224	23836	17929	7480	2665	328
U 95% CI								93.9	99	98.7	98.8	104.2	104.7	106.8	113.1	122.9
SCIR								90.9	97.3	97.2	97.5	102.9	103.2	104.4	108.9	110.3
L 95% CI								87.9	95.6	95.8	96.2	101.6	101.7	102	104.8	99
								Ages 50–84 years								
n	1697	8680	19935	35810	54052	62042	53589	60092	42996	28386	15676	2826	–	–	–	–
U 95% CI	89.7	90.9	92.6	93.9	97.5	98.8	98.1	99	109.3	117.7	130.7	152.9	–			
SCIR	85.5	89	91.3	93	96.7	98	97.3	98.2	108.3	116.4	128.7	147.4				
L 95% CI	81.5	87.1	90.1	92	95.9	97.2	96.5	97.4	107.3	115	126.7	142.1				

Table C16 Cancer of breast, male

(a) Mortality, males, 1960–97

Age		1960–4	1965–9	1970–4	1975–9	1980–4	1985–9	1990–4	1995–7
0–14	n	0	0	0	0	0	0	0	0
	Rate	0	0	0	0	0	0	0	0
15–34	n	3	1	1	6	1	1	0	0
	Rate	0.0095	0.003	0.0038	0.017	0.0028	0.0022	0	0
35–49	n	29	29	17	28	17	16	20	8
	Rate	0.1194	0.1256	0.0722	0.1259	0.0762	0.0644	0.0732	0.0455
50–69	n	176	234	178	202	192	155	161	70
	Rate	0.7458	0.9502	0.6949	0.7845	0.7634	0.6089	0.6401	0.4664
70–84	n	146	145	167	154	197	207	220	108
	Rate	2.47	2.3465	2.5429	2.0945	2.3447	2.2611	2.2699	1.8138
0–84	n	354	409	363	390	407	379	401	186
	Rate	0.4156	0.4483	0.401	0.393	0.3982	0.3542	0.3628	0.2777

(b) Incidence, males, 1971–92

Age		1971–4	1975–9	1980–4	1985–9	1990–2
0–14	n	1	0	0	0	0
	Rate	0.0042	0	0	0.0086	0
15–34	n	8	23	9	10	5
	Rate	0.029	0.0673	0.0246	0.0269	0.0205
35–49	n	72	112	63	66	51
	Rate	0.3907	0.5083	0.2818	0.277	0.3271
50–69	n	336	535	450	406	223
	Rate	1.6353	2.0647	1.7977	1.6112	1.4892
70–84	n	253	336	370	455	268
	Rate	4.7081	4.4712	4.3037	4.9495	4.6875
0–84	n	670	1006	892	939	547
	Rate	0.8723	0.9767	0.8493	0.8693	0.8235

(c) Birth cohort mortality, ages 35–84 years, males, 1960–97

Year of birth	1875–79	1880–84	1885–89	1890–94	1895–99	1900–4	1905–9	1910–14	1915–19	1920–24	1925–29	1930–34	1935–39	1940–44	1945–49	1950–54	1955–59	1960–64
n	22	51	111	187	250	343	382	441	329	309	197	124	57	41	23	7	2	0
U 95% CI	218.8	120.5	120.9	130.5	125.6	119	108.1	115.3	113.1	106.8	107.8	108.7	86.8	113.7	122.2	120.8	154.7	
SCMR	144.5	91.6	100.4	113.1	110.9	107.1	97.8	105	101.5	95.5	93.8	91.2	67	83.8	81.5	58.6	42.8	
L 95% CI	90.6	68.2	82.6	97.5	98	96.3	88.4	95.7	91.1	85.4	81.1	75.8	50.8	60.1	51.6	23.6	5.2	

(d) Birth cohort incidence, ages 35–84 years, males, 1971–92

Year of birth	1885–89	1890–94	1895–99	1900–4	1905–9	1910–14	1915–19	1920–24	1925–29	1930–34	1935–39	1940–44	1945–49	1950–54	1955–59
n	21	104	229	379	633	706	555	513	344	246	126	83	38	17	2
U 95% CI	162.7	130.7	119.2	98.6	109.3	113.2	115.6	105.9	110.1	120	99.1	117	103.5	156	349.6
SCIR	106.4	107.9	104.7	89.1	101.1	105.1	106.4	97.2	99	105.9	83.2	94.4	75.4	97.5	96.8
L 95% CI	65.9	88.2	92	80.6	93.6	97.7	97.9	89.1	89.1	93.5	69.3	75.2	53.4	56.8	11.8

Table C17 Cancer of cervix uteri

(a) Mortality, females, 1960–97

Age		1960–4	1965–9	1970–4	1975–9	1980–4	1985–9	1990–4	1995–7
0–14	n	2	1	0	0	0	1	0	0
	Rate	0.0066	0.0028	0	0	0	0.0039	0	0
15–34	n	203	171	233	402	578	600	442	252
	Rate	0.6911	0.5803	0.734	1.1421	1.6009	1.6724	1.1047	1.0023
35–49	n	3023	2692	1879	1441	1536	1888	1669	803
	Rate	12.4014	11.1159	8.0899	6.6956	6.9261	7.8184	6.456	4.9828
50–69	n	5864	5938	5801	5592	4530	3879	2653	1190
	Rate	20.5085	20.2201	19.6774	19.2828	16.0675	14.059	9.8915	7.4355
70–84	n	3150	2956	2836	2834	2755	2738	2611	1302
	Rate	30.5601	26.4265	23.3323	21.4797	19.4011	18.9377	17.8645	14.6854
0–84	n	12242	11758	10749	10269	9399	9106	7375	3547
	Rate	9.7411	9.0344	8.139	7.7584	7.0401	6.7364	5.3045	4.1785

(b) Incidence, females, 1971–92

Age		1971–4	1975–9	1980–4	1985–9	1990–2
0–14	n	3	4	4	5	0
	Rate	0.014	0.0159	0.0168	0.0206	0
15–34	n	1248	2201	3020	3474	1786
	Rate	4.8072	6.1866	8.3494	9.5212	7.5283
35–49	n	3901	4143	4983	6429	3501
	Rate	21.6904	19.5003	22.3546	26.5489	23.0659
50–69	n	8293	9805	8279	7523	3520
	Rate	35.2098	33.8102	29.4929	27.3976	21.9813
70–84	n	2649	3305	3542	3708	2145
	Rate	27.1566	25.1609	25.2172	26.0892	24.9379
0–84	n	16094	19458	19828	21139	10952
	Rate	15.5695	15.1095	15.3305	16.0522	13.5239

(c) Birth cohort mortality, ages 25–84 years, females, 1960–97

Year of birth	1875–79	1880–84	1885–89	1890–94	1895–99	1900–4	1905–9	1910–14	1915–19	1920–24	1925–29	1930–34	1935–39	1940–44	1945–49	1950–54	1955–59	1960–64	1965–69	1970–74
n	337	1211	2355	3755	4976	6306	7749	9711	8895	9587	5493	3355	2702	2274	2265	1704	975	458	151	10
U 95% CI	186.7	154.6	133.5	131.1	116.4	105.9	103	113.1	120.2	114.3	85.7	66.1	66.6	71.1	84.2	110.9	112	103.5	108.4	121.4
SCMR	167.8	146.1	128.2	127	113.2	103.3	100.7	110.9	117.8	112	83.4	63.9	64.1	68.3	80.8	105.7	105.2	94.4	92.4	66
L 95% CI	150.8	138.1	123.1	123	110.1	100.8	98.5	108.7	115.3	109.8	81.3	61.8	61.8	65.5	77.5	100.8	98.8	86.2	78.3	31.6

(d) Birth cohort incidence, ages 25–84 years, females, 1971–92

Year of birth	1885–89	1890–94	1895–99	1900–4	1905–9	1910–14	1915–19	1920–24	1925–29	1930–34	1935–39	1940–44	1945–49	1950–54	1955–59	1960–64	1965–69
n	166	966	2206	3973	6223	8954	9121	11530	8113	6050	6016	6339	6932	5436	3223	1167	123
U 95% CI	124.3	121.2	108.5	99.7	97.4	109.8	115.8	115.1	94.6	79.4	83.9	93	103.5	126.6	123.8	104.6	111.5
SCIR	106.8	113.8	104.1	96.6	95	107.5	113.4	113.1	92.6	77.5	81.8	90.7	101.1	123.3	119.6	98.7	93.4
L 95% CI	91.1	106.9	99.8	93.7	92.7	105.3	111.1	111	90.6	75.5	79.8	88.5	98.8	120.1	115.6	93.2	77.7

Table C18 Cancer of of corpus uteri plus uterus unspecified

(a) Mortality, females, 1960–97

Age		1960–4	1965–9	1970–4	1975–9	1980–4	1985–9	1990–4	1995–7
0–14	n	1	4	3	1	1	2	0	1
	Rate	0.0033	0.0127	0.0101	0.0041	0.0043	0.0078	0	0.0056
15–34	n	25	22	15	22	23	17	16	13
	Rate	0.0839	0.0741	0.0467	0.0641	0.0641	0.0485	0.0403	0.0537
35–49	n	449	387	346	236	234	232	171	97
	Rate	1.8173	1.5764	1.4519	1.0671	1.0712	0.9874	0.6568	0.5696
50–69	n	3793	3849	3642	3296	2996	2540	2215	1179
	Rate	13.5455	13.1304	12.2006	11.1939	10.5633	9.088	8.2043	7.3971
70–84	n	2620	2767	3171	3331	3513	3482	3252	1867
	Rate	25.4214	24.7307	26.02	25.1686	24.4478	23.3674	21.5028	20.7003
0–84	n	6888	7029	7177	6886	6767	6273	5654	3157
	Rate	5.6701	5.4714	5.3543	4.9901	4.7857	4.3426	3.9137	3.6519

(b) Incidence, females, 1971–92

Age		1971–4	1975–9	1980–4	1985–9	1990–2
0–14	n	2	3	2	4	1
	Rate	0.0082	0.0124	0.0084	0.0176	0.0061
15–34	n	94	150	122	147	92
	Rate	0.3779	0.4354	0.3384	0.4134	0.4062
35–49	n	1413	1674	1612	1628	1029
	Rate	7.6084	7.5929	7.3436	6.9306	6.677
50–69	n	8618	11305	11083	10731	6469
	Rate	36.4207	38.8942	39.4495	39.2488	40.3042
70–84	n	4110	5948	6550	6802	4272
	Rate	42.1164	45.2513	46.1931	47.046	48.7019
0–84	n	14237	19080	19369	19312	11863
	Rate	13.361	14.2096	14.3439	14.3295	14.6646

(c) Birth cohort mortality, ages 35–84 years, females, 1960–97

Year of birth	1875–79	1880–84	1885–89	1890–94	1895–99	1900–4	1905–9	1910–14	1915–19	1920–24	1925–29	1930–34	1935–39	1940–44	1945–49	1950–54	1955–59	1960–64
n	252	1042	2167	3622	4993	6662	7303	7267	5161	5012	2876	1608	933	452	220	73	20	2
U 95% CI	106.2	107.5	105.9	115.2	112.9	115.9	109.5	104.9	98.6	98.2	88.7	78.8	77.7	72.4	67.8	70.7	81.8	162.3
SCMR	93.9	101.2	101.5	111.5	109.9	113.2	107	102.5	95.9	95.5	85.5	75.1	72.9	66	59.4	56.3	53	44.9
L 95% CI	83	95.2	97.4	107.9	106.9	110.5	104.6	100.2	93.3	92.9	82.5	71.5	68.4	60.2	52.1	44.1	32.4	5.5

(d) Birth cohort incidence, ages 35–84 years, females, 1971–92

Year of birth	1885–89	1890–94	1895–99	1900–4	1905–9	1910–14	1915–19	1920–24	1925–29	1930–34	1935–39	1940–44	1945–49	1950–54	1955–59
n	268	1477	3793	7299	10687	12386	11506	13191	9624	6396	3743	1693	892	263	26
U 95% CI	96.5	93	98.7	102.3	100.4	99.2	103.5	104.7	107.5	104.2	100.9	95.7	105.9	109.5	114.3
SCIR	85.7	88.3	95.6	99.9	98.6	97.5	101.7	103	105.4	101.7	97.7	91.2	99.2	97	78
L 95% CI	76	83.9	92.6	97.7	96.7	95.8	99.8	101.2	103.3	99.2	94.6	87	92.9	86	50.9

Table C19 Cancer of ovary

(a) Mortality, females, 1960–97

Age		1960–4	1965–9	1970–4	1975–9	1980–4	1985–9	1990–4	1995–7
0–14	n	29	22	20	15	16	6	3	3
	Rate	0.1206	0.0922	0.0832	0.0573	0.0655	0.0275	0.0133	0.0228
15–34	n	250	259	254	244	207	184	184	93
	Rate	0.8371	0.8481	0.8072	0.7006	0.5732	0.5014	0.4742	0.3953
35–49	n	2224	2205	2277	1969	1635	1602	1499	845
	Rate	9.0417	9.0699	9.7356	8.9632	7.4629	6.8124	5.6931	5.0353
50–69	n	8712	9476	9669	9777	9473	9224	8738	5175
	Rate	30.6138	32.3297	32.6661	33.5294	33.6275	33.461	32.7131	32.5659
70–84	n	3711	4350	5142	5887	6516	7078	7444	4791
	Rate	36.069	39.1207	42.4585	44.7717	45.8652	48.7745	50.7071	54.4784
0–84	n	14926	16312	17362	17892	17847	18094	17868	10907
	Rate	11.9438	12.6049	13.09	13.3179	13.1366	13.2224	13.0256	13.2014

(b) Incidence, females, 1971–92

Age		1971–4	1975–9	1980–4	1985–9	1990–2
0–14	n	38	52	46	63	20
	Rate	0.187	0.2	0.1912	0.3014	0.1534
15–34	n	534	682	721	794	483
	Rate	2.0619	1.9432	1.9816	2.1397	2.0864
35–49	n	2831	3108	3091	3382	1995
	Rate	15.4524	14.2395	14.0575	14.2638	12.9104
50–69	n	8633	11312	11736	12174	7441
	Rate	36.4376	38.7788	41.7649	44.4414	46.3487
70–84	n	4021	5824	6982	7898	5004
	Rate	41.1879	44.3273	49.1753	54.5215	57.6008
0–84	n	16057	20978	22576	24311	14943
	Rate	15.2222	15.7776	16.8586	18.0472	18.4634

(c) Birth cohort mortality, ages 35–84 years, females, 1960–97

Year of birth	1875–79	1880–84	1885–89	1890–94	1895–99	1900–4	1905–9	1910–14	1915–19	1920–24	1925–29	1930–34	1935–39	1940–44	1945–49	1950–54	1955–59	1960–64
n	326	1339	3075	5485	8836	12944	15676	18172	15589	16860	11921	8166	5276	3106	1780	638	200	30
U 95% CI	89	82.5	82.8	89	95.7	101.6	100.1	105.8	110.2	111.4	111.2	106.2	97.5	88.2	77.9	72.1	76.1	116.3
SCMR	79.8	78.2	79.9	86.7	93.7	99.9	98.5	104.2	108.5	109.7	109.2	103.9	94.9	85.2	74.4	66.7	66.2	81.5
L 95% CI	71.6	74.1	77.1	84.5	91.8	98.2	97	102.7	106.8	108.1	107.3	101.7	92.4	82.2	71	61.8	57.4	55

(d) Birth cohort incidence, ages 35–84 years, females, 1971–92

Year of birth	1885–89	1890–94	1895–99	1900–4	1905–9	1910–14	1915–19	1920–24	1925–29	1930–34	1935–39	1940–44	1945–49	1950–54	1955–59
n	256	1414	3769	7535	11084	13264	12250	14498	11430	8287	5679	3308	1905	670	83
U 95% CI	84.7	82.4	91.2	98.6	97.2	99.9	104.4	106.3	110.1	107.1	104.5	99.2	98.4	109.8	122.7
SCIR	75	78.2	88.4	96.4	95.4	98.2	102.6	104.6	108.1	104.8	101.8	95.9	94.1	101.8	99
L 95% CI	66.3	74.3	85.6	94.3	93.7	96.6	100.8	102.9	106.1	102.6	99.2	92.6	90	94.4	78.8

Table C20 Cancer of prostate

(a) Mortality, males, 1960–97

Age		1960–4	1965–9	1970–4	1975–9	1980–4	1985–9	1990–4	1995–7
0–14	n	8	4	4	3	2	2	2	0
	Rate	0.0282	0.0142	0.0125	0.0099	0.0076	0.0071	0.008	0
15–34	n	5	7	4	4	2	2	4	1
	Rate	0.0165	0.0214	0.0118	0.0109	0.0053	0.0048	0.0108	0.0035
35–49	n	79	66	83	56	69	79	99	68
	Rate	0.3243	0.272	0.3472	0.2471	0.3133	0.3413	0.3797	0.3869
50–69	n	4545	4883	5257	5878	6200	7341	7808	4292
	Rate	22.0184	21.0317	20.979	23.1256	25.1081	29.447	31.1524	29.1098
70–84	n	12041	12309	12662	14561	17702	23395	26996	16032
	Rate	206.9797	203.3895	195.1755	200.8894	212.5761	255.3186	277.4434	264.8927
0–84	n	16678	17269	18010	20502	23975	30819	34909	20393
	Rate	23.9624	23.4041	22.6467	23.6265	25.1479	30.0411	32.4614	30.8542

(b) Incidence, males, 1971–92

Age		1971–4	1975–9	1980–4	1985–9	1990–2
0–14	n	5	9	11	9	3
	Rate	0.0183	0.0345	0.0428	0.037	0.0208
15–34	n	12	19	15	34	12
	Rate	0.046	0.0538	0.0405	0.0878	0.0593
35–49	n	138	153	181	210	148
	Rate	0.7315	0.6797	0.819	0.9033	0.9822
50–69	n	8797	12432	13979	16248	11246
	Rate	43.509	48.9857	56.5025	64.916	74.1553
70–84	n	15446	23186	30096	37527	26785
	Rate	291.3794	313.4975	356.0406	408.8269	466.381
0–84	n	24398	35799	44282	54028	38194
	Rate	36.5391	39.7766	45.3687	52.1065	59.4387

(c) Birth cohort mortality, ages 45–84 years, males, 1960–97

Year of birth	1875–79	1880–84	1885–89	1890–94	1895–99	1900–4	1905–9	1910–14	1915–19	1920–24	1925–29	1930–34	1935–39	1940–44	1945–49	1950–54
n	1623	6093	10461	13666	16070	21988	27413	31938	22310	17358	8191	3436	1288	412	113	10
U 95% CI	86.3	92.9	89.3	89.4	87	91.7	99.3	111	115.7	116.5	120.2	120.8	125.7	131.3	140.9	249.1
SCMR	82.2	90.6	87.6	87.9	85.6	90.5	98.1	109.8	114.2	114.8	117.7	116.9	119	119.2	117.2	135.5
L 95% CI	78.3	88.3	86	86.4	84.3	89.3	97	108.6	112.7	113.1	115.1	113	112.7	108.3	96.6	64.9

(d) Birth cohort incidence, ages 45–84 years, males, 1971–92

Year of birth	1885–89	1890–94	1895–99	1900–4	1905–9	1910–14	1915–19	1920–24	1925–29	1930–34	1935–39	1940–44	1945–49
n	1440	7102	15376	29303	42213	41419	26872	19551	8648	3177	1003	231	16
U 95% CI	84.1	81.8	84.1	90.9	99	106.2	114	114.8	122.2	123.2	129.2	143	168.6
SCIR	79.9	79.9	82.7	89.8	98.1	105.2	112.7	113.2	119.6	119	121.5	125.7	103.8
L 95% CI	75.9	78	81.4	88.8	97.1	104.2	111.4	111.6	117.1	114.9	114.2	110.5	59.3

Table C21 Cancer of testis

(a) Mortality, males, 1960–97

Age		1960–4	1965–9	1970–4	1975–9	1980–4	1985–9	1990–4	1995–7
0–14	n	13	20	28	20	6	2	3	0
	Rate	0.0436	0.062	0.0882	0.0725	0.0227	0.0072	0.014	0
15–34	n	468	485	605	600	354	275	186	86
	Rate	1.5266	1.491	1.7494	1.6368	0.9419	0.6954	0.4493	0.347
35–49	n	262	310	314	291	214	167	157	83
	Rate	1.1373	1.3772	1.4619	1.3844	0.9376	0.6797	0.6095	0.5191
50–69	n	235	207	221	193	146	113	102	48
	Rate	0.962	0.8086	0.8503	0.7304	0.5738	0.4498	0.4015	0.3073
70–84	n	66	90	91	87	86	66	70	38
	Rate	1.1163	1.4333	1.3298	1.115	1.0234	0.7171	0.7162	0.6213
0–84	n	1044	1112	1259	1191	806	623	518	255
	Rate	0.9906	1.0216	1.1204	1.0229	0.6787	0.4991	0.4023	0.3228

(b) Incidence, males, 1971–92

Age		1971–4	1975–9	1980–4	1985–9	1990–2
0–14	n	49	77	58	76	35
	Rate	0.1995	0.2928	0.2264	0.291	0.2294
15–34	n	1423	2061	2358	3191	2094
	Rate	5.1193	5.6275	6.2935	8.1066	8.3393
35–49	n	833	1148	1448	1967	1357
	Rate	4.8663	5.4218	6.345	7.991	8.939
50–69	n	377	516	545	592	398
	Rate	1.7795	1.9555	2.1125	2.3372	2.6176
70–84	n	100	134	160	167	92
	Rate	1.8234	1.7247	1.8357	1.8235	1.6209
0–84	n	2782	3936	4569	5993	3976
	Rate	3.0247	3.327	3.7251	4.6315	4.9012

247

(c) Birth cohort mortality, ages 15–49, 50–84 years, males, 1960–97

Year of birth	1875–79	1880–84	1885–89	1890–94	1895–99	1900–4	1905–9	1910–14	1915–19	1920–24	1925–29	1930–34	1935–39	1940–44	1945–49	1950–54	1955–59	1960–64	1965–69	1970–74	1975–79
												Ages 15–49 years									
n	–	–	–	–	–	–	–	40	109	223	360	525	631	717	791	564	413	289	126	57	10
U 95% CI								202.9	160	132	142.5	150.1	140.1	135	121.9	104.7	85.3	65.9	45	47.8	46.8
SCMR								149	132.6	115.8	128.5	137.8	129.6	125.5	113.7	96.4	77.5	58.8	37.8	36.9	25.4
L 95% CI								106.4	108.9	101.5	115.9	126.5	119.9	116.6	106	88.8	70.3	52.4	31.5	27.9	12.2
									Ages 50–84 years												
n	9	22	63	101	160	253	247	319	202	185	130	67	61	32	8	–					
U 95% CI	277.1	143.3	168.3	159	165	162	114.4	129.3	106.4	92.2	91	68.8	86.3	87.2	166.2						
SCMR	146	94.7	131.6	130.8	141.3	143.3	101	115.9	92.7	79.9	76.7	54.2	67.2	61.8	84.3						
L 95% CI	66.7	59.3	101.1	106.6	120.3	126.7	89.1	103.8	80.8	68.8	64.1	42	51.4	42.2	36.4						

(d) Birth cohort incidence, ages 15–49, 50–84 years, males, 1971–92

Year of birth	1885–89	1890–94	1895–99	1900–4	1905–9	1910–14	1915–19	1920–24	1925–29	1930–34	1935–39	1940–44	1945–49	1950–54	1955–59	1960–64	1965–69	1970–74	1975–79
											Ages 15–49 years								
n	–	–	–	–	–	–	–	74	336	744	1376	2355	3404	3082	2866	2307	1042	281	13
U 95% CI								92.4	81.4	84.2	87.8	96.7	100.7	104.5	116.3	124.7	121.4	140.2	190.2
SCIR								73.6	73.2	78.4	83.3	92.9	97.4	100.9	112.1	119.7	114.3	124.7	111.2
L 95% CI								57.8	65.8	73	79	89.2	94.2	97.4	108.1	114.9	107.5	111	59.2
									Ages 50–84 years									
n	9	31	82	193	256	376	394	516	487	386	296	54	–						
U 95% CI	260.4	130.2	126.3	131	104.6	109.5	101.8	91	112.8	119.7	151.1	176.1							
SCIR	137.2	91.7	101.7	113.7	92.6	98.9	92.3	83.5	103.2	108.4	134.9	134.9							
L 95% CI	62.7	62.3	80.9	98.3	81.9	89.4	83.6	76.6	94.5	98.1	120.3	101.4							

Table C22 Cancer of penis

(a) Mortality, males, 1960-97

Age		1960-4	1965-9	1970-4	1975-9	1980-4	1985-9	1990-4	1995-7
0-14	n	0	0	0	0	0	0	0	0
	Rate	0	0	0	0	0	0	0	0
15-34	n	1	2	4	2	4	8	2	3
	Rate	0.0038	0.0066	0.0142	0.0051	0.011	0.0219	0.0055	0.0108
35-49	n	34	29	41	29	29	30	40	18
	Rate	0.1438	0.1252	0.1786	0.1339	0.1307	0.1264	0.1529	0.1092
50-69	n	205	186	185	188	181	163	164	86
	Rate	0.9019	0.7555	0.7263	0.7253	0.7135	0.6502	0.6662	0.5552
70-84	n	230	180	174	197	233	247	226	109
	Rate	3.962	2.9641	2.684	2.6862	2.7647	2.6877	2.3218	1.7921
0-84	n	470	397	404	416	447	448	432	216
	Rate	0.5898	0.4633	0.4429	0.4322	0.438	0.4196	0.3892	0.3098

(b) Incidence, males, 1971-92

Age		1971-4	1975-9	1980-4	1985-9	1990-2
0-14	n	0	0	1	0	0
	Rate	0	0	0.0039	0	0
15-34	n	28	26	26	31	14
	Rate	0.1066	0.0736	0.0713	0.0807	0.0568
35-49	n	120	113	136	154	118
	Rate	0.6494	0.5153	0.6106	0.6375	0.7648
50-69	n	509	638	589	571	375
	Rate	2.4575	2.4746	2.3468	2.27	2.4751
70-84	n	344	492	591	617	352
	Rate	6.4052	6.5025	6.9118	6.6991	6.1418
0-84	n	1001	1269	1343	1373	859
	Rate	1.2782	1.2571	1.2836	1.254	1.2632

(c) Birth cohort mortality, ages 35-84 years, males, 1960-97

Year of birth	1875-79	1880-84	1885-89	1890-94	1895-99	1900-4	1905-9	1910-14	1915-19	1920-24	1925-29	1930-34	1935-39	1940-44	1945-49	1950-54	1955-59	1960-64
n	40	109	163	216	254	382	417	464	295	330	174	142	88	67	40	17	6	0
U 95% CI	249.9	175.9	138	129.4	114.2	119.3	106.9	109.7	94.6	109.4	92.1	114.6	111.8	137.1	129.8	134.2	165.9	
SCMR	183.5	145.8	118.4	113.2	101	108	97.2	100.2	84.4	98.2	79.4	97.2	90.7	108	95.3	83.8	76.2	
L 95% CI	131.1	119.7	100.9	99.1	89.3	97.7	88.3	91.5	75.3	88.2	68	81.9	72.8	83.7	68.1	48.8	28	

(d) Birth cohort incidence, ages 35-84 years, males, 1971-92

Year of birth	1885-89	1890-94	1895-99	1900-4	1905-9	1910-14	1915-19	1920-24	1925-29	1930-34	1935-39	1940-44	1945-49	1950-54	1955-59
n	32	139	294	601	937	1005	683	731	435	319	234	154	106	41	8
U 95% CI	150.1	112.5	102.2	107.3	112.8	114.1	103	108	97.5	104.3	113.3	119.8	136.6	162.9	349
SCIR	106.3	95.2	91.2	99.1	105.8	107.3	95.6	100.5	88.7	93.4	99.7	102.3	112.9	120.1	177.1
L 95% CI	72.7	80.1	81.3	91.4	99.2	100.9	88.7	93.5	80.8	83.7	87.7	86.2	92.4	86.2	76.5

Table C23 Cancer of bladder and urethra

(a) Mortality, males, 1960-97

Age		1960-4	1965-9	1970-4	1975-9	1980-4	1985-9	1990-4	1995-7
0-14	n	14	11	9	4	4	2	2	3
	Rate	0.0449	0.032	0.0274	0.0139	0.0156	0.0076	0.0075	0.0195
15-34	n	17	13	11	11	19	13	9	6
	Rate	0.0557	0.0421	0.0343	0.0304	0.0519	0.0369	0.0219	0.0236
35-49	n	414	407	350	289	228	232	209	123
	Rate	1.7231	1.6885	1.4899	1.2972	1.0227	0.9818	0.7847	0.7314
50-69	n	5043	5795	5920	5577	5123	4917	4567	2372
	Rate	22.7772	23.9854	23.2262	21.8791	20.5912	19.573	18.3293	16.0432
70-84	n	5132	5660	6706	7661	8541	9190	9268	5266
	Rate	86.6559	91.8098	100.3419	102.5576	100.9758	100.3009	95.3604	86.6288
0-84	n	10620	11886	12996	13542	13915	14354	14055	7770
	Rate	13.3205	14.0478	14.6273	14.4964	14.0255	13.7258	12.9578	11.6446

(b) Incidence, males, 1971-92

Age		1971-4	1975-9	1980-4	1985-9	1990-2
0-14	n	7	9	15	21	5
	Rate	0.0261	0.033	0.0582	0.082	0.0354
15-34	n	181	246	209	276	121
	Rate	0.6817	0.6828	0.5668	0.7327	0.5069
35-49	n	1262	1398	1514	1689	963
	Rate	6.8517	6.3072	6.7946	7.1314	6.1982
50-69	n	11479	14447	15521	16805	10025
	Rate	55.6361	56.1334	61.6904	66.6015	66.264
70-84	n	8691	13019	16550	19029	12328
	Rate	159.2564	171.5341	192.7612	207.2075	214.8691
0-84	n	21620	29119	33809	37820	23442
	Rate	28.3324	29.4768	32.7098	35.2356	35.6222

(c) Mortality, females, 1960-97

Age		1960-4	1965-9	1970-4	1975-9	1980-4	1985-9	1990-4	1995-7
0-14	n	7	7	3	4	4	0	2	0
	Rate	0.024	0.0206	0.0096	0.0147	0.0164	0	0.0091	0
15-34	n	4	2	9	10	14	15	11	1
	Rate	0.0133	0.0064	0.0285	0.0282	0.0389	0.0408	0.0281	0.004
35-49	n	172	151	153	133	81	96	109	64
	Rate	0.6988	0.6144	0.6511	0.6094	0.367	0.4043	0.4144	0.3843
50-69	n	1600	1739	1824	1897	1792	1724	1524	761
	Rate	5.789	5.9914	6.1252	6.4462	6.3217	6.1498	5.6072	4.7901
70-84	n	2451	2829	3161	3497	3763	4191	4329	2468
	Rate	23.6892	25.0326	25.7528	26.2427	25.8815	27.5036	28.01	26.3686
0-84	n	4234	4728	5150	5541	5654	6026	5975	3294
	Rate	3.5874	3.7378	3.8445	3.9538	3.8537	3.969	3.8959	3.5504

(d) Incidence, females, 1971-92

Age		1971-4	1975-9	1980-4	1985-9	1990-2
0-14	n	3	12	4	12	5
	Rate	0.0137	0.0447	0.0165	0.0471	0.0336
15-34	n	37	67	78	110	62
	Rate	0.1472	0.1963	0.2165	0.3005	0.2617
35-49	n	369	410	405	555	317
	Rate	1.9746	1.8808	1.844	2.3427	2.0727
50-69	n	3300	4414	5149	5468	3107
	Rate	13.8169	14.9557	18.1417	19.5952	18.8701
70-84	n	3819	5278	6496	7964	5014
	Rate	38.7998	39.7964	45.1248	53.4382	55.0231
0-84	n	7528	10181	12132	14109	8505
	Rate	7.0103	7.3574	8.5429	9.7483	9.672

250

(e) Birth cohort mortality, ages 35–84 years, males, 1960–97

Year of birth	1875–79	1880–84	1885–89	1890–94	1895–99	1900–4	1905–9	1910–14	1915–19	1920–24	1925–29	1930–34	1935–39	1940–44	1945–49	1950–54	1955–59	1960–64
n	551	2202	4389	6806	9694	13770	15107	15678	10977	9591	5314	2660	1314	580	242	88	26	1
U 95% CI	85.7	91.4	93.8	101.2	110	114.6	107.1	105.4	100.7	96.3	92.9	85.1	82.9	79.4	69.8	83	99.4	129.5
SCMR	78.8	87.6	91.1	98.8	107.8	112.7	105.4	103.8	98.8	94.4	90.5	82	78.6	73.2	61.5	67.4	67.8	23.2
L 95% CI	72.5	84	88.4	96.5	105.7	110.8	103.7	102.2	97	92.5	88.1	78.9	74.4	67.4	54.2	54.1	44.3	0.6

(f) Birth cohort mortality, ages 35–84 years, females, 1960–97

Year of birth	1875–79	1880–84	1885–89	1890–94	1895–99	1900–4	1905–9	1910–14	1915–19	1920–24	1925–29	1930–34	1935–39	1940–44	1945–49	1950–54	1955–59	1960–64
n	346	1232	2336	3316	4304	5174	5972	6415	4153	3634	1857	927	432	219	127	42	18	4
U 95% CI	99.5	96	96.5	100.5	102.4	101.1	104.2	110.6	105.7	110.9	105.2	95.8	84.6	85.3	91.7	89.6	129.5	447.4
SCMR	89.6	90.8	92.7	97.2	99.4	98.4	101.6	108	102.5	107.3	100.6	89.9	77	74.8	77.1	66.3	82	174.7
L 95% CI	80.6	85.8	89	93.9	96.5	95.7	99.1	105.3	99.4	103.9	96.1	84.2	70.1	65.5	64.2	47.8	48.6	47.6

(g) Birth cohort incidence, ages 35–84 years, males, 1971–92

Year of birth	1885–89	1890–94	1895–99	1900–4	1905–9	1910–14	1915–19	1920–24	1925–29	1930–34	1935–39	1940–44	1945–49	1950–54	1955–59
n	567	3108	8084	16784	24753	27107	20548	19176	11782	6458	3498	1710	853	261	30
U 95% CI	80.6	81.8	91.3	97.4	99.2	102.9	105.6	105.7	110.5	105.7	105.7	105.5	104.4	108.6	128.6
SCIR	74.3	79	89.3	95.9	98	101.7	104.1	104.3	108.5	103.2	102.2	100.7	97.6	96.2	90.1
L 95% CI	68.4	76.2	87.4	94.5	96.8	100.5	102.7	102.8	106.6	100.7	98.9	96	91.2	85.2	60.8

(h) Birth cohort incidence, ages 35–84 years, females, 1971–92

Year of birth	1885–89	1890–94	1895–99	1900–4	1905–9	1910–14	1915–19	1920–24	1925–29	1930–34	1935–39	1940–44	1945–49	1950–54	1955–59
n	386	1709	3930	6611	9246	9339	6751	6423	3699	1990	1026	524	313	110	7
U 95% CI	94.4	84	90.9	93.5	99.5	105.5	108.9	114.9	115.4	108.4	102.7	111.5	126.2	140.3	143.6
SCIR	85.4	80.1	88.1	91.3	97.5	103.4	106.4	112.1	111.7	103.7	96.6	102.4	112.9	116.4	69.7
L 95% CI	77.3	76.4	85.4	89.1	95.5	101.3	103.9	109.4	108.2	99.2	90.9	94	101.1	95.6	28

Table C24 Cancer of kidney and ureter

(a) Mortality, males, 1960–97

Age		1960–4	1965–9	1970–4	1975–9	1980–4	1985–9	1990–4	1995–7
0–14	n	149	148	93	62	47	20	29	20
	Rate	0.488	0.4462	0.2934	0.2243	0.1831	0.0774	0.1071	0.1229
15–34	n	58	60	56	61	60	48	50	27
	Rate	0.1897	0.1901	0.1675	0.1656	0.1606	0.1269	0.1242	0.1049
35–49	n	382	414	400	438	436	434	542	313
	Rate	1.5939	1.7268	1.7225	1.9867	1.9533	1.8259	2.0413	1.8677
50–69	n	2249	2630	2709	2902	3048	3381	3540	2099
	Rate	9.6174	10.542	10.4704	11.2512	12.0689	13.4038	14.1732	13.9843
70–84	n	1078	1182	1384	1854	2194	2726	3083	2010
	Rate	17.9474	18.875	20.25	24.158	25.1129	29.7038	31.8034	33.1921
0–84	n	3916	4434	4642	5317	5785	6609	7244	4469
	Rate	4.2098	4.5139	4.5856	5.1492	5.4012	6.0629	6.469	6.5217

(b) Incidence, males, 1971–92

Age		1971–4	1975–9	1980–4	1985–9	1990–2
0–14	n	159	184	188	149	117
	Rate	0.6291	0.668	0.7218	0.5522	0.6771
15–34	n	72	115	96	131	83
	Rate	0.2693	0.3212	0.2604	0.3607	0.3513
35–49	n	655	795	867	950	700
	Rate	3.5731	3.5945	3.89	3.986	4.5093
50–69	n	3179	4431	4923	5559	3740
	Rate	15.2746	17.1553	19.4326	21.9704	24.8187
70–84	n	1524	2443	3185	3994	2818
	Rate	27.4121	31.618	36.3027	43.4201	49.2136
0–84	n	5589	7968	9259	10783	7458
	Rate	6.7309	7.5595	8.5369	9.7633	11.0392

(c) Mortality, females, 1960–97

Age		1960–4	1965–9	1970–4	1975–9	1980–4	1985–9	1990–4	1995–7
0–14	n	136	144	100	62	39	39	34	20
	Rate	0.4816	0.4527	0.3341	0.232	0.1602	0.1632	0.1323	0.1296
15–34	n	33	34	34	48	56	36	54	23
	Rate	0.11	0.1093	0.1034	0.1367	0.1536	0.0943	0.1422	0.0973
35–49	n	227	201	171	200	209	236	285	139
	Rate	0.9312	0.8357	0.7425	0.9147	0.9467	0.9928	1.0765	0.8358
50–69	n	1162	1229	1331	1352	1532	1640	1726	1021
	Rate	4.1752	4.2109	4.4916	4.62	5.4298	5.9307	6.4221	6.4466
70–84	n	928	1059	1213	1343	1551	1957	2216	1439
	Rate	8.9905	9.444	9.9839	10.1734	10.8322	13.2602	14.845	16.0316
0–84	n	2486	2667	2849	3005	3387	3908	4315	2642
	Rate	2.0443	2.0708	2.1395	2.205	2.4399	2.7643	3.0415	3.0991

(d) Incidence, females, 1971–92

Age		1971–4	1975–9	1980–4	1985–9	1990–2
0–14	n	152	197	160	179	104
	Rate	0.622	0.7589	0.6474	0.6935	0.6368
15–34	n	70	93	114	98	89
	Rate	0.269	0.2606	0.3102	0.2679	0.3878
35–49	n	280	398	394	532	363
	Rate	1.552	1.8239	1.7869	2.2579	2.3241
50–69	n	1548	2087	2452	2712	1901
	Rate	6.5321	7.1123	8.6868	9.773	11.6993
70–84	n	1190	1751	2168	2766	1932
	Rate	12.1427	13.2899	15.2256	18.8818	21.8797
0–84	n	3240	4526	5288	6287	4389
	Rate	3.0408	3.3479	3.8582	4.5141	5.2506

(e) Birth cohort mortality, ages 35–84 years, males, 1960–97

Year of birth	1875–79	1880–84	1885–89	1890–94	1895–99	1900–4	1905–9	1910–14	1915–19	1920–24	1925–29	1930–34	1935–39	1940–44	1945–49	1950–54	1955–59	1960–64
n	89	352	788	1606	2386	3904	5125	6141	5094	5479	4069	2716	1751	977	617	246	81	7
U 95% CI	80.7	70.5	69.4	84.6	85.3	93.3	98.5	107.7	109.7	110.9	119.4	118.5	118.5	112.3	116.8	121.8	130.9	135.6
SCMR	65.6	63.5	64.7	80.5	81.9	90.4	95.9	105	106.7	108	115.8	114.2	113.1	105.5	108	107.5	105.3	65.8
L 95% CI	52.7	57.2	60.3	76.7	78.7	87.6	93.3	102.4	103.8	105.2	112.3	109.9	107.9	99.1	99.8	94.9	83.6	26.5

(f) Birth cohort mortality, ages 35–84 years, females, 1960–97

Year of birth	1875–79	1880–84	1885–89	1890–94	1895–99	1900–4	1905–9	1910–14	1915–19	1920–24	1925–29	1930–34	1935–39	1940–44	1945–49	1950–54	1955–59	1960–64
n	101	417	786	1298	1857	2444	3050	3538	2832	3037	1944	1270	843	460	315	130	37	8
U 95% CI	95.5	91	80.2	86.9	89.5	90.9	97.2	107.2	112.3	123	123	124.2	129.2	119.1	126.9	129.2	110.4	244
SCMR	78.6	82.7	74.8	82.3	85.5	87.4	93.8	103.8	108.2	118.7	117.6	117.6	120.8	108.7	113.7	108.8	80.1	123.8
L 95% CI	64	75.1	69.8	77.9	81.7	84	90.5	100.4	104.3	114.6	112.5	111.3	112.9	99.2	101.8	90.9	56.4	53.5

(g) Birth cohort incidence, ages 35–84 years, males, 1971–92

Year of birth	1885–89	1890–94	1895–99	1900–4	1905–9	1910–14	1915–19	1920–24	1925–29	1930–34	1935–39	1940–44	1945–49	1950–54	1955–59
n	69	503	1322	3048	5304	6615	5558	6136	4448	3045	1896	973	614	210	22
U 95% CI	73.5	80.7	81.6	87.9	97.4	103.4	104.2	107.3	113.6	116.5	115	107	122.2	135.1	156.9
SCIR	58.1	73.9	77.3	84.8	94.9	100.9	101.5	104.7	110.3	112.4	110	100.5	112.9	118	103.6
L 95% CI	45.2	67.7	73.2	81.9	92.3	98.5	98.9	102.1	107.2	108.5	105.1	94.3	104.3	103.1	65

(h) Birth cohort incidence, ages 35–84 years, females, 1971–92

Year of birth	1885–89	1890–94	1895–99	1900–4	1905–9	1910–14	1915–19	1920–24	1925–29	1930–34	1935–39	1940–44	1945–49	1950–54	1955–59
n	105	481	1166	2181	3331	3690	2953	3208	2100	1418	890	490	318	131	12
U 95% CI	101.8	81.6	84.9	89.9	98.2	103.8	107.1	115.5	116.6	118.7	118	113.8	126.4	159.1	167.4
SCIR	84.1	74.6	80.1	86.2	94.9	100.5	103.3	111.6	111.7	112.7	110.5	104.2	113.2	134.1	95.9
L 95% CI	68.8	68.2	75.7	82.6	91.8	97.3	99.7	107.8	107	107	103.4	95.3	101.4	112.1	49.5

Table C25 Cancer of eye

(a) Mortality, males, 1960–97

Age		1960–4	1965–9	1970–4	1975–9	1980–4	1985–9	1990–4	1995–7
0–4	n	24	20	15	10	10	9	7	3
	Rate	0.0797	0.0612	0.0476	0.0336	0.0377	0.0332	0.0261	0.0191
15–34	n	11	9	9	7	6	11	7	1
	Rate	0.0376	0.0292	0.0273	0.0198	0.0163	0.0284	0.0177	0.0035
35–49	n	43	33	26	24	29	28	32	11
	Rate	0.1794	0.1398	0.1137	0.11	0.128	0.1155	0.1199	0.063
50–69	n	169	187	203	214	164	198	133	47
	Rate	0.7363	0.7539	0.7714	0.829	0.6468	0.7854	0.536	0.3133
70–84	n	76	90	111	105	147	114	103	53
	Rate	1.2653	1.4338	1.6131	1.3545	1.703	1.2392	1.052	0.8703
0–84	n	323	339	364	360	356	360	282	115
	Rate	0.3382	0.3442	0.3566	0.3396	0.3345	0.3229	0.2469	0.1652

(b) Incidence, males, 1971–92

Age		1971–4	1975–9	1980–4	1985–9	1990–2
0–14	n	98	140	99	86	66
	Rate	0.3901	0.5374	0.3856	0.3197	0.3949
15–34	n	38	37	53	55	42
	Rate	0.1433	0.1027	0.1432	0.1423	0.175
35–49	n	107	125	106	132	110
	Rate	0.5819	0.569	0.4713	0.5477	0.7228
50–69	n	366	443	404	461	291
	Rate	1.7351	1.7107	1.5819	1.8262	1.9169
70–84	n	135	199	221	286	210
	Rate	2.4306	2.5091	2.5427	3.1139	3.6467
0–84	n	744	944	883	1020	719
	Rate	0.8328	0.8503	0.7888	0.8949	1.0204

(c) Mortality, females, 1960–97

Age		1960–4	1965–9	1970–4	1975–9	1980–4	1985–9	1990–4	1995–7
0–14	n	14	11	18	18	12	7	9	2
	Rate	0.0476	0.0333	0.0557	0.0703	0.0491	0.0284	0.033	0.0118
15–34	n	12	5	8	8	9	7	3	1
	Rate	0.0387	0.0156	0.0232	0.0228	0.0249	0.0211	0.0085	0.0047
35–49	n	45	34	35	28	29	28	17	7
	Rate	0.1835	0.1416	0.1525	0.1282	0.1314	0.1192	0.0641	0.0434
50–69	n	155	180	201	174	172	156	117	37
	Rate	0.551	0.6141	0.6754	0.5886	0.6063	0.5547	0.4425	0.2343
70–84	n	96	108	166	154	138	141	139	56
	Rate	0.9334	0.9703	1.3741	1.1617	0.9762	0.9581	0.929	0.6322
0–84	n	322	338	428	382	360	339	285	103
	Rate	0.2613	0.2612	0.3207	0.2806	0.2643	0.2437	0.2037	0.1213

(d) Incidence, females, 1971–92

Age		1971–4	1975–9	1980–4	1985–9	1990–2
0–14	n	95	95	96	72	60
	Rate	0.4009	0.3875	0.3926	0.2833	0.3715
15–34	n	25	62	55	42	31
	Rate	0.0895	0.1798	0.1499	0.1144	0.1347
35–49	n	102	105	101	133	102
	Rate	0.5625	0.4931	0.4576	0.5624	0.6619
50–69	n	328	370	378	404	277
	Rate	1.3715	1.272	1.3378	1.471	1.7175
70–84	n	171	212	246	303	209
	Rate	1.7451	1.6086	1.7332	2.0588	2.4132
0–84	n	721	844	876	954	679
	Rate	0.6721	0.65	0.6616	0.7063	0.8351

(e) Birth cohort mortality, ages 35–84 years, males, 1960–97

Year of birth	1875–79	1880–84	1885–89	1890–94	1895–99	1900–4	1905–9	1910–14	1915–19	1920–24	1925–29	1930–34	1935–39	1940–44	1945–49	1950–54	1955–59	1960–64
n	6	19	68	111	173	275	347	308	267	317	176	114	65	48	34	7	5	0
U 95% CI	198.9	111.1	142.3	128.9	127.9	131.2	131.3	106.8	112.5	120.4	97.6	95	87.3	107.6	122.5	81.4	167.3	
SCMR	91.4	71.1	112.2	107	110.2	116.6	118.2	95.5	99.8	107.8	84.2	79.1	68.5	81.2	87.7	39.5	71.7	
L 95% CI	33.5	42.8	87.2	88	94.4	103.6	106.4	85.4	88.5	96.6	72.2	65.2	52.9	59.9	60.7	15.9	23.3	

(f) Birth cohort mortality, ages 35–84 years, females, 1960–97

Year of birth	1875–79	1880–84	1885–89	1890–94	1895–99	1900–4	1905–9	1910–14	1915–19	1920–24	1925–29	1930–34	1935–39	1940–44	1945–49	1950–54	1955–59	1960–64
n	6	29	93	155	235	286	325	342	272	280	172	91	62	31	21	11	2	0
U 95% CI	132.6	104.8	131.9	131	133.8	121.6	116.6	115.7	116.8	116.2	108.4	90.3	97.1	86.9	87.6	116.1	103.1	
SCMR	60.9	73	107.7	111.9	117.8	108.3	104.6	104	103.7	103.3	93.3	73.6	75.8	61.2	57.3	64.9	28.5	
L 95% CI	22.4	48.9	86.9	95	103.6	96.4	93.8	93.6	92.1	91.9	79.9	59.2	58.1	41.6	35.5	32.4	3.5	

(g) Birth cohort incidence, ages 35–84 years, males, 1971–92

Year of birth	1885–89	1890–94	1895–99	1900–4	1905–9	1910–14	1915–19	1920–24	1925–29	1930–34	1935–39	1940–44	1945–49	1950–54	1955–59
n	7	31	126	216	478	505	484	548	421	291	206	143	97	36	7
U 95% CI	165.2	84.9	119	91.7	121.3	105	114	111.6	115.1	108.7	108.9	123.3	129.9	146.1	284.8
SCIR	80.2	59.8	100	80.2	110.9	96.2	104.3	102.6	104.6	96.9	95	104.7	106.5	105.5	138.2
L 95% CI	32.2	40.6	83.3	70.2	101.4	88.2	95.4	94.4	95.1	86.3	82.9	88.2	86.3	73.9	55.6

(h) Birth cohort incidence, ages 35–84 years, females, 1971–92

Year of birth	1885–89	1890–94	1895–99	1900–4	1905–9	1910–14	1915–19	1920–24	1925–29	1930–34	1935–39	1940–44	1945–49	1950–54	1955–59
n	12	68	155	282	420	508	448	493	359	232	194	146	83	38	3
U 95% CI	156.6	116.6	107.3	105.6	103.8	109.3	116.3	114.1	114	104.2	120	135.9	121.6	154.6	187.5
SCIR	89.7	92	91.7	94	94.4	100.2	106	104.4	102.8	91.6	104.3	115.5	98.1	112.6	64.2
L 95% CI	46.3	71.4	77.8	83.6	85.8	91.9	96.6	95.6	92.7	80.5	90.1	97.5	78.1	79.7	13.2

Table C26 Tumours of nervous system (benign and malignant)

(a) Mortality, males, 1960–97

Age		1960–4	1965–9	1970–4	1975–9	1980–4	1985–9	1990–4	1995–7
0–14	n	517	517	535	450	354	295	315	143
	Rate	1.8735	1.7659	1.7713	1.5853	1.3884	1.1976	1.2536	0.9233
15–34	n	613	635	638	655	596	554	574	305
	Rate	2.0121	1.9875	1.8995	1.8203	1.5974	1.4584	1.4572	1.242
35–49	n	1618	1529	1424	1326	1271	1397	1441	856
	Rate	6.8726	6.5118	6.2721	6.0581	5.6746	5.8243	5.5191	5.1489
50–69	n	4063	4175	4284	4397	4538	4628	4474	2665
	Rate	16.4991	16.1599	16.2573	16.9353	17.8414	18.2842	17.8961	17.5726
70–84	n	433	528	721	1055	1639	2211	2699	1879
	Rate	6.9671	8.2	9.9841	13.0041	18.3158	24.0356	27.8401	31.0967
0–84	n	7244	7384	7602	7883	8398	9085	9503	5848
	Rate	6.4918	6.4369	6.5542	6.881	7.3928	7.9616	8.1832	8.2125

(b) Incidence, males, 1971–92

Age		1971–4	1975–9	1980–4	1985–9	1990–2
0–14	n	698	803	695	732	453
	Rate	2.8846	2.8258	2.7229	2.9714	2.9775
15–34	n	815	1209	1247	1308	863
	Rate	2.9775	3.3453	3.3312	3.4072	3.6433
35–49	n	1452	1908	1915	2146	1405
	Rate	8.1043	8.7633	8.5181	8.8658	9.1521
50–69	n	3826	5227	5523	5655	3536
	Rate	18.0998	20.0572	21.6748	22.3117	23.4591
70–84	n	627	1209	1960	2430	1786
	Rate	10.7938	14.935	21.9484	26.4203	31.1301
0–84	n	7418	10356	11340	12271	8043
	Rate	7.917	8.946	9.8785	10.5662	11.3763

(c) Mortality, females, 1960–97

Age		1960–4	1965–9	1970–4	1975–9	1980–4	1985–9	1990–4	1995–7
0–14	n	420	409	389	346	270	251	241	132
	Rate	1.5975	1.4589	1.3556	1.2813	1.1177	1.0721	1.0116	0.881
15–34	n	542	465	452	496	408	419	374	236
	Rate	1.7949	1.5033	1.3914	1.4212	1.1175	1.1421	0.9769	1.0323
35–49	n	1155	1011	953	915	891	891	924	557
	Rate	4.7717	4.2632	4.2081	4.233	4.0189	3.7143	3.5406	3.3928
50–69	n	3043	3128	3355	3455	3443	3483	3266	1919
	Rate	10.6502	10.6219	11.3827	11.8593	12.2052	12.6275	12.2331	12.031
70–84	n	523	616	781	1139	1759	2374	2900	1979
	Rate	5.1206	5.5972	6.5123	8.7615	12.6416	16.6353	19.9054	22.4304
0–84	n	5683	5629	5930	6351	6771	7418	7705	4823
	Rate	4.5383	4.3683	4.5549	4.865	5.134	5.5385	5.659	5.8107

(d) Incidence, females, 1971–92

Age		-1971–4	1975–9	1980–4	1985–9	1990–2
0–14	n	532	660	580	588	400
	Rate	2.3299	2.4628	2.3961	2.5017	2.7985
15–34	n	723	1011	999	1052	705
	Rate	2.745	2.8839	2.7409	2.8407	3.1147
35–49	n	1185	1530	1643	1935	1335
	Rate	6.6364	7.1341	7.4015	8.0788	8.7013
50–69	n	3273	4622	4991	5019	3059
	Rate	13.8596	15.9154	17.753	18.2533	19.0375
70–84	n	759	1462	2381	2924	2080
	Rate	7.827	11.2035	17.1095	20.5585	24.0692
0–84	n	6472	9285	10594	11518	7579
	Rate	6.2651	7.1863	8.1246	8.7245	9.4753

(e) Birth cohort mortality, ages 0–14, 15–44, 45–84 years, males, 1960–97

Year of birth	1875–79	1880–84	1885–89	1890–94	1895–99	1900–4	1905–9	1910–14	1915–19	1920–24	1925–29	1930–34	1935–39	1940–44	1945–49	1950–54	1955–59	1960–64	1965–69	1970–74	1975–79	1980–84	1985–89	1990–94
Ages 0–14 years																								
n	–	–	–	–	–	–	–	–	–	–	–	–	–	–	60	235	424	532	537	393	305	328	203	91
U 95% CI															123.3	147.5	135.5	122.2	124.1	105.6	98.4	99.9	80	71.5
SCMR															95.8	129.8	123.2	112.3	114.1	95.7	88	89.6	69.7	58.3
L 95% CI															73.1	114.2	112	103.1	104.8	86.7	78.6	80.4	60.7	46.9
Ages 15–44 years																								
n	–	–	–	–	–	–	–	–	243	761	990	1007	1130	1265	1497	1354	920	647	385	192	72	–	–	–
U 95% CI									127.5	123.2	125.4	111.1	110.4	108.4	102.6	105.2	97.1	92.2	92.8	94.6	95.4			
SCMR									112.5	114.8	117.8	104.5	104.1	102.6	97.6	99.8	91	85.4	84	82.1	75.7			
L 95% CI									99.2	106.9	110.7	98.2	98.3	97.1	92.8	94.6	85.3	79	76	70.9	59.3			
Ages 45–84 years																								
n	17	72	293	815	1929	3905	6098	7722	6762	7501	5484	3835	2544	1471	799	108	–	–	–	–	–	–	–	–
U 95% CI	41.7	29.3	40.9	55.6	75	90.3	105.5	115.5	117.2	114.7	110.7	104.3	100.6	96.8	98.4	111.4								
SCMR	26.1	23.2	36.5	51.9	71.7	87.6	102.9	112.9	114.4	112.2	107.8	101.1	96.7	92	91.9	92.2								
L 95% CI	15.2	18.2	32.5	48.5	68.6	84.9	100.3	110.4	111.7	109.7	105	97.9	93	87.4	85.7	75.7								

(f) Birth cohort mortality, ages 0–14, 15–44, 45–84 years, females, 1960–97

Year of birth	1875–79	1880–84	1885–89	1890–94	1895–99	1900–4	1905–9	1910–14	1915–19	1920–24	1925–29	1930–34	1935–39	1940–44	1945–49	1950–54	1955–59	1960–64	1965–69	1970–74	1975–79	1980–84	1985–89	1990–94
Ages 0–14 years																								
n	–	–	–	–	–	–	–	–	–	–	–	–	–	–	62	163	327	429	370	322	261	268	166	79
U 95% CI															174.4	137	135.8	126	110.1	111.5	108.4	104.7	82.6	78.7
SCMR															136	117.5	121.9	114.6	99.5	100	96	92.9	71	63.2
L 95% CI															104.3	100.2	109.4	104.3	89.8	89.7	85.1	82.4	60.6	50
Ages 15–44 years																								
n								–	166	540	654	746	799	901	1126	867	634	485	276	134	49	–		
U 95% CI									132.1	129.3	122.2	121.7	114.5	111.5	109.9	96.3	93.7	95.5	90.7	91.6	89.6			
SCMR									113.5	118.8	113.1	113.3	106.9	104.5	103.7	90.1	86.7	87.3	80.6	77.3	67.8			
L 95% CI									96.9	109.2	104.8	105.4	99.7	97.9	97.8	84.3	80.2	79.9	71.7	64.8	50.2			
Ages 45–84 years																								
n	20	107	375	915	1925	3408	5141	6804	5791	6061	3958	2754	1632	965	549	62	–	–	–	–	–	–	–	–
U 95% CI	34.6	31.6	41.4	54.7	71.1	87.2	104.2	123.5	126.2	122.8	111.8	108.9	95	94.1	103.5	106.1								
SCMR	22.4	26.1	37.4	51.2	68	84.3	101.4	120.6	123	119.8	108.4	104.9	90.5	88.4	95.2	82.8								
L 95% CI	13.7	21.4	33.8	48	65.1	81.5	98.7	117.7	119.8	116.8	105.1	101	86.2	83	87.6	63.5								

(g) Birth cohort incidence, ages 0–14, 15–44, 45–84 years, males, 1971–92

Year of birth	1885–89	1890–94	1895–99	1900–4	1905–9	1910–14	1915–19	1920–24	1925–29	1930–34	1935–39	1940–44	1945–49	1950–54	1955–59	1960–64	1965–69	1970–74	1975–79	1980–84	1985–89
Ages 0–14 years																					
n	–	–	–	–	–	–	–	–	–	–	–	–	–	–	84	344	690	745	592	563	311
U 95% CI															137.2	108.4	110.9	103.3	99.9	117.4	116.8
SCIR															110.8	97.5	102.9	96.2	92.2	108.1	104.5
L 95% CI															88.4	87.7	95.5	89.5	85	99.6	93.5
Ages 15–44 years																					
n	–	–	–	–	–	–	–	–	198	697	1188	1606	2180	1637	1337	932	571	237	46	–	–
U 95% CI									106.7	101	104.8	103.9	103.4	105.4	111.2	104.8	113.7	118	196.6		
SCIR									92.9	93.7	99	99	99.2	100.4	105.4	98.3	104.7	103.9	147.4		
L 95% CI									80.4	87	93.5	94.2	95.1	95.7	99.9	92.2	96.5	91.5	107.9		
Ages 45–84 years																					
n	21	107	514	1626	3649	5632	5601	6622	5095	3345	2062	959	185	–	–	–	–	–	–	–	–
U 95% CI	69.8	44.2	63.8	78.6	96.2	108.6	111.3	106.2	107.4	105.9	108.1	109.1	132.7								
SCIR	45.7	36.6	58.5	74.8	93.1	105.8	108.5	103.7	104.5	102.3	103.5	102.4	114.9								
L 95% CI	28.3	30	53.7	71.3	90.1	103	105.7	101.2	101.7	98.9	99.1	96.1	98.9								

(h) Birth cohort incidence, ages 0–14, 15–44, 45–84 years, females, 1971–92

Year of birth	1885–89	1890–94	1895–99	1900–4	1905–9	1910–14	1915–19	1920–24	1925–29	1930–34	1935–39	1940–44	1945–49	1950–54	1955–59	1960–64	1965–69	1970–74	1975–79	1980–84	1985–89
Ages 0–14 years																					
n	–	–	–	–	–	–	–	–	–	–	–	–	–	–	56	306	490	594	530	467	269
U 95% CI															122.1	122.4	98.7	101.9	110.1	118.7	120.9
SCIR															94	109.5	90.3	94.1	101.1	108.4	107.2
L 95% CI															71	97.9	82.7	86.8	92.8	99	95.2
Ages 15–44 years																					
n	–	–	–	–	–	–	–	–	156	584	910	1370	2005	1442	1020	763	467	191	44	–	
U 95% CI									97.5	99.7	95.3	104.6	112.1	110.5	103.3	106.3	114.1	115	218.8		
SCIR									83.3	92	89.3	99.2	107.3	105	97.2	99	104.2	99.8	163		
L 95% CI									70.8	84.8	83.7	94.1	102.7	99.7	91.4	92.2	95.2	86.1	118.4		
Ages 45–84 years																					
n	35	209	745	2056	3921	5571	5197	5951	4375	2871	1728	922	155	–				–	–	–	–
U 95% CI	58.6	48.5	61.4	82.3	97.3	110.7	112.4	108.4	108.5	108	107.6	122	132.5								
SCIR	42.2	42.3	57.2	78.8	94.3	107.8	109.3	105.7	105.3	104.1	102.7	114.4	113.2								
L 95% CI	29.4	37	53.2	75.5	91.4	105	106.4	103	102.2	100.4	97.9	107.2	96.1								

Table C27 Cancer of thyroid

(a) Mortality, males, 1960–97

Age		1960–4	1965–9	1970–4	1975–9	1980–4	1985–9	1990–4	1995–7
0–14	n	0	0	0	0	1	0	0	0
	Rate	0	0	0	0	0.004	0	0	0
15–34	n	8	6	10	11	9	6	8	1
	Rate	0.0256	0.0218	0.0301	0.0297	0.0242	0.016	0.0206	0.0036
35–49	n	44	46	48	45	32	29	35	17
	Rate	0.188	0.1969	0.207	0.2032	0.1441	0.1206	0.1343	0.1019
50–69	n	267	270	283	273	257	231	206	124
	Rate	1.1349	1.0786	1.0953	1.0561	1.0249	0.9151	0.826	0.8246
70–84	n	173	193	194	229	184	243	182	128
	Rate	2.9249	3.1045	2.8431	3.0173	2.1468	2.6585	1.8701	2.1122
0–84	n	492	515	535	558	483	509	431	270
	Rate	0.5602	0.5647	0.5487	0.5553	0.4569	0.4724	0.384	0.3951

(b) Incidence, males, 1971–92

Age		1971–4	1975–9	1980–4	1985–9	1990–2
0–14	n	6	7	8	15	5
	Rate	0.0267	0.0246	0.0318	0.0659	0.0345
15–34	n	69	98	135	160	108
	Rate	0.2584	0.2707	0.3621	0.422	0.4388
35–49	n	126	162	199	175	144
	Rate	0.7016	0.7458	0.8825	0.7165	0.9258
50–69	n	341	431	479	513	275
	Rate	1.633	1.6534	1.8952	2.0162	1.8335
70–84	n	172	270	273	295	162
	Rate	3.1043	3.5105	3.1603	3.2284	2.8391
0–84	n	714	968	1094	1158	694
	Rate	0.854	0.907	0.9816	1.0103	0.9701

(c) Mortality, females, 1960–97

Age		1960–4	1965–9	1970–4	1975–9	1980–4	1985–9	1990–4	1995–7
0–14	n	0	1	0	0	0	0	0	0
	Rate	0	0.0041	0	0	0	0	0	0
15–34	n	17	13	11	6	6	3	9	1
	Rate	0.0563	0.042	0.0344	0.0181	0.0164	0.0082	0.024	0.0036
35–49	n	74	63	70	55	43	28	36	15
	Rate	0.3019	0.2627	0.2996	0.2507	0.1965	0.1175	0.1381	0.0915
50–69	n	586	572	550	543	384	362	301	124
	Rate	2.1173	1.9606	1.8475	1.8201	1.3452	1.2877	1.1156	0.7699
70–84	n	647	658	714	716	622	600	578	287
	Rate	6.2693	5.8307	5.8385	5.3938	4.2723	3.9724	3.7891	3.1243
0–84	n	1324	1307	1345	1320	1055	993	924	427
	Rate	1.1138	1.0285	1.0077	0.9471	0.7292	0.6724	0.6261	0.4743

(d) Incidence, females, 1971–92

Age		1971–4	1975–9	1980–4	1985–9	1990–2
0–14	n	15	18	21	17	8
	Rate	0.0765	0.0687	0.0873	0.0851	0.0641
15–34	n	246	392	514	511	372
	Rate	0.9317	1.1277	1.4016	1.3622	1.5612
35–49	n	278	425	514	599	451
	Rate	1.5686	2.0089	2.3032	2.4838	2.9583
50–69	n	742	977	988	863	599
	Rate	3.1137	3.3236	3.5158	3.1578	3.7357
70–84	n	638	907	883	766	522
	Rate	6.4851	6.862	6.1027	5.2355	5.9237
0–84	n	1919	2719	2920	2756	1952
	Rate	1.8604	2.0776	2.1896	2.0506	2.3817

(e) Birth cohort mortality, ages 15–44, 45–84 years, males, 1960–97

Year of birth	1875–79	1880–84	1885–89	1890–94	1895–99	1900–4	1905–9	1910–14	1915–19	1920–24	1925–29	1930–34	1935–39	1940–44	1945–49	1950–54	1955–59	1960–64	1965–69	1970–74	1975–79
											Ages 15–44 years										
n	–	–	–	–	–	–	–	–	5	21	20	32	17	32	27	24	14	4	5	1	1
U 95% CI									204.3	193	156.6	214.9	119.5	181.6	130	135.1	138	101	217.8	238.9	777.3
SCMR									87.6	126.2	101.4	152.2	74.6	128.7	89.4	90.8	82.2	39.4	93.3	42.9	139.5
L 95% CI									28.4	78.1	61.9	104.1	43.5	88	58.9	58.2	45	10.7	30.3	1.1	3.6
									Ages 45–84 years												
n	21	61	144	221	291	444	500	507	445	388	255	154	95	45	16	2	–	–	–	–	–
U 95% CI	220	134.4	138.6	130.8	119.7	123.8	112.2	104.2	116.6	100.8	102.3	98.8	101.5	94.8	93.5	228.8					
SCMR	143.9	104.6	117.7	114.6	106.7	112.8	102.8	95.5	106.2	91.2	90.5	84.3	83	70.8	57.6	63.3					
L 95% CI	89.1	80	99.3	100.5	95.1	102.8	94.2	87.6	96.8	82.6	80	71.5	67.2	51.7	32.9	7.7					

(f) Birth cohort mortality, ages 15–44, 45–84 years, females, 1960–97

Year of birth	1875–79	1880–84	1885–89	1890–94	1895–99	1900–4	1905–9	1910–14	1915–19	1920–24	1925–29	1930–34	1935–39	1940–44	1945–49	1950–54	1955–59	1960–64	1965–69	1970–74	1975–79
											Ages 15–44 years										
n	–	–	–	–	–	–	–	–	8	28	35	40	32	24	34	22	10	7	1	1	1
U 95% CI									214.8	186.9	202.7	217	170	121.1	130.6	105	93.3	130.2	93.8	205.5	466.8
SCMR									109	129.3	145.7	159.4	120.4	81.4	93.4	69.4	50.7	63.2	16.8	36.9	83.8
L 95% CI									47.1	85.9	101.5	113.9	82.4	52.1	64.7	43.5	24.3	25.4	0.4	1	2.2
									Ages 45–84 years												
n	84	263	559	819	993	1179	1156	1220	770	675	376	198	103	38	17	1	–	–	–	–	–
U 95% CI	175	131.5	137.2	138.7	126.2	118.8	102	104.3	92.3	90.2	86.8	78.4	74.7	61.2	73.5	130.7					
SCMR	141.3	116.5	126.3	129.5	118.6	112.2	96.3	98.6	86	83.7	78.4	68.2	61.6	44.6	45.9	23.4					
L 95% CI	112.7	103.3	116.3	120.9	111.4	106	90.9	93.2	80.2	77.6	70.9	59	50.3	31.6	26.8	0.6					

(g) Birth cohort incidence, ages 15–44, 45–84 years, males, 1971–92

Year of birth	1885-89	1890-94	1895-99	1900-4	1905-9	1910-14	1915-19	1920-24	1925-29	1930-34	1935-39	1940-44	1945-49	1950-54	1955-59	1960-64	1965-69	1970-74	1975-79
									Ages 15–44 years										
n	–	–	–	–	–	–	–	–	16	74	106	157	232	193	127	106	66	22	1
U 95% CI									125.6	123.2	102	105.9	112	124.3	114.4	138	172.4	215.4	407.8
SCIR									77.4	98.2	84.3	90.6	98.4	108	96.2	114.1	135.5	142.3	73.2
L 95% CI									44.2	77.1	69	77	86.6	93.3	80.2	93.4	104.8	89.2	1.9
									Ages 45–84 years										
n	9	62	152	330	443	523	496	570	406	250	165	65	16	–	–	–	–	–	–
U 95% CI	150.2	130.8	124.5	121.2	100	100.9	110.6	112.2	115.4	112.1	126.4	117.6	190.3						
SCIR	79.1	102	106.2	108.8	91.1	92.6	101.2	103.4	104.7	99.1	108.5	92.3	117.2						
L 95% CI	36.2	78.2	90	97.7	83	85	92.7	95.2	95	87.5	92.6	71.2	67						

(h) Birth cohort incidence, ages 15–44, 45–84 years, females, 1971–92

Year of birth	1885-89	1890-94	1895-99	1900-4	1905-9	1910-14	1915-19	1920-24	1925-29	1930-34	1935-39	1940-44	1945-49	1950-54	1955-59	1960-64	1965-69	1970-74	1975-79
									Ages 15–44 years										
n	–	–	–	–	–	–	–	–	29	168	286	511	735	658	495	381	223	69	6
U 95% CI									80.4	96.7	89.4	105.9	104.8	116.8	113.9	122.8	141.8	151.1	254.7
SCIR									56	83.1	79.6	97.1	97.5	108.2	104.3	111.1	124.3	119.4	117
L 95% CI									37.5	71	70.9	89.1	90.7	100.3	95.5	100.5	109	92.9	43
									Ages 45–84 years										
n	64	294	624	1025	1186	1314	1003	1063	775	578	402	244	54	–	–	–	–	–	–
U 95% CI	159	126.2	118.2	114.5	97.3	104.2	102	99.2	99.9	111.7	120.3	145.8	210						
SCIR	124.5	112.6	109.3	107.7	91.9	98.7	95.9	93.4	93.1	103	109.1	128.6	161						
L 95% CI	95.9	100.4	101	101.3	86.9	93.5	90.2	88	86.8	94.9	98.9	113.5	120.9						

Table C28 Hodgkin's disease

(a) Mortality, males, 1960–97

Age		1960–4	1965–9	1970–4	1975–9	1980–4	1985–9	1990–4	1995–7
0–14	n	65	44	37	22	7	7	4	1
	Rate	0.2572	0.1761	0.1401	0.0799	0.0273	0.0323	0.0175	0.0081
15–34	n	623	679	529	450	352	322	226	96
	Rate	2.0196	2.0859	1.5121	1.2189	0.9357	0.8288	0.5538	0.3814
35–49	n	652	637	484	402	331	290	215	101
	Rate	2.7644	2.7716	2.1848	1.8687	1.4657	1.1931	0.8385	0.6234
50–69	n	966	1024	981	792	589	386	348	161
	Rate	3.9844	3.9877	3.7511	3.0382	2.3085	1.5128	1.384	1.0605
70–84	n	293	365	379	326	304	251	204	117
	Rate	4.8734	5.8632	5.527	4.098	3.4795	2.7416	2.1031	1.9483
0–84	n	2599	2749	2410	1992	1583	1256	997	476
	Rate	2.4848	2.5814	2.2119	1.7656	1.3794	1.0564	0.8195	0.6413

(b) Incidence, males, 1971–92

Age		1971–4	1975–9	1980–4	1985–9	1990–2
0–14	n	139	224	205	150	94
	Rate	0.6226	0.7882	0.8125	0.6728	0.6923
15–34	n	1234	1567	1481	1474	892
	Rate	4.4202	4.3118	3.918	3.7427	3.7476
35–49	n	690	805	814	765	465
	Rate	3.9367	3.7542	3.5967	3.1191	3.0408
50–69	n	1160	1226	1009	838	448
	Rate	5.4872	4.6796	3.944	3.3042	2.9645
70–84	n	338	438	384	332	180
	Rate	6.0279	5.5131	4.3944	3.6131	3.1308
0–84	n	3561	4260	3893	3559	2079
	Rate	3.9366	3.6801	3.2722	2.8925	2.765

(c) Mortality, females, 1960–97

Age		1960–4	1965–9	1970–4	1975–9	1980–4	1985–9	1990–4	1995–7
0–14	n	28	20	8	8	5	7	0	2
	Rate	0.1201	0.0869	0.0309	0.0316	0.0212	0.0327	0	0.014
15–34	n	344	384	304	232	214	187	181	77
	Rate	1.1396	1.2107	0.9173	0.6589	0.5816	0.4943	0.4631	0.3309
35–49	n	290	298	248	177	136	159	102	51
	Rate	1.2192	1.2834	1.1291	0.8351	0.6085	0.6571	0.3989	0.3175
50–69	n	592	578	537	465	322	239	198	94
	Rate	2.0764	1.9721	1.8098	1.5844	1.1433	0.8529	0.7284	0.6022
70–84	n	387	393	437	371	314	286	209	114
	Rate	3.7559	3.5213	3.5976	2.829	2.2213	1.9	1.4154	1.2211
0–84	n	1641	1673	1534	1253	991	878	690	338
	Rate	1.3912	1.3729	1.2158	0.9647	0.7458	0.6366	0.5025	0.405

(d) Incidence, females, 1971–92

Age		1971–4	1975–9	1980–4	1985–9	1990–2
0–14	n	62	74	92	68	40
	Rate	0.2956	0.2836	0.3846	0.3206	0.3316
15–34	n	737	984	1098	1215	704
	Rate	2.7591	2.79	2.9746	3.1951	3.1019
35–49	n	335	393	389	411	240
	Rate	1.9249	1.882	1.7397	1.6932	1.6011
50–69	n	680	729	610	483	267
	Rate	2.8514	2.5191	2.1549	1.7727	1.6571
70–84	n	431	464	476	353	183
	Rate	4.4186	3.5378	3.358	2.3789	2.1478
0–84	n	2245	2644	2665	2530	1434
	Rate	2.2776	2.1228	2.0778	1.9493	1.8601

(e) Birth cohort mortality, ages 0–14, 15–44, 45–84 years, males, 1960–97

Year of birth	1875–79	1880–84	1885–89	1890–94	1895–99	1900–4	1905–9	1910–14	1915–19	1920–24	1925–29	1930–34	1935–39	1940–44	1945–49	1950–54	1955–59	1960–64	1965–69	1970–74	1975–79	1980–84	1985–89	1990–94
Ages 0–14 years																								
n	–	–	–	–	–	–	–	–	–	–	–	–	–	–	20	42	60	31	15	10	5	3	1	0
U 95% CI															307.5	306.3	319.2	156.2	88.5	75.3	56.1		58.5	
SCMR															199.1	226.6	248	110	53.6	40.9	24	14.4	10.5	
L 95% CI															121.6	163.3	189.2	74.8	30	19.6	7.8	3	0.3	
Ages 15–44 years																								
n	–	–	–	–	–	–	–	–	95	362	449	599	709	768	812	564	407	292	153	92	12	–	–	–
U 95% CI									196.7	188.3	159.7	158.2	145.2	133.3	113.9	89.3	74.9	61.8	48.9	63.6	41.4			
SCMR									160.9	169.9	145.5	146	134.9	124.2	106.3	82.2	67.9	55.1	41.8	51.9	23.7			
L 95% CI									130.2	153.3	132.7	134.8	125.3	115.7	99.2	75.7	61.7	49.1	35.4	41.8	12.2			
Ages 45–84 years																								
n	19	108	239	454	624	1027	1253	1379	1059	942	591	380	257	146	77	6	–	–	–	–	–	–	–	–
U 95% CI	184.2	182.4	159.7	167.8	142.2	144.1	132.2	123	110.4	89.1	76	66.2	63.7	56.4	53	52								
SCMR	117.9	151	140.7	153	131.5	135.6	125.1	116.7	103.9	83.6	70.1	59.8	56.4	47.9	42.4	23.9								
L 95% CI	71	123.9	123.9	139.6	121.6	127.5	118.3	110.7	97.9	78.4	64.7	54.1	49.9	40.5	33.5	8.8								

(f) Birth cohort mortality, ages 0–14, 15–44, 45–84 years, females, 1960–97

Year of birth	1875–79	1880–84	1885–89	1890–94	1895–99	1900–4	1905–9	1910–14	1915–19	1920–24	1925–29	1930–34	1935–39	1940–44	1945–49	1950–54	1955–59	1960–64	1965–69	1970–74	1975–79	1980–84	1985–89	1990–94
Ages 0–14 years																								
n	–	–	–	–	–	–	–	–	–	–	–	–	–	–	13	19	14	14	7	5	3	1	2	0
U 95% CI															437	361.8	232.3	199.6	123.6	115	101.5	65.9	214	–
SCMR															255.6	231.7	138.4	119	60	49.3	34.7	11.8	59.2	
L 95% CI															136.1	139.5	75.7	65	24.1	16	7.2	0.3	7.2	
Ages 15–44 years																								
n	–	–	–	–	–	–	–	–	44	150	227	314	365	428	401	317	246	200	126	62	15	–	–	–
U 95% CI									200.2	169.4	167.4	168.8	148.4	140.1	105.9	94.5	83.4	75.4	70	72.4	75.1			
SCMR									149.1	144.4	146.9	151.1	133.9	127.4	96.1	84.6	73.6	65.6	58.8	56.5	45.6			
L 95% CI									108.3	122.2	129	135.3	120.9	115.9	87.1	75.8	65	56.9	49	43.3	25.5			
Ages 45–84 years																								
n	39	149	301	462	634	844	898	821	621	565	306	161	123	64	33	4	–	–	–	–	–			
U 95% CI	226.5	177.5	154	146.7	139.3	138.7	123.3	104	98.8	89.8	74.8	59.8	69.6	60.9	56.8	83								
SCMR	165.7	151.2	137.6	133.9	128.9	129.7	115.5	97.1	91.4	82.7	66.9	51.3	58.3	47.7	40.4	32.4								
L 95% CI	117.8	127.9	122.9	122.3	119.2	121.2	108.2	90.7	84.5	76.1	59.8	43.7	48.5	36.7	27.8	8.8								

(g) Birth cohort incidence, ages 0–14, 15–44, 45–84 years, males, 1971–92

Ages 0–14 years

Year of birth	1885–89	1890–94	1895–99	1900–4	1905–9	1910–14	1915–19	1920–24	1925–29	1930–34	1935–39	1940–44	1945–49	1950–54	1955–59	1960–64	1965–69	1970–74	1975–79	1980–84	1985–89
n	–	–	–	–	–	–	–	–	–	–	–	–	–	–	39	126	214	208	143	65	17
U 95% CI															137.2	102.5	122.7	131.1	115.7	103.9	135.8
SCIR															100.4	86.1	107.3	114.4	98.2	81.5	84.8
L 95% CI															71.4	71.7	93.8	99.9	82.8	62.9	49.4

Ages 15–44 years

Year of birth	1885–89	1890–94	1895–99	1900–4	1905–9	1910–14	1915–19	1920–24	1925–29	1930–34	1935–39	1940–44	1945–49	1950–54	1955–59	1960–64	1965–69	1970–74	1975–79	1980–84	1985–89
n	–	–	–	–	–	–	–	–	–	–	97	346	665	1040	1649	1559	1406	1208	803	314	25
U 95% CI											145.4	118.2	118.4	113.3	109.5	105.3	99.6	97.1	103.1	109.8	124.4
SCIR											119.2	106.4	109.7	106.6	104.3	100.2	94.6	91.8	96.2	98.3	84.3
L 95% CI											96.6	95.7	101.7	100.3	99.4	95.3	89.7	86.7	89.8	88	54.6

Ages 45–84 years

Year of birth	1885–89	1890–94	1895–99	1900–4	1905–9	1910–14	1915–19	1920–24	1925–29	1930–34	1935–39	1940–44	1945–49	1950–54	1955–59	1960–64	1965–69	1970–74	1975–79	1980–84	1985–89
n	14	100	231	549	864	1025	1016	1221	993	675	468	214	58	–	–	–	–	–	–	–	–
U 95% CI	202.8	175	137.3	136	123.1	108.8	110.3	100.3	98.4	93.8	97.9	88.7	152.4								
SCIR	120.9	143.9	120.7	125	115.2	102.3	103.8	94.8	92.5	87	89.4	77.6	117.9								
L 95% CI	66.1	117.1	106.1	115	107.8	96.2	97.6	89.6	86.9	80.7	81.6	67.8	89.5								

(h) Birth cohort incidence, ages 0–14, 15–44, 45–84 years, females, 1971–92

Year of birth	1885–89	1890–94	1895–99	1900–4	1905–9	1910–14	1915–19	1920–24	1925–29	1930–34	1935–39	1940–44	1945–49	1950–54	1955–59	1960–64	1965–69	1970–74	1975–79	1980–84	1985–89
Ages 0–14 years																					
n	–	–	–	–	–	–	–	–	–	–	–	–	–	–	19	62	88	76	61	25	5
U 95% CI															126	121	131.8	127.4	136.1	151.5	150.4
SCIR															80.7	94.4	107	101.8	105.9	102.7	64.5
L 95% CI															48.6	72.4	85.8	80.2	81	66.4	20.9
Ages 15–44 years																					
n	–	–	–	–	–	–	–	–	34	171	326	543	848	1030	1035	988	718	298	19	–	–
U 95% CI									125.1	128.5	115.8	110.2	96.9	105.9	104.3	107.7	115.5	123.2	111.9		
SCIR									89.5	110.6	103.9	101.3	90.6	99.6	98.1	101.2	107.3	109.9	71.7		
L 95% CI									62	94.6	93.2	93.1	84.7	93.7	92.3	95.1	99.8	98.1	43.1		
Ages 45–84 years																					
n	24	146	331	598	757	783	662	705	532	310	201	101	22	–	–	–	–	–			
U 95% CI	178.1	151.5	134.4	131.2	113.8	104.6	105.6	100.4	103.4	92.7	96.3	99.4	141.3								
SCIR	119.7	128.8	120.7	121.1	106	97.5	97.9	93.2	95	82.9	83.9	81.8	93.4								
L 95% CI	76.7	108.8	108.3	111.7	98.7	90.9	90.7	86.6	87.2	74.2	73	66.6	58.5								

Table C29 Non-Hodgkin's lymphoma

(a) Mortality, males, 1960–97

Age		1960–4	1965–9	1970–4	1975–9	1980–4	1985–9	1990–4	1995–7
0–14	n	194	243	187	169	96	66	59	31
	Rate	0.7148	0.8547	0.6228	0.5865	0.3773	0.2761	0.2464	0.2037
15–34	n	348	362	361	368	373	297	407	221
	Rate	1.1296	1.1101	1.0708	1.0197	0.996	0.7819	1.0131	0.9026
35–49	n	551	603	549	531	624	793	972	549
	Rate	2.3433	2.5904	2.4336	2.4377	2.7902	3.303	3.723	3.3137
50–69	n	1762	2129	2227	2406	2864	3474	3698	2409
	Rate	7.5066	8.5444	8.578	9.3096	11.3252	13.7946	14.7404	15.9763
70–84	n	794	938	1185	1631	2270	3431	4066	2566
	Rate	13.1423	15.0963	17.5288	21.3355	26.2714	37.366	41.9353	42.4577
0–84	n	3649	4275	4509	5105	6227	8061	9202	5776
	Rate	3.7691	4.244	4.3878	4.8769	5.7872	7.3567	8.1244	8.3293

(b) Incidence, males, 1971–92

Age		1971–4	1975–9	1980–4	1985–9	1990–2
0–14	n	183	324	298	268	186
	Rate	0.7638	1.1329	1.1642	1.1167	1.2571
15–34	n	494	730	779	925	707
	Rate	1.8415	2.011	2.0811	2.4083	2.9734
35–49	n	811	1118	1487	2002	1492
	Rate	4.5316	5.1409	6.6323	8.2964	9.671
50–69	n	2569	3962	4900	6290	4310
	Rate	12.3	15.3173	19.299	24.8768	28.5918
70–84	n	1234	2186	3330	4823	3585
	Rate	22.4385	28.3057	38.3327	52.5203	62.3657
0–84	n	5291	8320	10794	14308	10280
	Rate	6.2954	7.7352	9.8271	12.746	14.9149

(c) Mortality, females, 1960–97

Age		1960–4	1965–9	1970–4	1975–9	1980–4	1985–9	1990–4	1995–7
0–14	n	104	89	81	67	48	25	21	12
	Rate	0.3922	0.3194	0.2854	0.2536	0.1987	0.1033	0.0879	0.0855
15–34	n	154	185	181	191	184	196	177	115
	Rate	0.5102	0.5889	0.5516	0.5367	0.5018	0.5358	0.4473	0.5016
35–49	n	324	329	345	339	388	435	519	319
	Rate	1.3367	1.3748	1.5209	1.5735	1.7584	1.821	1.9936	1.9367
50–69	n	1263	1520	1643	1802	2006	2495	2730	1608
	Rate	4.4837	5.1938	5.5193	6.1329	7.0659	8.9805	10.1382	10.0709
70–84	n	962	1299	1477	1960	2631	3615	4286	2635
	Rate	9.3454	11.6296	12.1448	14.8096	18.309	24.2427	28.2998	29.1433
0–84	n	2807	3422	3727	4359	5257	6766	7733	4689
	Rate	2.3204	2.7027	2.8294	3.208	3.7463	4.7157	5.3444	5.4131

(d) Incidence, females, 1971–92

Age		1971–4	1975–9	1980–4	1985–9	1990–2
0–14	n	105	133	125	104	81
	Rate	0.4701	0.4998	0.5186	0.4552	0.5679
15–34	n	310	383	462	550	375
	Rate	1.1719	1.087	1.2686	1.4666	1.6331
35–49	n	510	770	980	1349	915
	Rate	2.8373	3.5928	4.4335	5.6401	5.9065
50–69	n	2046	3123	3796	4907	3266
	Rate	8.6384	10.6384	13.4099	17.7594	20.1161
70–84	n	1519	2549	3770	5280	3680
	Rate	15.5387	19.3074	26.43	35.9257	41.4123
0–84	n	4490	6958	9133	12190	8317
	Rate	4.2891	5.1906	6.6646	8.7575	9.9024

(e) Birth cohort mortality, ages 35–84 years, males, 1960–97

Year of birth	1875–79	1880–84	1885–89	1890–94	1895–99	1900–4	1905–9	1910–14	1915–19	1920–24	1925–29	1930–34	1935–39	1940–44	1945–49	1950–54	1955–59	1960–64
n	48	265	674	1273	2023	3432	4974	6318	5535	5990	4169	2976	2120	1451	1006	492	244	32
U 95% CI	39.3	46.2	53.6	63.7	70.9	82	95.7	110.1	118.5	120.9	121.6	125.8	130.3	133.1	126.7	125.1	143.8	146.3
SCMR	29.6	41	49.7	60.3	67.9	79.3	93	107.4	115.4	117.8	118	121.4	124.9	126.4	119.1	114.5	126.8	103.6
L 95% CI	21.8	36.3	46.1	57	65	76.6	90.5	104.8	112.4	114.9	114.4	117.1	119.7	120.1	112	104.8	111.9	70.9

(f) Birth cohort mortality, ages 35–84 years, females, 1960–97

Year of birth	1875–79	1880–84	1885–89	1890–94	1895–99	1900–4	1905–9	1910–14	1915–19	1920–24	1925–29	1930–34	1935–39	1940–44	1945–49	1950–54	1955–59	1960–64
n	82	406	909	1567	2346	3478	4845	5806	4833	4636	2898	1948	1306	881	578	282	113	16
U 95% CI	46.3	53.1	56.6	66	73.1	85.1	102	116.4	128.4	128	126.9	131.5	132.7	137.4	128	131.4	129.5	169.6
SCMR	37.3	48.2	53.1	62.8	70.2	82.3	99.2	113.5	124.8	124.3	122.4	125.8	125.7	128.7	118	116.9	107.7	104.5
L 95% CI	29.7	43.7	49.7	59.7	67.4	79.7	96.4	110.6	121.4	120.8	118	120.3	119.1	120.4	108.7	104.1	88.8	59.7

(g) Birth cohort incidence, ages 35–84 years, males, 1971–92

Year of birth	1885–89	1890–94	1895–99	1900–4	1905–9	1910–14	1915–19	1920–24	1925–29	1930–34	1935–39	1940–44	1945–49	1950–54	1955–59
n	78	398	1221	2929	5345	6721	5867	6433	4792	3567	2715	1933	1377	631	92
U 95% CI	66.4	54.5	67.5	78.6	93.5	102.8	109.2	110.3	113.7	113	116.6	124.2	127	147.9	168.5
SCIR	53.2	49.4	63.8	75.8	91	100.4	106.4	107.7	110.5	109.3	112.3	118.8	120.5	136.8	137.4
L 95% CI	42	44.8	60.3	73.1	88.6	98	103.7	105.1	107.4	105.8	108.1	113.6	114.3	126.6	110.8

(h) Birth cohort incidence, ages 35–84 years, females, 1971–92

Year of birth	1885–89	1890–94	1895–99	1900–4	1905–9	1910–14	1915–19	1920–24	1925–29	1930–34	1935–39	1940–44	1945–49	1950–54	1955–59
n	101	674	1707	3409	5581	6304	5139	5085	3397	2582	1827	1325	932	351	46
U 95% CI	55.1	63.8	70.5	82	97.6	107.7	114.9	113	111.5	118.6	117.7	131.3	135.3	135.2	155.9
SCIR	45.4	59.1	67.2	79.3	95.1	105	111.8	109.9	107.8	114.1	112.5	124.4	126.8	121.8	116.8
L 95% CI	37	54.8	64.1	76.7	92.6	102.5	108.7	106.9	104.2	109.8	107.4	117.9	119	109.7	85.5

Table C30 Multiple myeloma

(a) Mortality, males, 1960–97

Age		1960–4	1965–9	1970–4	1975–9	1980–4	1985–9	1990–4	1995–7
0–14	n	1	0	0	0	0	0	0	0
	Rate	0.0035	0	0	0	0	0	0	0
15–34	n	11	6	13	12	11	16	6	3
	Rate	0.0364	0.0196	0.039	0.0341	0.0299	0.0448	0.0168	0.0138
35–49	n	181	161	159	184	163	182	177	102
	Rate	0.7486	0.675	0.684	0.8261	0.7344	0.7772	0.6688	0.5984
50–69	n	1077	1360	1588	1848	1852	2082	1999	1120
	Rate	4.6128	5.462	6.1662	7.1586	7.3352	8.2481	8.0069	7.5206
70–84	n	477	675	966	1365	1933	2648	2639	1667
	Rate	7.8745	10.8332	14.2551	18.0141	22.5599	28.8048	27.221	27.5844
0–84	n	1747	2202	2726	3409	3959	4928	4821	2892
	Rate	1.8848	2.3251	2.8025	3.3906	3.8303	4.618	4.3914	4.3044

(b) Incidence, males, 1971–92

Age		1971–4	1975–9	1980–4	1985–9	1990–2
0–14	n	0	3	3	1	2
	Rate	0	0.01	0.0115	0.0043	0.0135
15–34	n	18	32	20	26	19
	Rate	0.0639	0.0924	0.0552	0.0715	0.0827
35–49	n	213	308	283	296	220
	Rate	1.1599	1.3871	1.2725	1.2522	1.4168
50–69	n	1738	2410	2520	2871	1787
	Rate	8.3603	9.3283	10.0357	11.3302	11.8363
70–84	n	890	1725	2463	3187	1933
	Rate	16.1261	22.5361	28.7299	34.7207	33.766
0–84	n	2859	4478	5289	6381	3961
	Rate	3.5498	4.4038	5.0982	5.9343	5.9924

(c) Mortality, females, 1960–97

Age		1960–4	1965–9	1970–4	1975–9	1980–4	1985–9	1990–4	1995–7
0–14	n	1	0	0	0	0	0	0	0
	Rate	0.0033	0	0	0	0	0	0	0
15–34	n	11	8	7	6	5	2	4	2
	Rate	0.0357	0.0256	0.023	0.0171	0.0143	0.006	0.0099	0.0078
35–49	n	102	115	104	121	123	112	121	65
	Rate	0.4147	0.4736	0.4467	0.5469	0.563	0.4815	0.4599	0.3829
50–69	n	1060	1239	1343	1448	1435	1570	1498	905
	Rate	3.8003	4.2138	4.5147	4.9085	5.0222	5.6065	5.5278	5.6547
70–84	n	672	1018	1416	1764	2220	2851	2876	1683
	Rate	6.5325	9.1157	11.6517	13.3479	15.3786	18.9778	18.8863	18.519
0–84	n	1846	2380	2870	3339	3783	4535	4499	2655
	Rate	1.5229	1.8583	2.1524	2.4112	2.6251	3.0679	3.0395	3.0193

(d) Incidence, females, 1971–92

Age		1971–4	1975–9	1980–4	1985–9	1990–2
0–14	n	1	1	0	0	0
	Rate	0.0057	0.0041	0	0.008	0
15–34	n	13	16	11	26	3
	Rate	0.0503	0.0473	0.0302	0.0751	0.0121
35–49	n	144	206	184	213	150
	Rate	0.7815	0.9354	0.841	0.9024	0.9694
50–69	n	1427	1909	1954	2256	1284
	Rate	5.9806	6.5043	6.89	8.0905	7.853
70–84	n	1329	2137	2834	3290	2058
	Rate	13.5746	16.1842	19.7151	22.0031	22.8496
0–84	n	2914	4269	4983	5787	3495
	Rate	2.721	3.1025	3.4895	3.9905	4.0072

(e) Birth cohort mortality, ages 45–84 years, males, 1960–97

Year of birth	1875–79	1880–84	1885–89	1890–94	1895–99	1900–4	1905–9	1910–14	1915–19	1920–24	1925–29	1930–34	1935–39	1940–44	1945–49	1950–54
n	33	148	459	893	1560	2709	3809	4657	3512	3519	2212	1335	757	319	142	13
U 95% CI	36.3	35.6	49.9	62.2	76.9	93	107.9	122.7	120.2	122.2	121.7	120.7	122.3	106.9	115.7	141.5
SCMR	25.8	30.3	45.5	58.3	73.1	89.6	104.5	119.2	116.3	118.2	116.8	114.4	113.9	95.7	98.2	82.7
L 95% CI	17.8	25.7	41.6	54.6	69.6	86.3	101.3	115.9	112.5	114.4	112	108.4	106.1	85.8	82.7	44.1

(f) Birth cohort mortality, ages 45–84 years, females, 1960–97

Year of birth	1875–79	1880–84	1885–89	1890–94	1895–99	1900–4	1905–9	1910–14	1915–19	1920–24	1925–29	1930–34	1935–39	1940–44	1945–49	1950–54
n	48	272	701	1345	2123	3186	3929	4377	3232	2806	1668	1021	512	225	95	6
U 95% CI	36.9	47.2	57.5	73.8	86.4	102.9	111.4	120.7	122.7	117.1	119.5	127.4	118.3	111.3	116.1	107.7
SCMR	27.9	41.9	53.4	69.9	82.8	99.4	108	117.2	118.5	112.9	113.9	119.8	108.5	97.6	95	49.5
L 95% CI	20.5	37.2	49.6	66.3	79.3	96	104.6	113.8	114.5	108.8	108.6	112.7	99.5	85.7	76.8	18.2

(g) Birth cohort incidence, ages 45–84 years, males, 1971–92

Year of birth	1885–89	1890–94	1895–99	1900–4	1905–9	1910–14	1915–19	1920–24	1925–29	1930–34	1935–39	1940–44	1945–49
n	51	299	975	2276	3849	4327	3302	3180	2009	1161	614	211	33
U 95% CI	60.7	58.1	78.1	92	105.2	109.5	109.9	108.6	112.6	116	122.8	115.1	150.1
SCIR	46.2	51.9	73.4	88.3	101.9	106.3	106.2	104.9	107.8	109.5	113.4	100.6	106.9
L 95% CI	34.4	46.3	68.9	84.8	98.8	103.2	102.7	101.3	103.2	103.4	104.8	87.9	73.6

(h) Birth cohort incidence, ages 45–84 years, females, 1971–92

Year of birth	1885–89	1890–94	1895–99	1900–4	1905–9	1910–14	1915–19	1920–24	1925–29	1930–34	1935–39	1940–44	1945–49
n	102	557	1433	2878	3953	3947	2856	2413	1476	818	398	149	19
U 95% CI	73.7	72.3	84.3	100.8	104.9	109.1	112.3	106.1	115.8	117.7	117.7	125.5	140.4
SCIR	60.7	66.5	80.1	97.2	101.7	105.8	108.2	101.9	110	109.9	106.7	106.9	89.9
L 95% CI	49.5	61.2	76	93.7	98.6	102.5	104.3	97.9	104.5	102.6	96.7	90.5	54.1

Table C31 Leukaemia*

(a) Mortality, males, 1960–97

Age		1960–4	1965–9	1970–4	1975–9	1980–4	1985–9	1990–4	1995–7
0–14	n	984	958	885	788	536	368	349	167
	Rate	3.4623	3.1558	2.8554	2.7438	2.1055	1.5455	1.395	1.0981
15–34	n	742	708	717	815	800	778	606	315
	Rate	2.4083	2.189	2.1214	2.276	2.1206	2.03	1.5959	1.4284
35–49	n	891	792	747	687	727	741	631	384
	Rate	3.7894	3.4258	3.3289	3.1651	3.2298	3.0811	2.4203	2.3311
50–69	n	2662	2992	3004	3065	2998	3029	2905	1629
	Rate	11.537	12.1146	11.6772	11.9073	11.8727	12.0445	11.6184	10.9011
70–84	n	1910	2204	2560	2977	3700	4081	4201	2562
	Rate	32.0837	35.6992	38.2897	39.6568	43.5589	44.4569	43.1863	42.3993
0–84	n	7189	7654	7913	8332	8761	8997	8692	5057
	Rate	7.6105	7.876	7.9186	8.0901	8.2745	8.2258	7.7346	7.3763

(b) Incidence, males, 1971–92

Age		1971–4	1975–9	1980–4	1985–9	1990–2
0–14	n	1023	1159	1071	1058	715
	Rate	4.0731	4.0859	4.1593	4.1473	4.4167
15–34	n	625	885	910	912	582
	Rate	2.3087	2.4606	2.4116	2.3928	2.5379
35–49	n	709	846	874	946	661
	Rate	3.9667	3.8819	3.8889	3.9373	4.2925
50–69	n	3231	4043	4273	4461	2720
	Rate	15.6329	15.7403	16.9576	17.6654	17.9771
70–84	n	2442	3809	4820	5472	3442
	Rate	45.1044	50.6136	56.5948	59.633	59.8565
0–84	n	8030	10742	11948	12849	8120
	Rate	9.8371	10.4015	11.2213	11.6571	11.909

(c) Mortality, females, 1960–97

Age		1960–4	1965–9	1970–4	1975–9	1980–4	1985–9	1990–4	1995–7
0–14	n	746	751	679	484	378	286	204	124
	Rate	2.7536	2.6209	2.2959	1.8039	1.5675	1.2355	0.8526	0.8698
15–34	n	516	528	506	548	489	443	370	227
	Rate	1.7116	1.673	1.5433	1.5908	1.3393	1.1912	0.9959	1.0924
35–49	n	717	697	596	569	538	631	513	300
	Rate	2.967	2.9642	2.6374	2.6641	2.4236	2.6419	1.9791	1.8371
50–69	n	2249	2243	2174	2207	2122	2132	1949	1085
	Rate	7.9736	7.6373	7.2948	7.4832	7.4979	7.7006	7.2473	6.8019
70–84	n	1926	2317	2488	2942	3400	3717	3589	2140
	Rate	18.6828	20.5809	20.3077	22.0959	23.393	24.2929	23.1734	23.2038
0–84	n	6154	6536	6443	6750	6927	7209	6625	3876
	Rate	5.0889	5.15	4.8851	5.0093	4.9639	5.0167	4.558	4.4705

(d) Incidence, females, 1971–92

Age		1971–4	1975–9	1980–4	1985–9	1990–2
0–14	n	704	877	835	816	527
	Rate	2.9328	3.295	3.4245	3.3457	3.4737
15–34	n	466	651	617	634	425
	Rate	1.7834	1.8755	1.6888	1.718	1.931
35–49	n	522	653	651	821	470
	Rate	2.9155	3.042	2.9411	3.3396	3.0613
50–69	n	2164	2799	2847	2970	1706
	Rate	9.0735	9.5055	10.0556	10.6926	10.4625
70–84	n	2307	3531	4328	4825	2760
	Rate	23.4281	26.5411	29.8323	31.7072	30.135
0–84	n	6163	8511	9278	10066	5888
	Rate	5.8173	6.3238	6.6996	7.0936	6.9223

* Cohort data not shown – see text

Table C32 Cancer of of unspecified primary site*

(a) Mortality, males, 1960–97

Age		1960–4	1965–9	1970–4	1975–9	1980–4	1985–9	1990–4	1995–7
0–14	n	23	27	40	18	14	8	12	8
	Rate	0.08	0.0883	0.132	0.0636	0.0543	0.0344	0.0439	0.0566
15–34	n	100	107	134	151	198	130	168	104
	Rate	0.3277	0.3408	0.387	0.4162	0.5347	0.334	0.4071	0.4143
35–49	n	436	526	547	584	756	834	1080	729
	Rate	1.8263	2.2085	2.3596	2.6492	3.3927	3.4931	4.1125	4.3266
50–69	n	3192	4245	5072	6269	8270	9161	10749	7068
	Rate	14.0843	17.1696	19.743	24.4162	32.8974	36.4549	42.9028	47.3768
70–84	n	2224	2928	4040	5858	10183	13846	16317	11021
	Rate	37.3923	47.3141	60.1942	77.4072	119.4956	150.8795	168.4309	182.4792
0–84	n	5975	7833	9833	12880	19421	23979	28326	18930
	Rate	6.982	8.6478	10.4494	13.1084	19.0147	22.6385	25.8072	28.1277

(b) Incidence, males, 1971–92

Age		1971–4	1975–9	1980–4	1985–9	1990–2
0–14	n	34	39	80	43	26
	Rate	0.1461	0.1438	0.3119	0.1696	0.164
15–34	n	208	233	259	273	190
	Rate	0.7725	0.6528	0.6978	0.7126	0.794
35–49	n	806	1063	1100	1234	873
	Rate	4.398	4.8237	4.9268	5.1545	5.6711
50–69	n	6502	9344	10643	11454	7113
	Rate	31.4039	36.3383	42.2037	45.6097	47.0181
70–84	n	4748	7812	11198	14150	8927
	Rate	87.7379	102.7481	130.4901	154.1441	155.3716
0–84	n	12298	18491	23280	27154	17129
	Rate	16.0333	18.5395	22.4502	25.3923	25.9307

(c) Mortality, females, 1960–97

Age		1960–4	1965–9	1970–4	1975–9	1980–4	1985–9	1990–4	1995–7
0–14	n	35	22	25	29	16	11	20	14
	Rate	0.1282	0.0757	0.0875	0.112	0.0651	0.0444	0.085	0.1003
15–34	n	87	94	80	103	122	86	133	114
	Rate	0.293	0.3076	0.2541	0.2953	0.3359	0.2363	0.3538	0.4812
35–49	n	465	544	597	567	694	737	931	689
	Rate	1.9035	2.2534	2.5674	2.5799	3.1544	3.1117	3.5387	4.1398
50–69	n	3017	3721	4326	5138	7125	7511	8187	5174
	Rate	10.8256	12.6906	14.5326	17.4798	25.0311	26.8358	30.123	32.4809
70–84	n	2954	3851	5092	7171	11489	14901	17189	11315
	Rate	28.5779	34.2102	41.6114	53.8406	79.1685	97.2953	111.5489	123.6455
0–84	n	6558	8232	10120	13008	19446	23246	26460	17306
	Rate	5.4665	6.4512	7.5796	9.3736	13.4714	15.4946	17.6498	19.4307

(d) Incidence, females, 1971–92

Age		1971–4	1975–9	1980–4	1985–9	1990–2
0–14	n	29	34	68	58	32
	Rate	0.1324	0.1357	0.2799	0.2377	0.2005
15–34	n	133	210	227	200	151
	Rate	0.5196	0.6039	0.6255	0.5505	0.6572
35–49	n	844	1024	1047	1093	771
	Rate	4.5954	4.6739	4.7622	4.6135	4.9809
50–69	n	5415	7857	9138	9489	5759
	Rate	22.6996	26.7794	32.1925	33.9489	35.0565
70–84	n	5612	9441	12790	15440	10035
	Rate	56.9841	71.0958	88.4627	102.0969	109.4822
0–84	n	12033	18566	23270	26280	16748
	Rate	11.2424	13.4794	16.321	17.9044	18.9179

* Cohort data not shown – see text

References

Adelstein, A., White, G. (1976). Leukaemia 1911–1973: cohort analysis. *Population Trends*, 3, 9–13.

Agricultural Research Council (1978). *Annual Report 1977*. HMSO, London.

Ahlbom, A. (1990). Some notes on brain tumor epidemiology. In: Davis, D. L., Hoel, D. (eds.) Trends in Cancer Mortality in Industrial Countries. *Ann. N. Y. Acad. Sci.*, 609, 179–85.

Ahlbom, A., Day, N., Feychting, M., Roman, E., Skinner, J., Dockerty, J., Linet, M., McBride, M., Michaelis, J., Olsen, J. H., Tynes, T., Verkasalo, P. K. (2000). A pooled analysis of magnetic fields and childhood leukaemia. *Br. J. Cancer*, 83, 692–8.

Akslen, L. A., Haldorsen, T., Thoresen, S. Ø., Glattre, E. (1993). Incidence pattern of thyroid cancer in Norway: influence of birth cohort and time period. *Int. J. Cancer*, 53, 183–7.

Alberman, E. (1974). Stillbirths and neonatal mortality in England and Wales by birthweight, 1953–71. *Health Trends*, 6, 14–17.

Alberman, E. (1977). Sociobiologic factors and birthweight in Great Britain. In: Reed, D. M., Stanley, F. J. (eds) *The Epidemiology of Prematurity*. Urban & Schwarzenberg, Baltimore, 145–56.

Alderson, M., Donnan, S. (1978). Hysterectomy rates and their influence upon mortality from carcinoma of the cervix. *J. Epidemiol. Community Health*, 32, 175–7.

Anderson, K. E., Potter, J. D., Mack, T. M. (1996). Pancreatic cancer. In: Schottenfeld, D., Fraumeni, J. F. Jr. (eds) *Cancer Epidemiology and Prevention*. Second edition. Oxford University Press, New York, 725–71.

Armstrong, B., Doll, R. (1974). Bladder cancer mortality in England and Wales in relation to cigarette smoking and saccharin consumption. *Br. J. Prev. Soc. Med.*, 28, 233–40.

Armstrong, B., Doll, R. (1975). Environmental factors and cancer incidence and mortality in different countries, with special reference to dietary practices. *Int. J. Cancer*, 15, 617–31.

Armstrong, B., Garrod, A., Doll, R. (1976). A retrospective study of renal cancer with special reference to coffee and animal protein consumption. *Br. J. Cancer*, 33, 127–36.

Bacon, R., Sayer Bain, G., Pimlott, J. (1972). The economic environment. In: Halsey, A. H. (ed.). *Trends in British Society Since 1900. A Guide to the Changing Social Structure of Britain*. St Martin's Press, London, 65–95.

Bailar, J. C. III., Ederer, F. (1964). Significance factors for the ratio of a Poisson variable to its expectation. *Biometrics*, 20, 639–44.

Baines, A. H. J., Hollingsworth, D. F., Leitch, I. (1963). Diets of working-class families with children before and after the Second World War. *Nutr. Abstr. Rev.*, 33, 653–68.

Banatvala, N., Mayo, K., Megraud, F., Jennings, R., Deeks, J. J., Feldman, R. A. (1993). The cohort effect and *helicobacter pylori*. *J. Infect. Dis.*, 168, 219–21.

Banks, P. M. (1992). Changes in diagnosis of non-Hodgkin's lymphoma over time. *Cancer Res.*, 52 suppl., 5453S–55S.

Banks, E., Crossley, B., English, R., Richardson, A. (1996). High prevalence of use is not confined to women doctors. *Br. Med. J.*, 312, 638.

Barker, D. J. P. (1989) Rise and fall of Western diseases. *Nature*, 338, 371–2.

Barnes, N., Cartwright, R. A., O'Brien, C., Richards, I. D. G., Roberts, B., Bird, C. C. (1986). Rising incidence of lymphoid malignancies—true or false? *Br. J. Cancer*, 53, 393–8.

Baxter, P. J., Werner, J. B. (1980). *Mortality in the British Rubber Industries 1967–76*. HMSO, London.

Bengtsson, U., Angervall, L., Ekman, H., Lehmann, L. (1968). Transitional cell tumors of the renal pelvis in analgesic abusers. *Scand. J. Urol. Nephrol.*, 2, 145–50.

Benn, R. T., Leck, I., Nwene, U. P. (1982). Estimation of completeness of cancer registration. *Int. J. Epidemiol.*, 11, 362–7.

Bennett, N., Dodd, T., Flatley, J., Freeth, S., Bolling, K. (1995). *The Health Survey for England 1993*. HMSO, London.

Beral, V. (1974). Cancer of the cervix. A sexually transmitted infection? *Lancet*, i, 1037–40.

Beral, V., Fraser, P. Chilvers, C. (1978). Does pregnancy protect against ovarian cancer? *Lancet*, i, 1083–7.

Bergström, R., Adami, H.-O., Möhner, M., Zatonski, W., Storm, H., Ekbom, A., Tretli, S., Teppo, L., Akre, O., Hakulinen, T. (1996). Increase in testicular cancer incidence in six European countries: a birth cohort phenomenon. *J. Natl. Cancer Inst.*, 88, 727–33.

Bernstein, L., Henderson, B. E., Hanisch, R., Sullivan-Halley, J., Ross, R. K. (1994). Physical exercise and reduced risk of breast cancer in young women. *J. Natl. Cancer Inst.*, 86, 1403–8.

Bingham. S., Cummings, J. H. (1980). Sources and intakes of dietary fiber in man. In: Spiller, G. A., Kay, R. M. (eds.) *Medical Aspects of Dietary Fiber*. Plenum, New York, 261–84.

Bingham, S., Cummings, J. H., McNeil, N. I. (1979). Intakes and sources of dietary fiber in the British population. *Am. J. Clin. Nutr.*, 32, 1313–9.

Blot, W. J. (1980). Changing patterns of breast cancer among American women. *Am. J. Public Health*, 70, 833–5.

Blot, W. J., Devesa, S. S., Kneller, R. W., Fraumeni, J. F. Jr. (1991). Rising incidence of adenocarcinoma of the esophagus and gastric cardia. *J. Am. Med. Assoc.*, 265, 1287–9.

Blot, W. J., Devesa, S. S., McLaughlin J. K., Fraumeni, J. F. Jr. (1994). Oral and pharyngeal cancers. In: Doll, R., Fraumeni, J. F. Jr., Muir, C. S. (eds.) *Trends in Cancer Incidence and Mortality. Cancer Surveys.* Vols. 19/20. Cold Spring Harbor Laboratory Press, New York, 23–42.

Bost, L., Primatesta, P., Dong, W. (1997). Anthropometric measures and children's iron status. In: Prescott-Clarke, P., Primatesta, P. (eds.) *Health Survey for England 1995. Volume I: Findings*. HMSO, London, 305–45.

Boyd, J. T., Doll, R., Hill, G. B., Sissons, H. A. (1969). Mortality from primary tumours of bone in England and Wales, 1961–63. *Br. J. Prev. Soc. Med.*, 23, 12–22.

Boyko, R. W., Cartwright, R. A., Glashan, R. W. (1985). Bladder cancer in dye manufacturing workers. *J. Occup. Med.*, 27, 799–803.

Brawley, O. W. (1997). Prostate carcinoma incidence and patient mortality. The effects of screening and early detection. *Cancer*, 80, 1857–63.

Breslow, N. E., Day, N. E. (1987). *Statistical Methods in Cancer Research. Volume II. The Design and Analysis of Cohort Studies.* IARC Scientific Publications No. 82. IARC, Lyon.

Breslow, N., Chan, C. W., Dhom, G., Drury, R. A. B., Franks, L. M., Gellei, B., Lee, Y. S., Lundberg, S., Sparke, B., Sternby, N. H., Tulinius, H. (1977). Latent carcinoma of prostate at autopsy in seven areas. *Int. J. Cancer*, 20, 680–8.

Brewers and Licensed Retailers Association (1993, 1998). *Statistical Handbook.* 1993 and 1998 editions. Brewing Publications Limited, London.

Bulman, A. (1995). People are overusing sunbeds. *Br. Med. J.*, 310, 1327.

Bülow, S. (1980). Colorectal cancer in patients less than 40 years of age in Denmark, 1943–1967. *Dis. Colon Rectum*, 23, 327–36.

Bülow, S., Holm, N. V., Hauge, M. (1986). The incidence and prevalence of familial polyposis coli in Denmark. *Scand. J. Soc. Med.*, 14, 67–74.

Butlin, H. T. (1892). Three lectures on cancer of the scrotum in chimney-sweeps and others. Lecture III—Tar and paraffin cancer. *Br. Med. J.*, ii, 66–71.

Campbell, H. (1965). *Changes in Mortality Trends: England and Wales, 1931–61.* National Center for Health Statistics, Series 3, no. 3. US Department of Health, Education and Welfare. Public Health Service, Washington DC.

Campbell, H., Doll, W. R. S., Letchner, J. (1963). The incidence of thyroid cancer in England and Wales. *Br. Med. J.*, ii, 1370–3.

Casagrande, J. T., Hanisch, R., Pike, M. C., Ross, R. K., Brown, J. B., Henderson, B. E. (1988). A case-control study of male breast cancer. *Cancer Res.*, 48, 1326–30.

Case, R. A. M. (1956a). Cohort analysis of mortality rates as an historical or narrative technique. *Br. J. Prev. Soc. Med.*, 10, 159–71.

Case, R. A. M. (1956b). Cohort analysis of cancer mortality in England and Wales, 1911–1954 by site and sex. *Br. J. Prev. Soc. Med.*, 10, 172–99.

Case, R. A. M., Hosker, M. E., McDonald, D. B., Pearson, J. T. (1954). Tumours of the urinary bladder in workmen engaged in the manufacture and use of certain dyestuff intermediates in the British chemical industry. Part I. The role of aniline, benzidine, alpha-naphthylamine, and beta-naphthylamine. *Br. J. Indust. Med.*, 11, 75–104.

Case, R. A. M., Coghill, C., Davies, J. M., Harley, J. L., Hytten, C. A., Pearson, J. T., Willard, S. R., Alderson, M. R. (1976). Serial mortality tables. *Neoplastic Diseases Volume 1. England and Wales, 1911–70. Deaths and Death Rates by Sex, Age, Site and Calendar Period.* Division of Epidemiology, Institute of Cancer Research, London.

Census of England and Wales (1893). *Census of England and Wales, 1891. Ages, Condition as to Marriage, Occupations, Birth-Places and Infirmities.* Vol. III. HMSO, London.

Census of England and Wales (1911). *Census of England and Wales, 1911. Vol. X. Occupations and Industries.* Part II. HMSO, London.

Census of England and Wales (1921). *Census of England and Wales, 1921. Preliminary Report.* HMSO, London.

Census of England and Wales (1924). *Census of England and Wales, 1921. Occupation Tables.* HMSO, London.

Census of England and Wales (1931). *Census of England and Wales, 1931. Preliminary Report.* HMSO, London.

Census of England and Wales (1934). *Census of England and Wales, 1931. Occupation Tables.* HMSO, London.

Central Statistical Office (1970, 1971, 1974, 1975, 1977, 1983, 1990, 1993, 1996). *Social Trends*, nos. 1, 2, 5, 6, 8, 13, 20, 23, 26. HMSO, London.

Central Statistical Office (1995). *UK Social and Economic Statistics*, 95/96 edition. HMSO, London.

Chamberlain, J., Moss, S. M., Kirkpatrick, A. E., Michell, M., Johns, L. (1993). National Health Service breast screening programme results for 1991–2. *Br. Med. J.*, 307, 353–6.

Charlton, J., Quaife, K. (1997). Trends in diet 1841–1994. In: Charlton, J., Murphy, M. (eds.) *The Health of Adult Britain 1841–1994.* Volume 1. The Stationery Office, London, 93–113.

Chow, W.-H., Blaser, M. J., Blot, W. J., Gammon, M. D., Vaughan, T. L., Risch, H. A., Perez-Perez, G. I., Schoenberg, J. B., Stanford, J. L., Rotterdam, H., West, A. B., Fraumeni, J. F. Jr. (1998). An inverse relationship between cagA⁺ strains of *Helicobacter pylori* infection and risk of esophageal and gastric cardia adenocarcinoma. *Cancer Res.*, 58, 588–90.

Coleman, D. (1993). Britain in Europe: international and regional comparisons of fertility levels and trends. In: Ni Bhrolchain, M. (ed.). *New Perspectives on Fertility in Britain.* Studies on Medical and Population Subjects, no. 55. HMSO, London, 67–93.

Coleman, M. P., Estève, J., Damiecki, P., Arslan, A., Renard, H. (1993). *Trends in Cancer Incidence and Mortality*. IARC Scientific Publication no. 121. IARC, Lyon.

Colhoun, J., Lampe, F., Dong, W. (1996). Obesity and other anthropometric measures. In: Colhoun, H., Prescott-Clarke, P. (eds.) *The Health Survey for England 1994*. HMSO, London, 235–302.

Collaborative Group on Hormonal Factors in Breast Cancer (CGHFBC) (1996). Breast cancer and hormonal contraceptives: collaborative reanalysis of individual data on 53297 women with breast cancer and 100239 women without breast cancer from 54 epidemiological studies. *Lancet*, 347, 1713–27.

Collaborative Group on Hormonal Factors in Breast Cancer (CGHFBC) (1997). Breast cancer and hormone replacement therapy: collaborative reanalysis of data from 51 epidemiological studies of 52 705 women with breast cancer and 108 411 women without breast cancer. *Lancet*, 350, 1047–59.

Conard, R. A., Dobyns, B. M., Sutow, W. W. (1970). Thyroid neoplasia as late effect of exposure to radioactive iodine in fallout. *J. Am. Med. Assoc.*, 214, 316–24.

Corder, E. H., Chute, C. G., Guess, H. A., Beard, C. M., O'Fallon, M., Lieber, M. M. (1994). Prostate cancer in Rochester, Minnesota (USA), from 1935 to 1989: increases in incidence related to more complete ascertainment. *Cancer Causes Control*, 5, 207–14.

Correa, P., O'Conor, G. T. (1971). Epidemiologic patterns of Hodgkin's disease. *Int. J. Cancer*, 8, 192–201.

Court Brown, W. M., Doll, R. (1959). Adult leukaemia. Trends in mortality in relation to aetiology. *Br. Med. J.*, 1, 1063–9.

Court Brown, W. M., Doll, R. (1961). Leukaemia in childhood and young adult life. Trends in mortality in relation to aetiology. *Br. Med. J.*, i, 981–8.

Cruickshank, C. N. D., Squire, J. R. (1950). Skin cancer in the engineering industry from the use of mineral oil. *Br. J. Industr. Med.*, 7, 1–11.

Cuzick, J. (1994). Multiple myeloma. In: Doll, R., Fraumeni, J. F. Jr., Muir, C. S. (eds.) *Trends in Cancer Incidence and Mortality*. *Cancer Surveys*. Vols. 19/20. Cold Spring Harbor Laboratory Press, New York, 455–74.

Dann, T. C., Roberts, D. F. (1993). Menarcheal age in University of Warwick young women. *J. Biosoc. Sci.*, 25, 531–8.

Darby, S. C., Olsen, J. H., Doll, R., Thakrar, B., de Nully Brown, P., Storm, H. H., Barlow, L., Langmark, F., Teppo, L., Tulinius, H. (1992). Trends in childhood leukaemia in the Nordic countries in relation to fallout from atmospheric nuclear weapons testing. *Br. Med. J.*, 304, 1005–9.

Darby, S., Whitley, E., Silcocks, P., Thakrar, B., Green, M., Lomas, P., Miles, J., Reeves, G., Fearn, T., Doll, R. (1998). Risk of lung cancer associated with residential radon exposure in south-west England: a case-control study. *Br. J. Cancer*, 78, 394–408.

Davie, R., Butler, N., Goldstein, H. (1972). *From Birth to Seven. The Second Report of the National Child Development Study (1958 cohort) with Full Statistical Appendix*. Longman, London.

Davis, D. L., Hoel, D. (eds.) (1990). Trends in cancer mortality in industrial countries. *Ann. N. Y. Acad. Sci.*, 609: 1–345.

Day, N. E. (1991). Screening for breast cancer. *Br. Med. Bull.*, 47, 400–15.

Day, N. E., Varghese, C. (1994). Oesophageal cancer. In: Doll, R., Fraumeni, J. F. Jr., Muir, C. S. (eds.) *Trends in Cancer Incidence and Mortality*. *Cancer Surveys*. Vols. 19/20. Cold Spring Harbor Laboratory Press, New York, 43–54.

Department of the Environment (1978). *Digest of Environmental Pollution Statistics*. Pollution Report no. 4. HMSO, London.

Department of Health (1994–99). *Cervical screening programme, England: 1992/93–1997/98. (Statistical Bulletin)*. Government Statistical Service, London.

Department of Health and Social Security, Office of Population Censuses and Surveys (1970–74). *Reports on Hospital In-Patient Enquiry for the years 1967–72. Part I. Tables*. HMSO, London.

Department of Health and Social Security, Office of Population Censuses and Surveys, Welsh Office (1975–89). *Reports on Hospital In-Patient Enquiry for the years 1973–85. Tables*. HMSO, London.

Desmeules, M., Mikkelsen, T., Mao, Y. (1992). Increasing incidence of primary malignant brain tumors: influence of diagnostic methods. *J. Natl. Cancer Inst.*, 84, 442–5.

De Stavola, B. L., Hardy, R., Kuh, D., dos Santos Silva, I., Wadsworth, M., Swerdlow, A. J. (2000). Birthweight, childhood growth and risk of breast cancer in a British cohort. *Br. J. Cancer*, 83: 964–8.

Devesa, S. S., Fears, T. (1992). Non-Hodgkin's lymphoma time trends: United States and international data. *Cancer Res. (Suppl.)*, 52, 5432s–40s.

Devesa, S. S., Silverman, D. T., Young, J. L. Jr., Pollack, E. S., Brown, C. C., Horm, J. W., Percy, C. L., Myers, M. H., McKay, F. W., Fraumeni, J. F. Jr. (1987). Cancer incidence and mortality trends among whites in the United States, 1947–84. *J. Natl. Cancer Inst.*, 79, 701–70.

Devesa, S. S., Blot, W. J., Fraumeni, J. F. Jr. (1990). Cohort trends in mortality from oral, esophageal, and laryngeal cancers in the United States. *Epidemiology*, 1, 116–21.

Devesa, S. S., Blot, W. J., Stone, B. J., Miller, B. A., Tarone, R. E., Fraumeni, J. F. Jr. (1995). Recent cancer trends in the United States. *J. Natl. Cancer Inst.*, 87, 175–82.

Devesa, S. S., Blot, W. J., Fraumeni, J. F. Jr. (1998). Changing patterns in the incidence of esophageal and gastric carcinoma in the United States. *Cancer*, 83, 2049–53.

Dolin, P. J. (1992). *Epidemiological Investigations of Cancer of the Bladder*. D. Phil. Thesis, Oxford University, Oxford.

Doll, R. (1967). *Prevention of Cancer. Pointers from Epidemiology*. The Rock Carling Fellowship. Nuffield Provincial Hospitals Trust, London.

Doll, R. (1975). Part III: 7th Walter Hubert Lecture. Pott and the prospects for prevention. *Br. J. Cancer*, 32, 263–72.

Doll, R. (1989). The epidemiology of childhood leukaemia. *J. R. Statist. Soc. A.*, 152, 341–51.

Doll, R. (1991). Urban and rural factors in the aetiology of cancer. *Int. J. Cancer*, 47, 803–10.

Doll, R. (1996). Cancers weakly related to smoking. *Br. Med. Bull.*, 52, 35–49.

Doll, R. (1998). Uncovering the effects of smoking: historical perspective. *Stat. Methods Med. Res.*, 7, 87–117.

Doll, R., Darby, S. (1990). Childhood leukaemia in the United Kingdom. *Radiat. Protect. Australia*, 8, 55–61.

Doll, R., Hill, A. B. (1950). Smoking and carcinoma of the lung: preliminary report. *Br. Med. J.*, ii, 739–48.

Doll, R., Peto, R. (1976). Mortality in relation to smoking: 20 years' observations on male British doctors. *Br. Med. J.*, 2, 1525–36.

Doll, R, Peto, R. (1981). *The Causes of Cancer. Quantitative Estimates of Avoidable Risks of Cancer in the United States Today*. Oxford University Press, Oxford.

Doll, R., Wakeford, R. (1997). Risk of childhood cancer from fetal irradiation. *Br. J. Radiol.*, 70, 130–9.

Doll, R., Hill, A. B., Gray, P. G., Parr, E. A. (1959). Lung cancer mortality and the length of cigarette ends. An international comparison. *Br. Med. J.*, i, 322–5.

Doll, R., Vessey, M. P., Beasley, R. W. R., Buckley, A. R., Fear, E. C., Fisher, R. E. W., Gammon, E. J., Gunn, W., Hughes, G. O., Lee, K., Norman-Smith, B. (1972). Mortality of gasworkers—final report of a prospective study. *Br. J. Indust. Med.*, 29, 394–406.

Doll, R., Gray, R., Hafner, B., Peto, R. (1980). Mortality in relation to smoking: 22 years' observations on female British doctors. *Br. Med. J.*, 280, 967–71.

Doll, R., Fraumeni, J. F., Jr., Muir, C. S. (eds.) (1994). *Trends in Cancer Incidence and Mortality. Cancer Surveys*. Vols. 19/20. Cold Spring Harbor Laboratory Press, New York.

dos Santos Silva, I., Swerdlow, A. J. (1991). Ovarian germ cell malignancies in England: epidemiological parallels with testicular cancer. *Br. J. Cancer*, 63, 814–18.

dos Santos Silva, I., Swerdlow, A. J. (1993). Sex differences in the risks of hormone-dependent cancers. *Am. J. Epidemiol.*, 138, 10–28.

dos Santos Silva, I., Swerdlow, A. J. (1995). Recent trends in incidence of and mortality from breast, ovarian and endometrial cancers in England and Wales and their relation to changing fertility and oral contraceptive use. *Br. J. Cancer*, 72, 485–92.

dos Santos Silva, I., Swerdlow, A. J. (1996). Sex differences in time trends of colorectal cancer in England and Wales: the possible effect of female hormonal factors. *Br. J. Cancer*, 73, 692–7.

Douglas, J. W. B. (1950). The extent of breast feeding in Great Britain in 1946, with special reference to the health and survival of children. *Br. J. Obstet. Gynaecol. Br. Empire*, 57, 335–61.

Draper, G. (1995). Cancer. In: Botting, B. (ed.) *The Health of Our Children. Decennial Supplement*. OPCS Series DS no. 11. HMSO, London, 135–47.

Draper, G. J., Birch, J. M., Bithell, J. F., Kinnier Wilson, L. M., Leck, I., Marsden, H. B., Morris Jones, P. H., Stiller, C. A., Swindell, R. (1982). *Childhood Cancer in Britain. Incidence, Survival and Mortality*. Studies on Medical and Population Subjects no. 37. HMSO, London.

Draper, G. J., Stiller, C. A., Fearnley, H, Lennox, E. L., Roberts, E. M., Sanders, B. M. (1988). United Kingdom—England and Wales. National Registry of Childhood Tumours, 1971–1980. In: Parkin, D. M., Stiller, C. A., Draper, G. J., Bieber, C. A., Terracini, B., Young, J. L. (eds.) *International Incidence of Childhood Cancer*. IARC Scientific Publications no. 87. IARC, Lyon, 295–8.

Draper, G. J., Kroll, M. E., Stiller, C. A. (1994). Childhood cancer. In: Doll, R., Fraumeni, J. F. Jr., Muir, C. S. (eds.) *Trends in Cancer Incidence and Mortality. Cancer Surveys*. Vols. 19/20. Cold Spring Harbor Laboratory Press, New York, 493–517.

Dubrow, R., Bernstein, J., Holford, T. R. (1993). Age-period-cohort modelling of large-bowel-cancer incidence by anatomic sub-site and sex in Connecticut. *Int. J. Cancer*, 53, 907–13.

Early Breast Cancer Trialists' Collaborative Group (EBCTCG) (1992). Systemic treatment of early breast cancer by hormonal, cytotoxic, or immune therapy: 133 randomised trials involving 31 000 recurrences and 24 000 deaths among 75 000 women. *Lancet*, 339, 1–15, 71–85.

Early Breast Cancer Trialists' Collaborative Group (EBCTCG) (1998). Tamoxifen for early breast cancer: an overview of the randomised trials. *Lancet*, 351, 1451–67.

Elwood, J. M., Pearson, J. C. G., Skippen, D. H., Jackson, S. M. (1984). Alcohol, smoking, social and occupational factors in the aetiology of cancer of the oral cavity, pharynx and larynx. *Int. J. Cancer*, 34, 603–12.

Evans, B. G., Catchpole, M. A., Heptonstall, J., Mortimer, J. Y., McGarrigle, C. A., Nicoll, A. G., Waight, P., Gill, O. N., Swan, A. V. (1993). Sexually transmitted diseases and HIV-1 infection among homosexual men in England and Wales. *Br. Med. J.*, 306, 426–8.

Farr, W. (1839). Letter to the Registrar-General. In: *First Annual Report of the Registrar-General of Births, Deaths, and Marriages, in England*. HMSO, London, 63–123.

Fletcher, W., Loulit, J. F., Papworth, D. G. (1966). Interpretation of levels of strontium-90 in human bone. *Br. Med. J.*, 2, 1225–30.

Floud, R., Wachter, K., Gregory, A. (1990). *Height, Health and History. Nutritional Status in the United Kingdom, 1750–1980*. Cambridge University Press, Cambridge.

Franssila, K. O., Harach, H. R. (1986). Occult papillary carcinoma of the thyroid in children and young adults. A systemic [sic] autopsy study in Finland. *Cancer*, 58, 715–19.

Fraumeni, J. F. Jr. (1967). Stature and malignant tumors of bone in childhood and adolescence. *Cancer*, 20, 967–73.

Fukunaga, F. H., Yatani, R. (1975). Geographic pathology of occult thyroid carcinomas. *Cancer*, 36, 1095–9.

Gail, M. H., Pluda, J. M., Rabkin, C. S., Biggar, R. J., Goedert, J. J., Horm, J. W., Sondik, E. J., Yarchoan, R., Broder, S. (1991). Projections of the incidence of non-Hodgkin's lymphoma related to acquired immunodeficiency syndrome. *J. Natl. Cancer Inst.*, 83, 695–701.

Gatter, K. C., Alcock, C., Heryet, A., Mason, D. Y. (1985). Clinical importance of analysing malignant tumours of uncertain origin with immunohistological techniques. *Lancet*, i, 1302–5.

Giles, G. G., Armstrong, B. K., Burton, R. C., Staples, M. P., Thursfield, V. J. (1996). Has mortality from melanoma stopped rising in Australia? Analysis of trends between 1931 and 1994. *Br. Med. J.*, 312, 1121–5.

Gilliland, F. D., Samet, J. M. (1994). Lung cancer. In: Doll, R., Fraumeni, J. F. Jr., Muir, C. S. (eds.) *Trends in Cancer Incidence and Mortality. Cancer Surveys*. Vols. 19/20. Cold Spring Harbor Laboratory Press, New York, 175–95.

Gilman, E. A., Stewart, A. M., Knox, E. G., Kneale, G. W. (1989). Trends in obstetric radiography, 1939–81. *J. Radiol. Prot.* 9, 93–101.

Giovannucci, E., Colditz, G. A., Stampfer, M. J. (1993). A meta-analysis of cholecystectomy and risk of colorectal cancer. *Gastroenterology*, 105, 130–41.

Glaser, S. L. (1994). Reproductive factors in Hodgkin's disease in women: a review. *Am. J. Epidemiol.*, 139, 237–46.

Glaser, S. L., Swartz, W. G. (1990). Time trends in Hodgkin's disease incidence. The role of diagnostic accuracy. *Cancer*, **66**, 2196–204.

Glass, A. G., Fraumeni, J. F. Jr. (1970). Epidemiology of bone cancer in children. *J. Natl. Cancer Inst.*, **44**, 187–99.

Glass, D. V., Grebenik, E. (1954). *The Trend and Pattern of Fertility in Great Britain. A Report of the Family Census of 1946. Papers of the Royal Commission on Population*. Vol. VI. HMSO, London.

Godfrey, B. E., Vennart, J. (1968). Measurements of caesium-137 in human beings in 1958–67. *Nature*, **218**, 741–6.

Golding, J., Butler, N. R. (1986). The first months. In: Butler, N. R., Golding, J. (eds.) *From Birth to Five. A Study of the Health and Behaviour of Britain's 5-year-olds*. Pergamon, Oxford, 46–63.

Grady, D., Ernster, V. L. (1996). Endometrial cancer. In: Schottenfeld, D., Fraumeni, J. F. Jr. (eds.) *Cancer Epidemiology and Prevention*. Second edition. Oxford University Press, New York, 1058–89.

Graham, S., Priore, R., Graham, M., Browne, R., Burnett, W., West, D. (1979). Genital cancer in wives of penile cancer patients. *Cancer*, **44**, 1870–4.

Graunt, J. (1662). *Natural and Political Observations Mentioned in a Following Index, and Made Upon the Bills of Mortality*. Printed by Tho. Roycroft, for John Martin, James Allestry and Tho. Dicas, London.

Gray, G. E., Pike, M. C., Henderson, B. E. (1979). Breast-cancer incidence and mortality rates in different countries in relation to known risk factors and dietary practices. *Br. J. Cancer*, **39**, 1–7.

Gray, R. (1996). Physical activity. In: Colhoun, H., Prescott-Clarke, P. (eds.) *Health Survey for England, 1994*. HMSO, London, 175–203.

Greaves, M. F. (1997). Aetiology of acute leukaemia. *Lancet*, **349**, 344–9.

Greaves, J. P., Hollingsworth, D. F. (1966). Trends in food consumption in the United Kingdom. *World Rev. Nutr. Diet*, **6**, 34–89.

Greenberg, M., Lloyd Davies, T. A. (1974). Mesothelioma register 1967–68. *Br. J. Indust. Med.*, **31**, 91–104.

Greenwood, M. (1935). *Epidemics and Crowd Diseases, An Introduction to the Study of Epidemiology*. Macmillan, New York.

Gregory, J., Foster, K., Tyler, H., Wiseman, M. (1990). *The Dietary and Nutritional Survey of British Adults*. HMSO, London.

Greig, N. H., Ries, L. G., Yancik, R., Rapoport, S. (1990). Increasing annual incidence of primary malignant brain tumors in the elderly. *J. Natl. Cancer Inst.*, **82**, 1621–4.

Griffiths, F., Convery, B. (1995). Women's use of hormone replacement therapy for relief of menopausal symptoms, for prevention of osteoporosis, and after hysterectomy. *Br. J. Gen. Pract*, **45**, 355–8.

Grulich, A. E., Swerdlow, A. J., dos Santos Silva, I., Beral, V. (1995). Is the apparent rise in cancer mortality in the elderly real? Analysis of changes in certification and coding of cause of death in England and Wales, 1970–1990. *Int. J. Cancer*, **63**, 164–8.

Gulliford, M. C., Bell, J., Bourne, H. M., Petruckevitch, A. (1993). The reliability of cancer registry records. *Br. J. Cancer*, **67**, 819–21.

Gunby, J. A., Darby, S. C., Miles, J. C. H., Green, B. M. R., Cox, D. R. (1993). Factors affecting indoor radon concentrations in the United Kingdom. *Health Phys.*, **64**, 2–12.

Gutensohn, N., Cole, P. (1977). Epidemiology of Hodgkin's disease in the young. *Int. J. Cancer*, **19**, 595–604.

Gutensohn, N., Cole, P. (1981). Childhood social environment and Hodgkin's disease. *New Engl. J. Med.*, **304**, 135–40.

Haenszel, W. (1982). Migrant studies. In: Schottenfeld, D., Fraumeni, J. F. Jr. (eds.) *Cancer Epidemiology and Prevention*. Saunders, Philadelphia, 194–207.

Hakulinen, T., Teppo, L., Saxén, E. (1978). Cancer of the eye, a review of trends and differentials. *World Health Stats. Q.*, **31**, 143–58.

Hansen, N. E., Karle, H., Jensen, O. M. (1983). Trends in the incidence of leukemia in Denmark, 1943–77: an epidemiologic study of 14,000 patients. *J. Natl. Cancer Inst.*, **71**, 697–701.

Hansen, S., Melby, K. K., Aase, S., Jellum, E., Vollset, S. E. (1999). *Helicobacter pylori* infection and risk of cardia cancer and non-cardia gastric cancer. A nested case-control study. *Scand. J. Gastroenterol.*, **4**, 353–60.

Harach, H. R., Franssila, K. O., Wasenius, V.-M. (1985). Occult papillary carcinoma of the thyroid. A 'normal' finding in Finland. A systematic autopsy study. *Cancer*, **56**, 531–8.

Hartge, P., Devesa, S. S. (1992). Quantification of the impact of known risk factors on time trends in non-Hodgkin's lymphoma incidence. *Cancer Res.*, **52** (Suppl.), 5566s–9s.

Hasle, H., Mellemgaard, A. (1993). Hodgkin's disease diagnosed post mortem: a population based study. *Br. J. Cancer*, **67**, 185–9.

Hawkins, M. M., Swerdlow, A. J. (1992) Completeness of cancer and death follow-up obtained through the National Health Service Central Register for England and Wales. *Br. J. Cancer*, **66**, 408–13.

Health and Safety Executive (HSE) (1993). *Analysis of Doses Reported to the Health and Safety Executive's Central Index of Dose Information*. Health and Safety Executive, London.

Health and Safety Executive (HSE) (1997). *Central Index of Dose Information. Summary of Statistics for 1996*. Health and Safety Executive, London.

Heasman, M. A., Lipworth, L. (1966). *Accuracy of Certification of Cause of Death*. SMPS no. 20. HMSO, London.

Helseth, A., Langmark, F., Mørk, S. J. (1988). Neoplasms of the central nervous system in Norway. II. Descriptive epidemiology of intracranial neoplasms 1955–1984. *Acta Path Microbiol Immunol Scand*, **96**, 1066–74.

Hems, G. (1980). Associations between breast-cancer mortality rates, child-bearing and diet in the United Kingdom. *Br. J. Cancer*, **41**, 429–37.

Henderson, B. E., Ross, R. K., Pike, M. C. Depue, R. H. (1983). Epidemiology of testis cancer. In: Skinner, D. G. (ed.) *Urological Cancer*. Grune & Stratton, New York, 237–50.

Henderson, B., Ross, R. K., Yu, M. C., Bernstein, L. (1997). An explanation for the increasing incidence of testis cancer: decreasing age at first full-term pregnancy. *J. Natl. Cancer Inst.*, **89**, 818–20.

Hewitt, D. (1955). Some features of leukaemia mortality. *Br. J. Prev. Soc. Med.*, 9, 81–8.

Houghton, A. N., Viola, M. V. (1981). Solar radiation and malignant melanoma of the skin. *J. Am. Acad. Dermatol.*, 5, 477–83.

Houghton, A. N., Munster, E. W., Viola, M. V. (1978). Increased incidence of malignant melanoma after peaks of sunspot activity. *Lancet*, i, 759–60.

Hrubec, Z., Robinette, C. D. (1984). The study of human twins in medical research. *New Engl. J. Med.*, 310, 435–41.

Huang, T., Watt, H., Wald, N., Morris, J., Mutton, D., Alberman, E., Kelekun, C. (1998). Birth prevalence of Down's syndrome in England and Wales 1990 to 1997. *J. Med. Screen.*, 5, 213–14.

Hughes, J. S., O'Riordan, M. C. (1993). *Radiation Exposure of the UK Population—1993 Review*. (NRPB-R263). National Radiological Protection Board, Chilton.

Hughes, J. S., Shaw, K. B., O'Riordan, M. C. (1989). *Radiation Exposure of the UK Population—1988 Review*. (NRPB-R227). National Radiological Protection Board, Chilton.

Hutchings, S., Jones, J., Hodgson, J. (1995). Asbestos-related diseases. In: Drever, F. (ed.) *Occupational Health Decennial Supplement*. Series DS no. 10. HMSO, London, 127–52.

International Agency for Research on Cancer (1980). Phenacetin. In: International Agency for Research on Cancer (ed.) *Some Pharmaceutical Drugs*. IARC Monograph no. 24. IARC, Lyon, 135–61.

Isaacs, A. J., Britton, A. R., McPherson, K. (1995). Utilization of hormone replacement therapy by women doctors. *Br. Med. J.*, 311, 1399–401.

Järvinen, H. J. (1992). Epidemiology of familial adenomatous polyposis in Finland: impact of family screening on the colorectal cancer rate and survival. *Gut*, 33, 357–60.

Jensen, O. M., Estève, J., Møller, H., Renard, H. (1990). Cancer in the European Community and its member states. *Eur. J. Cancer*, 26, 1167–256.

John Radcliffe Hospital Cryptorchidism Study Group (1992). Cryptorchidism: a prospective study of 7500 consecutive male births, 1984–8. *Arch. Dis. Childhood*, 67, 892–9.

Johnson, A. M., Wadsworth, J., Wellings, K., Field, J. (1994). *Sexual Attitudes and Lifestyles*. Blackwell Scientific Publications, Oxford.

Kendall, G. M., Dar, S. C., Harries, S. V., Rae, S. (1980). *A Frequency Survey of Radiological Examinations Carried Out in National Health Service Hospitals in Great Britain in 1977 for Diagnostic Purposes*. (NRPB-R104). National Radiological Protection Board, Harwell.

Kennaway, E. L., Kennaway, N. M. (1947). A further study of the incidence of cancer of the lung and larynx. *Br. J. Cancer*, 1, 260–98.

Kinlen, L. J. (1994). Leukaemia. In: Doll, R., Fraumeni, J. F. Jr., Muir, C. S. (eds.) *Trends in Cancer Incidence and Mortality. Cancer Surveys*. Vols. 19/20. Cold Spring Harbor Laboratory Press, New York, 475–91.

Kinlen, L. J. (1996). Epidemiological evidence for an infective basis in childhood leukaemia. *J. R. Soc. Health*, 116, 393–9.

Kinlen, L. J., Hudson, C. (1991). Childhood leukaemia and poliomyelitis in relation to military encampments in England and Wales in the period of national military service, 1950–63. *Br. Med. J.*, 303, 1357–64.

Kinlen, L. J., John, S. M. (1994). Wartime evacuation and mortality from childhood leukaemia in England and Wales in 1945–9. *Br. Med. J.*, 309, 1197–202.

Kinlen, L. J., Badaracco, M. A., Moffett, J., Vessey, M. P. (1974). A survey of the use of oestrogens during pregnancy in the United Kingdom and of the genito-urinary cancer mortality and incidence rates in young people in England and Wales. *J. Obstet. Gynaecol. Br. Commonwealth*, 81, 849–55.

Knight, I. (1984). *The Heights and Weights of Adults in Great Britain*. HMSO, London.

Ko, C. B., Walton, S., Keczkes, K., Bury, H. P. R., Nicholson, C. (1994). The emerging epidemic of skin cancer. *Br. J. Dermatol.*, 130, 269–72.

Kravdal, Ø., Hansen, S. (1993). Hodgkin's disease: the protective effect of childbearing. *Int. J. Cancer*, 55, 909–14.

Kuh, D. L., Power, C., Rodgers, B. (1991). Secular trends in social class and sex differences in adult height. *Int. J. Epidemiol.*, 20, 1001–9.

Kurihara, M., Aoki, K., Hisamichi, S. (1989). *Cancer Mortality Statistics in the World, 1950–1985*. University of Nagoya Press, Nagoya.

Lancaster, G., Moran, T., Woodman, C. (1994). Towards achieving the Health of the Nation target for cervical cancer: accuracy of cancer registration. *J. Publ. Health Med.*, 16, 50–2.

Lancet (1965). Bladder tumours in industry. *Lancet*, ii, 1173.

La Vecchia, C., Lucchini, F., Negri, E., Boyle, P., Maisonneuve, P., Levi, F. (1992). Trends of cancer mortality in Europe, 1955–1989. *Eur. J. Cancer*, 28, 132–235, 514–99, 28A, 927–98, 1210–81, 1509–81.

Leach, J. F., Beadle, P. C., Pingstone, A. R., Aughton, P. (1979). Some effects of the variation of atmospheric particulates on disease in Great Britain. *Aviat. Space Environ. Med.*, 50, 72–9.

Lee, J. A. H. (1961). Acute myeloid leukaemia in adolescents. *Br. Med. J.*, i: 988–92.

Lee, P. N. (1976) (ed.). *Statistics of Smoking in the United Kingdom. Research Paper I*, 7th edition. Tobacco Research Council, London.

Lee, P. N., Fry, J. S., Forey, B. A. (1990). Trends in lung cancer, chronic obstructive lung disease, and emphysema death rates for England and Wales 1941–85 and their relation to trends in cigarette smoking. *Thorax*, 45, 657–65.

Levi, F., La Vecchia, C., Lucchini, F., Negri, E., Boyle, P. (1992). Patterns of childhood cancer incidence and mortality in Europe. *Eur. J. Cancer*, 28A, 2028–49.

Levi, F., Lucchini, F., Negri, E., La Vecchia, C. (2000). Recent trends in prostate cancer mortality in the European Union. Epidemiology, 11, 612.

Levy, I. G., Gibbons, L., Collins, J. P., Perkins, D. G., Mao, Y. (1993). Prostate cancer trends in Canada: rising incidence or increased detection? *Can. Med. Assoc. J.*, 149, 617–24.

Linos, A., Kyle, R. A., Elvelback, L. R., Kurland, L. T. (1978). Leukemia in Olmsted County, Minnesota, 1965–1974. *Mayo Clin. Proc.*, 53, 714–18.

Linos, A., Kyle, R. A., O'Fallon, W. M., Kurland, L. T. (1981). Incidence and secular trend of multiple myeloma in Olmsted County, Minnesota: 1965–77. *J. Natl. Cancer Inst.*, 66, 17–20.

Lloyd Roberts, D. (1990). Incidence of non-melanoma skin cancer in West Glamorgan, South Wales. *Br. J. Dermatol.*, **122**, 399–403.

Lynch, C. F., Platz, C. E., Jones, M. P., Gazzaniga, J. M. (1991). Cancer registry problems in classifying invasive bladder cancer. *J. Natl. Cancer Inst.*, **83**, 429–33.

Lynge, E., Storm, H. H., Jensen, O. M. (1987). The evaluation of trends in soft tissue sarcoma according to diagnostic criteria and consumption of phenoxy herbicides. *Cancer*, **60**, 1896–901.

MacKenzie, A., Court Brown, W. M., Doll, R., Sissons, H. A. (1961). Mortality from primary tumours of bone in England and Wales. *Br. Med. J.*, **i**, 1782–90.

MacMahon, B. (1966). Epidemiology of Hodgkin's disease. *Cancer Res.*, **26**, 1189–200.

Magnus, K. (ed.) (1982). *Trends in Cancer Incidence. Causes and Practical Implications.* Hemisphere Publishing, Washington.

Marshall, W. A., Tanner, J. M. (1986). Puberty. In: Falkner, F., Tanner, J. M. (eds.) *Human Growth. A Comprehensive Treatise. Vol 2. Postnatal Growth, Neurobiology.* Plenum Press, London, 171–209.

Martinez, I. (1969). Relationship of squamous cell carcinoma of the cervix uteri to squamous cell carcinoma of the penis among Puerto Rican women married to men with penile carcinoma. *Cancer*, **24**, 777–80.

Martinsson, U., Glimelius, B., Sandström, C. (1992). Lymphoma incidence in a Swedish county during 1969–1987. *Acta Oncol.*, **31**, 275–82.

McCredie, M., Ford, J. M., Taylor, J. S., Stewart, J. H. (1982). Analgesics and cancer of the renal pelvis in New South Wales. *Cancer*, **49**, 2617–25.

McDonald, A. D. (1979). Mesothelioma registries in identifying asbestos hazards. *Ann. N. Y. Acad. Sci.*, **330**, 441–54.

McKenzie, A., Case, R. A. M., Pearson, J. T. (1957). *Cancer Statistics for England and Wales 1901–1955. A Summary of Data Relating to Mortality and Morbidity.* SMPS no. 13. HMSO, London.

McKinlay, S., Jefferys, M., Thompson, B. (1972). An investigation of the age at menopause. *J. Biosoc. Sci.*, **4**, 161–73.

Medical Research Council (MRC) (1960). *The Hazards to Man of Nuclear and Allied Radiations. A Second Report to the Medical Research Council.* HMSO, London.

Medical Research Council (MRC) (1960–70). *Assay of Strontium-90 in Human Bone in the United Kingdom. Results for 1959–68.* Series no. 1–17. HMSO, London.

Medical Research Council (MRC) (1964). *The Exposure of the Population to Radiation from Fallout. A Report to the Medical Research Council by their Committee on Protection Against Ionizing Radiation.* HMSO, London.

Medical Research Council (MRC) (1966). *The Assessment of the Possible Risks to the Population from Environmental Contamination.* HMSO, London.

Michels, K. B., Trichopoulos, D., Robins, J. M., Rosner, B. A., Manson, J. E., Hunter, D. J., Colditz, G. A., Hankinson, S. E., Speizer, F. E., Willett, W. C. (1996). Birthweight as a risk factor for breast cancer. *Lancet*, **348**, 1542–6.

Miller, R. W., Boice, J. D. Jr., Curtis, R. E. (1996). Bone cancer. In: Schottenfeld, D., Fraumeni, J. F. Jr. (eds.) *Cancer Epidemiology and Prevention.* Second edition. Oxford University Press, New York, 971–83.

Ministry of Agriculture, Fisheries and Food (MAFF) (1991*a*). *Fifty Years of the National Food Survey 1940–1990. The Proceedings of a Symposium held in December 1990, London.* HMSO, London.

Ministry of Agriculture, Fisheries and Food (MAFF) (1991*b*). *Household Food Consumption and Expenditure 1990 With a Study of Trends Over the Period 1940–1990. Annual Report of the National Food Survey Committee.* HMSO, London.

Ministry of Agriculture, Fisheries and Food (MAFF) (1992). *Household Food Consumption and Expenditure 1991. Annual Report of the National Food Survey Committee.* HMSO, London.

Ministry of Agriculture, Fisheries and Food (MAFF) (1993–8). *National Food Survey, 1992–1997. Annual Report on Household Food Consumption and Expenditure.* HMSO, London.

Ministry of Health, General Register Office (1964, 1968). *Reports on Hospital In-Patient Enquiry for the Years 1961, 1966. Part II. Detailed Tables.* HMSO, London.

Ministry of Health, Scottish Home and Health Department (1966). *Radiological Hazards to Patients. Final Report of the Committee.* HMSO, London.

Mitchell, B. R. (1988). *British Historical Statistics.* Cambridge University Press, Cambridge.

Mobile Communications (1996–9). Numbers of cellular subscribers in West European countries, 1984–1995. *Mobile Communications*, **188** (and subsequent issues).

Moss, S. M., Michel, M., Patnick, J., Johns, L., Blanks, R., Chamberlain, J. (1995). Results from the NHS breast screening programme 1990–1993. *J. Med. Screening*, **2**, 186–90.

Mueller, N. E., Grufferman, S. (1999). The epidemiology of Hodgkin's disease. In: Mauch, P. M., Armitage, J. O., Diehl, V., Hoppe, R. T., Weiss, L. M. (eds.) *Hodgkin's Disease.* Lippincott Williams & Wilkins, Philadelphia, 61–77.

Muir, C. S. (1992). Classification. In: Parkin, D. M., Muir, C. S., Wheland, S. L., Gao, Y.-T., Ferlay, J., Powell, J. (eds.) *Cancer Incidence in Five Continents. Volume VI.* IARC Scientific Publication no. 120. IARC, Lyon, 25–30.

Muir, C., Waterhouse, J, Mack, T., Powell, J., Whelan, S. (eds.) (1987). *Cancer Incidence in Five Continents. Volume V.* IARC Scientific Publication no. 88. IARC, Lyon.

Muir, C. S., Storm, H. H., Polednak, A. (1994). Brain and other nervous system tumours. In: Doll, R., Fraumeni, J. F. Jr., Muir, C. S. (eds.) *Trends in Cancer Incidence and Mortality. Cancer Surveys* Vols. 19/20. Cold Spring Harbor Laboratory Press, New York, 369–92.

Murray, R. M. (1978). Genesis of analgesic nephropathy in the United Kingdom. *Kidney Int.*, **13**, 50–7.

Mutton, D., Ide, R. G., Alberman, E. (1998). Trends in prenatal screening for and diagnosis of Down's syndrome: England and Wales, 1989–97. *Br. Med. J.*, **317**, 922–3.

National Health Service Breast Screening Programme (NHSBSP) (1998). *Annual Review.* Department of Health, Sheffield.

National Radiological Protection Board (NRPB) (1980–1994). *NRPB Reports.* National Radiological Protection Board, Chilton.

National Radiological Protection Board (NRPB) (1995). *Board Statement on Effects of Ultraviolet Radiation on Human Health, and Health Effects from Ultraviolet Radiation, Report of an Advisory Group on Non-Ionising Radiation.* National Radiological Protection Board, Chilton.

Nectoux, J. (1976). Comparison of 7th and 8th revisions of the ICD. In: Waterhouse, J., Muir, C., Correa, P., Powell, J. (eds.) *Cancer Incidence in Five Continents. Volume III.* IARC Scientific Publication no. 15. IARC, Lyon, 25–38.

Newsholme, A. (1923). Cancer mortality. In: Newsholme, A. (ed.) *The Elements of Vital Statistics.* George Allen & Unwin, London, 489–500.

Newton, D., Eagle, M. C., Venn, J. B. (1977). The caesium-137 content of man related to fallout in rain, 1957–76. *Int. J. Environ. Studies,* **11**, 83–90.

Nobrega, F. T., Sedlack, J. D., Sedlack, R. E., Dockerty, M. B., Ilstrup, D. M., Kurland, L. T. (1983). A decline in carcinoma of the stomach. A diagnostic artifact? *Mayo Clin. Proc.,* **58**, 255–60.

Nugent, K. P., Northover, J. (1994). Total colectomy and ileorectal anastamosis. In: Phillips, R. K. S., Spigelman, A. D., Thomson, J. P. S. (eds.) *Familial Adenomatous Polyposis and Other Polyposis Syndromes.* Edward Arnold, London, 79–91.

Nwene, U., Smith, A. (1982). Assessing completeness of cancer registration in the North-Western region of England by a method of independent comparison. *Br. J. Cancer,* **46**, 635–9.

Office for National Statistics (ONS) (1997). *Birth Statistics. Review of the Registrar General on Births and Patterns of Family Building in England and Wales, 1995.* Series FM1 no.24. Stationery Office, London.

Office for National Statistics (ONS) (1998a). *Cancer Survival in England and Wales: 1981 and 1989 Registrations.* ONS Monitor MBI 98/1. ONS, London.

Office for National Statistics (ONS) (1998b). *Living in Britain. Results from the 1996 General Household Survey.* The Stationery Office, London.

Office for National Statistics (ONS) (1998c). *Annual Abstract of Statistics, 1998 Edition.* No. 134. The Stationery Office, London, 202.

Office of Population Censuses and Surveys (OPCS) (1972a). *The Registrar General's Statistical Review of England and Wales for the Year 1970. Part I. Tables. Medical.* HMSO, London.

Office of Population Censuses and Surveys (1972b). *The Registrar General's Statistical Review of England and Wales for the Year 1970. Part II. Population.* HMSO, London.

Office of Population Censuses and Surveys (OPCS) (1974a). *The Registrar General's Statistical Review of England and Wales for the Year 1972. Part II. Population.* HMSO, London.

Office of Population Censuses and Surveys (OPCS) (1974b). *The Registrar General's Statistical Review of England and Wales for the Year 1972. Part I. Tables, Medical.* HMSO, London.

Office of Population Censuses and Surveys (OPCS) (1975a). *Cancer Mortality. England and Wales 1911–1970.* SMPS no. 29. HMSO, London.

Office of Population Censuses and Surveys (OPCS) (1975b). *Census 1971. England and Wales. Household Composition. Tables. Part I (10% Sample).* HMSO, London.

Office of Population Censuses and Surveys (1975c). *Statistics of Infectious Diseases. Notifications of Infectious Diseases in England and Wales, 1974.* Series MB2 no.1. HMSO, London.

Office of Population Censuses and Surveys (OPCS) (1978). *Demographic Review. A Report on Population in Great Britain.* Series DR no.1. HMSO, London.

Office of Population Censuses and Surveys (OPCS) (1979). *Cancer Statistics Registrations. Cases of Diagnosed Cancer Registered in England and Wales, 1972–73.* Series MB1 no. 2. HMSO, London.

Office of Population Censuses and Surveys (OPCS) (1980–8). *Birthweight Statistics, 1977–86.* Monitor Series DH3. OPCS, London.

Office of Population Censuses and Surveys (OPCS) (1982). *A Comparison of the Registrar General's Annual Population Estimates for England and Wales with the Results of 1981 Census.* Occasional Paper 29. HMSO, London.

Office of Population Censuses and Surveys (OPCS) (1983a). *Mortality Statistics: Comparison of 8th and 9th Revision of the International Classification of Diseases, 1978 (Sample) England and Wales.* Series DH1, no. 10. HMSO, London.

Office of Population Censuses and Surveys (OPCS) (1983b). *Cancer Statistics Registrations. Cases of Diagnosed Cancer Registered in England and Wales, 1978.* Series MB1 no. 10. HMSO, London.

Office of Population Censuses and Surveys (OPCS) (1983c). *Census 1981. England and Wales. Housing and Households.* HMSO, London.

Office of Population Censuses and Surveys (OPCS) (1984). *Evaluation of the 1981 Census: Demographic Comparisons.* OPCS Monitor CEN84/1. OPCS, London.

Office of Population Censuses and Surveys (OPCS) (1985). *Mortality Statistics, Cause. Review of the Registrar General on Deaths by Cause, Sex and Age in England and Wales, 1984.* Series DH2, no. 11. HMSO, London.

Office of Population Censuses and Surveys (OPCS) (1986). *The General Household Survey, 1984.* Series GHS no. 14. HMSO, London.

Office of Population Censuses and Surveys (OPCS) (1987). *Birth Statistics. Historical Series of Births in England and Wales, 1837–1983.* Series FM1 no.13. HMSO, London.

Office of Population Censuses and Surveys (OPCS) (1990a). *Review of the National Cancer Registration System.* Series MB1 no. 17. HMSO, London.

Office of Population Censuses and Surveys (OPCS) (1990b). *The General Household Survey, 1988.* Series GHS no. 19. HMSO, London.

Office of Population Censuses and Surveys (OPCS) (1992). *Labour Force Survey 1990 and 1991.* HMSO, London.

Office of Population Censuses and Surveys (OPCS) (1994). *Mortality Statistics General. Review of the Registrar General on Deaths in England and Wales, 1992.* Series DH1 no. 27. HMSO, London.

Office of Population Censuses and Surveys (OPCS) (1995). *Mortality Statistics Cause. Review by the Registrar General on Deaths by Cause, Sex and Age, in England and Wales, 1993.* Series DH2 no. 20. HMSO, London.

Office of Population Censuses and Surveys (OPCS) (1996). *Living in Britain. Results from the 1994 General Household Survey.* HMSO, London.

Office of Population Censuses and Surveys, Communicable Disease Surveillance Centre of the Public Health Laboratory Service (1995). *Communicable Disease Statistics. Statistical Tables, 1993.* Series MB2 no.20. HMSO, London.

Office of Population Censuses and Surveys, Office for National Statistics (OPCS ONS) (1977–98). *Mortality Statistics by Cause, England and Wales, 1974–1996.* Series DH2 nos.1–23. HMSO, London.

Office of Population Censuses and Surveys, Office for National Statistics (OPCS, ONS) (1985–97). *Birth Statistics. England and Wales, 1984–1995.* Series FM1 nos.11–12, 15–24. HMSO, London.

Office of Population Censuses and Surveys, Office for National Statistics (OPCS, ONS) (1990–8). *Mortality Statistics, Childhood, Perinatal and Infant: Social and Biological Factors. Review of the Registrar General on Deaths in England and Wales, 1987–1996.* Series DH3, nos. 21–9. HMSO, London.

Office of Population Censuses and Surveys, Registrar General for Scotland (1974). *Census 1971. Great Britain. Migration Tables. Part I (10% Sample).* HMSO, London.

Office of Population Censuses and Surveys, Registrar General for Scotland (1975). *Census 1971. Great Britain. Economic Activity. Part II (10% Sample).* HMSO, London.

Office of Population Censuses and Surveys, Registrar General for Scotland (1983). *Census 1981. National Migration. Great Britain. Part 1 (100% Tables).* HMSO, London.

Office of Population Censuses and Surveys, Registrar General for Scotland (1984). *Census 1981. Economic Activity. Great Britain.* HMSO, London.

Office of Population Censuses and Surveys, Registrar General for Scotland (1993*a*). *1991 Census. Housing and Availability of Cars. Great Britain.* HMSO, London.

Office of Population Censuses and Surveys, Registrar General for Scotland (1993*b*). *1991 Census. Historical Tables.* HMSO, London.

Office of Population Censuses and Surveys, Registrar General for Scotland (1994*a*). *1991 Census. Economic Activity. Great Britain, Volume 1.* HMSO, London.

Office of Population Censuses and Surveys, Registrar General for Scotland (1994*b*). *1991 Census. Migration. Great Britain. Part 1 (100% Tables).* HMSO, London.

Osmond, C., Gardner, M. J., Acheson, E. D., Adelstein, A. M. (1983). *Trends in Cancer Mortality 1951–1980. Analyses by Period of Birth and Death.* OPCS Series DH1 no. 11. HMSO, London.

Parkin, D. M., Whelan, S. L., Ferlay, J., Raymond, L., Young, J. (eds.) (1997). *Cancer Incidence in Five Continents. Volume VII.* IARC Scientific Publication no. 143. IARC, Lyon.

Peach, C. (1996). *Ethnicity in the 1991 Census. Volume 2. The Ethnic Minority Populations of Great Britain.* HMSO, London.

Pendergrast, W. J., Milmore, B. K., Marcus, S. C. (1961). Thyroid cancer and thyrotoxicosis in the United States: their relation to endemic goiter. *J. Chron. Dis.,* **13,** 22–38.

Percy, A. K., Elveback, L. R., Okazaki, H., Kurland, L. T. (1972). Neoplasms of the central nervous system. Epidemiologic considerations. *Neurology,* **22,** 40–8.

Percy, C. (1987). Comparison of the 8th and 9th revisions of the International Classification of Diseases. In: Muir, C., Waterhouse, J., Mack, T., Powell, J., Whelan, S. (eds.) *Cancer Incidence in Five Continents. Volume V.* IARC Scientific Publication no. 88. IARC, Lyon, 33–41.

Percy, C. L., Horm, J. W., Young, J. L. Jr., Asire, A. J. (1983). Uterine cancers of unspecified origin—a reassessment. *Public Health Rep.,* **98,** 176–80.

Persky, V., Davis, F., Barrett, R., Ruby, E., Sailer, C., Levy, P. (1990). Recent time trends in uterine cancer. *Am. J. Public Health,* **80,** 935–9.

Peto, J., Hodgson, J. T., Matthews, F. E., Jones, J. R. (1995). Continuing increase in mesothelioma mortality in Britain. *Lancet,* **345,** 535–9.

Peto, R., Lopez, A. D., Boreham, J., Thun, M., Heath, C. Jr. (1992). Mortality from tobacco in developed countries: indirect estimation from national vital statistics. *Lancet,* **339,** 1268–78.

Pike, M. C., Chilvers, C. E. D., Bobrow, L. G. (1987). Classification of testicular cancer in incidence and mortality statistics. *Br. J. Cancer,* **56,** 83–5.

Piper, J. M., Tonascia, J., Matanoski, G. M. (1985). Heavy phenacetin use and bladder cancer in women aged 20 to 49 years. *New Engl. J. Med.,* **313,** 292–5.

Potosky, A. L., Kessler, L., Gridley, G., Brown, C. C., Horm, J. W. (1990). Rise in prostatic cancer incidence associated with increased use of transurethral resection. *J. Natl. Cancer Inst.,* **82,** 1624–8.

Pott, P. (1775). *Chirurgical Observations Relative to the Cataract, the Polypus of the Nose, the Cancer of the Scrotum, the Different Kinds of Ruptures and the Mortification of the Toes and Feet.* Hawes, Clarke, & Collins, London.

Pottern, L. M., Stone, B. J., Day, N. E., Pickle, L. W., Fraumeni, J. F. Jr. (1980). Thyroid cancer in Connecticut, 1935–1975: an analysis by cell type. *Am. J. Epidemiol.,* **112,** 764–74.

Powell, J., McConkey, C. C. (1992). The rising trend in oesophageal adenocarcinoma and gastric cardia [sic]. *Eur. J. Cancer Prev.,* **1,** 265–9.

Prior, G., Di Salvo, P. (1997). General health, psychosocial well-being and prescribed medicine. In: Prescott-Clarke P., Primatesta, P. (eds.) *Health Survey for England 1995. Volume I: Findings.* HMSO, London, 221–55.

Registrar General (1890). *Fifty-second Annual Report of the Registrar-General of Births, Deaths and Marriages in England (1889).* HMSO, London.

Registrar General (1892). *Fifty-fourth Annual Report of the Registrar-General of Births, Deaths, and Marriages in England (1891).* HMSO, London.

Registrar General (1899). *Sixtieth Annual Report of the Registrar-General of Births, Deaths, and Marriages in England (1897).* HMSO, London.

Registrar General (1903). *Sixty-fourth Annual Report of the Registrar-General of Births, Deaths, and Marriages in England and Wales (1901).* HMSO, London.

Registrar General (1912). *Seventy-third Annual Report of the Registrar-General of Births, Deaths, and Marriages in England and Wales (1910).* HMSO, London.

Registrar General (1919). *Eightieth Annual Report of the Registrar-General of Births, Deaths, and Marriages in England and Wales (1917).* HMSO, London.

Registrar General (1923). *The Registrar-General's Statistical Review of England and Wales, for the Year 1922. Tables. Part I. Medical.* HMSO, London.

Registrar General (1925). *The Registrar-General's Statistical Review of England and Wales for the Year 1924. Tables. Part I. Medical.* HMSO, London.

Registrar General (1930). *The Registrar General's Statistical Review of England and Wales, for the Year 1928. Text.* HMSO, London.

Registrar General (1932). *The Registrar-General's Statistical Review of England and Wales for the Year 1931. Tables. Part I. Medical.* HMSO, London.

Registrar General (1934). *The Registrar General's Statistical Review of England and Wales for the Year 1933. Tables. Part I. Medical.* HMSO, London.

Registrar General (1944a). *The Registrar-General's Statistical Review of England and Wales for the Year 1939. Tables. Part I. Medical.* HMSO, London.

Registrar General (1944b). *The Registrar General's Statistical Review of England and Wales for the Year 1940. Tables. Part I. Medical.* HMSO, London.

Registrar General (1947). *The Registrar-General's Statistical Review of England and Wales for the Years 1938 and 1939. Text.* HMSO, London.

Registrar General (1951). *Census 1951, England and Wales. Preliminary Tables.* HMSO, London.

Registrar General (1952). *The Registrar-General's Statistical Review of England and Wales for the Year 1950. Tables. Part I. Medical.* HMSO, London.

Registrar General (1953). *The Registrar-General's Statistical Review of England and Wales for the Two Years 1948–1949. Text, Medical.* HMSO, London.

Registrar General (1956). *Census 1951. Classification of Occupations.* HMSO, London.

Registrar General (1957). *The Registrar-General's Statistical Review of England and Wales for the Year 1954. Part III. Commentary.* HMSO, London.

Registrar General (1959). *The Registrar-General's Statistical Review of England and Wales for the Year 1957. Part III. Commentary.* HMSO, London.

Registrar General (1960). *The Registrar's Statistical Review of England and Wales for the Year 1959. Tables. Part III. Commentary.* HMSO, London.

Registrar General (1962). *The Registrar's Statistical Review of England and Wales for the Year 1960. Part I. Tables. Medical.* HMSO, London.

Registrar General (1966a). *Census 1961, England and Wales. Occupation Tables.* HMSO, London.

Registrar General (1966b). *Census 1961, England and Wales. Household Composition. Tables.* HMSO, London.

Registrar General (1968). *The Registrar General's Statistical Review of England and Wales for the Year 1965. Part III. Commentary.* HMSO, London.

Registrar General (1971). *The Registrar General's Statistical Review of England and Wales for the Year 1967. Part III. Commentary.* HMSO, London.

Ries, L. A. G. (1994). Colorectal cancer survival. *J. Natl. Cancer Inst.*, **86**, 415.

Roberts, A. (1982). Cervical cytology in England and Wales, 1965–80. *Health Trends*, **14**, 41–3.

Robertson, H. A., Falconer, I. R. (1959). Accumulation of radioactive iodine in thyroid glands subsequent to nuclear weapon tests and the accident at Windscale. *Nature*, **184**, 1699–702.

Rohr, L. R. (1987). Incidental adenocarcinoma in transurethral resections of the prostate. Partial versus complete microscopic examination. *Am. J. Surg. Pathol.*, **11**, 53–8.

Ron, E. (1996). Thyroid cancer. In: Schottenfeld, D., Fraumeni, J. F. Jr. (eds.) Cancer *Epidemiology and Prevention*. Second edition. Oxford University Press, New York, 1000–21.

Ron, E, Lubin, J. H., Shore, R. E., Mabuchi, K., Modan, B., Pottern, L. M., Schneider, A. B., Tucker, M. A., Boice, J. D. Jr. (1995). Thyroid cancer after exposure to external radia-tion: a pooled analysis of seven studies. *Radiation Res.*, **141**, 259–77.

Ross, R. K., Schottenfeld, D. (1996). Prostate cancer. In: Schottenfeld, D., Fraumeni, J. F. Jr. (eds.) *Cancer Epidemiology and Prevention*. Second edition. Oxford University Press, New York, 1180–206.

Rossing, M. A., Daling, J. R., Weiss, N. S., Moore, D. E., Self, S. G. (1994). Ovarian tumors in a cohort of infertile women. *New Engl. J. Med.*, **331**, 771–6.

Roush, G. C., McKay, L., Holford, T. R. (1992). A reversal in the long-term increase in deaths attributable to malignant melanoma. *Cancer*, **69**, 1714–20.

Royal College of General Practitioners' Manchester Research Unit (1986). New oral contraception study: pilot trial report. *J. R. Coll. Gen. Pract.*, **36**, 545–6.

Saxén, E. A. (1982). Trends: facts or fallacy. In: Magnus, K. (ed.) *Trends in Cancer Incidence: Causes and Practical Implications*. Hemisphere Publishing, Washington, 5–16.

Sayer Bain, G., Bacon, R., Pimlott, J. (1972). The labour force. In: Halsey, A. H. (ed.). *Trends in British Society Since 1900. A Guide to the Changing Social Structure of Britain*. Macmillan St Martin's Press, London, 97–119.

Schiffman, M. H., Brinton, L. A., Devesa, S. S., Fraumeni, J. F. Jr. (1996). Cervical cancer. In: Schottenfeld, D., Fraumeni, J. F. Jr. (eds.) *Cancer Epidemiology and Prevention*. Second edition. Oxford University Press, New York, 1090–116.

Schwartz, S. M., Daling, J. R., Doody, D. R., Wipf, G. C., Carter, J. J., Madeleine, M. M., Mao, E.-J., Fitzgibbons, E. D., Huang, S., Beckmann, A. M., McDougall, J. K., Galloway, D. A. (1998) Oral cancer risk in relation to sexual history and evidence of human papillomavirus infec-tion. *J. Natl. Cancer Inst*, **90**, 1626–36.

Seddon, D. J., Williams, E. M. I. (1997). Data quality in population-based cancer registration: an assessment of the Merseyside and Cheshire Cancer Registry. *Br. J. Cancer*, **76**, 667–74.

Sharpe, R. M., Skakkebaek, N. E. (1993). Are oestrogens involved in falling sperm counts and disorders of the male reproductive tract? *Lancet*, **341**, 1392–5.

Shrimpton, P. C., Wall, B. F. (1995). The increasing import-ance of X-ray computed tomography as a source of medical exposure. *Radiat. Prot. Dosim.*, **57**, 413–15.

Simmonds, J. R., Robinson, C. A., Phipps, A. W., Muirhead, C. R., Fry, F. A. (1995). *Risks of Leukaemia and Other Cancers in Seascale from all Sources of Ionising Radiation Exposure*. (NRPB-R276). National Radiological Protection Board, Chilton.

Simms, I., Hughes, G., Swan, A. V., Rogers, P. A., Catchpole, M. (1998). New cases seen at genitourinary medicine clinics: England 1996. *Communicable Disease Report*, Vol. 8, Suppl. 1. Communicable Disease Surveillance Centre, London.

Smans, M., Muir, C. S., Boyle, P. (eds.) (1992). *Atlas of Cancer Mortality in the European Economic Community*. IARC Scientific Publication No. 107. IARC, Lyon.

Smith, P. G., Kinlen, L. J., White, G. C., Adelstein, A. M., Fox, A. J. (1980). Mortality of wives of men dying with cancer of the penis. *Br. J. Cancer*, **41**, 422–8.

Southam, A. H., Wilson, S. R. (1922). Cancer of the scrotum: the etiology, clinical features, and treatment of the disease. *Br. Med. J.*, ii, 971–3.

Southgate, D. A. T., Bingham, S., Robertson, J. (1978). Dietary fibre in the British diet. *Nature*, **274**, 51–2.

Spring, J. A., Buss, D. H. (1977). Three centuries of alcohol in the British diet. *Nature*, **270**, 567–72.

Stalsberg, H. (1973). Lymphoreticular tumors in Norway and in other European countries. *J. Natl. Cancer Inst.*, **50**, 1685–702.

Stephen, A. M., Sieber, G. M. (1994). Trends in individual fat consumption in the United Kingdom 1900–1985. *Br. J. Nutr.*, **71**, 775–88.

Stevens, W., Thomas, D. C., Lyon, J. L., Till, J. E., Kerber, R. A., Simon, S. L., Lloyd, R. D., Elghany, N. A., Preston-Martin, S. (1990). Leukemia in Utah and radioactive fallout from the Nevada test site. *J. Am. Med. Assoc.*, **264**, 585–91.

Stewart, A., Kneale, G. W. (1969). Role of local infections in the recognition of haemopoietic neoplasms. *Nature*, **223**, 741–2.

Stiller, C. A. (1994). Population based survival rates for childhood cancer in Britain, 1980–91. *Br. Med. J.*, **309**, 1612–16.

Stiller, C. A., Bunch, K. J. (1990). Trends in survival for childhood cancer in Britain diagnosed 1971–85. *Br. J. Cancer*, **62**, 806–15.

Stiller, C. A., Draper, G. J., Vincent, T. J., O'Connor, C. M. (1991). Incidence rates nationally and in administratively defined areas. In: Draper, G. (ed.) *The Geographical Epidemiology of Childhood Leukaemia and Non-Hodgkin Lymphomas in Great Britain, 1966–83*. SMPS no. 53. HMSO, London, 25–35.

Stiller, C. A., Allen, M., Bayne, A., Brownbill, P., Draper, G., Eatock, E., Loach, M., Vincent, T. (1998). United Kingdom. National Registry of Childhood Tumours, England and Wales, 1981–1990. In: Parkin, D. M., Kramárová, E., Draper, G. J., Masuyer, E., Michaelis, J., Neglia, J., Qureshi, S., Stiller, C. A. (eds.) *International Incidence of Childhood Cancer*. Vol. II. IARC Scientific Publication no. 144. IARC, Lyon, 365–7.

Stocks, P. (1936). Distribution in England and Wales of cancer of various organs. In: *13th Annual Report of the British Empire Cancer Campaign*. British Empire Cancer Campaign, London, 240–74.

Stocks, P. (1939). Distribution in England and Wales of cancer of various organs. In: *16th Annual Report of the British Empire Cancer Campaign*. British Empire Cancer Campaign, London, 308–43.

Stocks, P. (1950). *Cancer Registration in England and Wales. An Enquiry into Treatment and its Results*. SMPS, No. 3. HMSO, London.

Stocks, P. (1953a). Studies of cancer death rates at different ages in England and Wales in 1921 to 1950: uterus, breast and lung. *Br. J. Cancer*, **7**, 283–302.

Stocks, P. (1953b). A study of the age curve for cancer of the stomach in connection with a theory of the cancer producing mechanism. *Br. J. Cancer*, **7**, 407–17.

Stocks, P. (1970). Breast cancer anomalies. *Br. J. Cancer*, **24**, 633–43.

Straus, S. E., Fleisher, G. R. (1990). Infectious mononucleosis epidemiology and pathogenesis. In: Scholssberg, D. (ed.) *Infectious Mononucleosis*. Second Edition. Springer, New York, 8–28.

Swanson, J. (1996). Long-term variations in the exposure of the population of England and Wales to power-frequency magnetic fields. *J. Radiol. Prot.*, **16**, 287–301.

Swerdlow, A. J. (1986). Cancer registration in England and Wales: some aspects relevant to interpretation of the data. *J. Royal. Stat. Soc. A.*, **149**, 146–60.

Swerdlow, A. J. (1987). 150 years of Registrar Generals' medical statistics. *Pop. Trends*, **48**, 20–6.

Swerdlow, A. J. (1989). Interpretation of England and Wales cancer mortality data: the effect of enquiries to certifiers for further information. *Br. J. Cancer*, **59**, 787–91.

Swerdlow, A. J. (1990). Effectiveness of primary prevention of occupational exposures on cancer risk. In: Hakama, M., Beral, V., Cullen, J. W., Parkin, D. M. (eds.) *Evaluating Effectiveness of Primary Prevention of Cancer*. IARC Scientific Publication no. 103. IARC, Lyon, 23–56.

Swerdlow, A. J., dos Santos Silva, I. (1991). Geographic distribution of lung and stomach cancers in England and Wales over 50 years: changing and unchanging patterns. *Br. J. Cancer*, **63**, 773–81.

Swerdlow, A., dos Santos Silva, I. (1993). *Atlas of Cancer Incidence in England and Wales 1968–85*. Oxford University Press, Oxford.

Swerdlow, A. J., Douglas, A. J., Vaughan Hudson, G., Vaughan Hudson, B. (1993). Completeness of cancer registration in England and Wales: an assessment based on 2,145 patients with Hodgkin's disease independently registered by the British National Lymphoma Investigation. *Br. J. Cancer*, **67**, 326–9.

Swerdlow, A. J., Marmot, M. G., Grulich, A. E., Head, J. (1995). Cancer mortality in Indian and British ethnic immigrants from the Indian subcontinent to England and Wales. *Br. J. Cancer*, **72**, 1312–19.

Swerdlow, A. J., dos Santos Silva, I., Reid, A., Qiao, Z. Brewster, D. H., Arrundale, J. (1998). Trends in cancer incidence and mortality in Scotland: description and possible explanations. *Br. J. Cancer*, **77** (Suppl. 3), 1–54.

Tanner J. M. (1981). Menarcheal age. *Science*, **214**, 604.

Tanner, J. M. (1989). *Foetus into Man. Physical Growth from Conception to Maturity*. Second edition. Castlemead Publications, Ware, England.

Tarone, R. E., Chu, K. C., Brawley, O. W. (2000). Implications of stage-specific survival rates in assessing recent declines in prostate cancer mortality rates. Epidemiology, 11, 167–70.

Thomas, D. B., Jimenez, L. M., McTiernan, A., Rosenblatt, K., Stalsberg, H., Stemhagen, A., Thompson, W. D., Curnen, M. G. M., Satariano, W., Austin, D. F., Greenberg, R. S., Key, C., Kolonel, L. N., West, D. W. (1992). Breast cancer in men: risk factors with hormonal implications. *Am. J. Epidemiol.*, **135**, 734–48.

Thörn, M., Sparén, P., Bergström, R., Adami, H.-O. (1992). Trends in mortality rates from malignant melanoma in Sweden 1953–1987 and forecasts up to 2007. *Br. J. Cancer*, **66**, 563–7.

Thorogood, M., Vessey, M. P. (1990). Trends in use of oral contraceptives in Britain. *Br. J. Fam. Planning*, **16**, 41–53.

Toms, J. R., Draper, G. J., Stiller, C. A., Adelstein, A. M., Donnan, S. P. B., Fox, A. J., Macdonald Davies, I. M., White, G. C. (1981). *Cancer Statistics. Incidence, Survival and Mortality in England and Wales*. SMPS no. 43. HMSO, London.

Tretli, S., Gaard, M. (1996). Lifestyle changes during adolescence and risk of breast cancer: an ecologic study of the effect of World War II in Norway. *Cancer Causes Control*, 7, 507–12.

Trichopoulos, D. (1990). Hypothesis: does breast cancer originate *in utero*? *Lancet*, 335, 939–40.

Tucker, M. A., D'Angio, G. J., Boice, J. D. Jr., Strong, L. C., Li, F. P., Stovall, M., Stone, B. J., Green, D. M., Lombardi, F., Newton, W., Hoover, R. N., Fraumeni, J. F. Jr. for the Late Effects Study Group (1987). Bone sarcomas linked to radiotherapy and chemotherapy in children. *New Engl. J. Med.*, 317, 588–93.

Tucker, M. A., Morris Jones, P. H., Boice, J. D. Jr., Robison, L. L., Stone, B. J., Stovall, M., Jenkin, R. D. T., Lubin, J. H., Baum, E. S., Siegel, S. E., Meadows, A. T., Hoover, R. N., Fraumeni, J. F. Jr. for the Late Effects Study Group (1991). Therapeutic radiation at a young age is linked to secondary thyroid cancer. *Cancer Res.*, 51, 2885–8.

Turesson, I., Zettervall, O., Cuzick, J., Waldenstrom, J. G., Velez, R. (1984). Comparison of trends in the incidence of multiple myeloma in Malmö, Sweden, and other countries, 1950–1979. *New Engl. J. Med.*, 310, 421–4.

Tuyns, A. J., Audigier, J. C. (1976). Double wave cohort increase for oesophageal and laryngeal cancer in France in relation to reduced alcohol consumption during the Second World War. *Digestion*, 14, 197–208.

UK Childhood Cancer Study Investigators (1999). Exposure to power-frequency magnetic fields and the risk of childhood cancer. *Lancet*, 354, 1925–31.

UK Testicular Cancer Study Group (1994). Aetiology of testicular cancer: association with congenital abnormalities, age at puberty, infertility, and exercise. *Br. Med. J.*, 308, 1393–9.

UK Trial of Early Detection of Breast Cancer Group (1988). First results on mortality reduction in the UK Trial of Early Detection of Breast Cancer. *Lancet*, 2, 411–16.

UNSCEAR (1977). *Sources and Effects of Ionising Radiation. United Nations Scientific Committee on the Effects of Atomic Radiation. 1977 Report to the General Assembly.* United Nations, New York.

Ursin, G., Bernstein, L., Pike, M. C. (1994). Breast cancer. In: Doll, R., Fraumeni, J. F. Jr., Muir, C. S. (eds.). *Trends in Cancer Incidence and Mortality. Cancer Surveys.* Vols. 19/20. Cold Spring Harbor Laboratory Press, New York, 241–64.

van der Esch, E. P., Muir, C. S., Nectoux, J., Macfarlane, G., Maisonneuve, P., Bharucha, H., Briggs, J., Cooke, R. A., Dempster, A. G., Essex, W. B., Hofer, P. A., Hood, A. F., Ironside, P., Larsen, T. E., Little, J. H., Philips, R., Pfau, R. S., Prade, M., Pozharisski, K. M., Rilke, F., Schafler, K. (1991). Temporal change in diagnostic criteria as a cause of the increase of malignant melanoma over time is unlikely. *Int. J. Cancer*, 47, 483–90.

Velez, R., Beral, V., Cuzick, J. (1982). Increasing trends of multiple myeloma mortality in England and Wales, 1950–79: are the changes real? *J. Natl. Cancer Inst.*, 69, 387–92.

Villard-Mackintosh, L., Coleman, M. P., Vessey, M. P. (1988). The completeness of cancer registration in England: an assessment from the Oxford-FPA contraceptive study. *Br. J. Cancer*, 58, 507–11.

Vineis, P., Simonato, L. (1986). Estimates of the proportion of bladder cancers attributable to occupation. *Scand. J. Work Environ. Health*, 12, 55–60.

Wald, N., Nicolaides-Bouman, A. (1991). *UK Smoking Statistics*, Second Edition. Oxford University Press, Oxford.

Wald, N., Kiryluk, S., Darby, S., Doll, R., Pike, M., Peto, R. (1988). *UK Smoking Statistics*. Oxford University Press, Oxford.

Waldron, H. A., Waterhouse, J. A. H., Tessema, N. (1984). Scrotal cancer in the West Midlands 1936–76. *Br. J. Indust. Med.*, 41, 437–44.

Walker, A. M., Jick, H. (1980). Declining rates of endometrial cancer. *Obstet. Gynecol.*, 56, 733–6.

Walker, A. H., Ross, R. K., Haile, R. W. C., Henderson, B. E. (1988). Hormonal factors and risk of ovarian germ cell cancer in young women. *Br. J. Cancer*, 57, 418–22.

Wall, B. F., Hillier, M. C., Kendall, G. M. (1986). *An Update on the Frequency of Medical and Dental X-ray Examinations in Great Britain—1983.* (NRPB-R201). National Radiological Protection Board, Chilton.

Walt, R., Katschinski, B., Logan, R., Ashley, J., Langman, M. (1986). Rising frequency of ulcer perforation in elderly people in the United Kingdom. *Lancet*, 1, 489–92.

Waterhouse, J., Muir, C., Correa, P., Powell, J. (eds.) (1976). *Cancer Incidence in Five Continents. Volume III.* IARC Scientific Publication no. 15. IARC, Lyon.

Welsh Cervical Screening Office (1994–99). *Cervical Screening Programme, Wales: 1992/93–1997/98.* Welsh Cervical Screening Office, Wales.

Wenlock, R. W., Buss, D. H., Moxon, R. E., Bunton, N. G. (1982). Trace nutrients 4. Iodine in British food. *Br. J. Nutr.*, 47, 381–90.

West, R. R. (1976). Accuracy of cancer registration. *Br. J. Prev. Soc. Med.*, 30, 187–92.

Westergaard, T., Melbye, M., Pedersen, J. B., Frisch, M., Olsen, J. H., Anderson, P. K. (1997). Birth order, sibship size and risk of Hodgkin's disease in children and young adults: a population-based study of 31 million person-years. *Int. J. Cancer*, 72, 977–81.

White, A., Nicolaas, G., Foster, K., Browne, F., Carey, S. (1993). *The Health Survey for England 1991.* HMSO, London.

Whitehead, R. Paul, A. (1987). Changes in infant feeding during the last century. In: MRC Environmental Epidemiology Unit (eds.) *Infant Nutrition and Cardiovascular Disease.* Scientific Report no. 8. Proceedings of a Meeting held on 29th October 1986 at the MRC Environmental Epidemiology Unit (Southampton, England). Southampton General Hospital, Southampton.

Whittemore, A. S., Harris, R., Intyre, J., and the Collaborative Ovarian Cancer Group. (1992). Characteristics relating to ovarian cancer risk: collaborative analysis of 12 US case-control studies. IV. The pathogenesis of epithelial ovarian cancer. *Am. J. Epidemiol.*, 136, 1212–20.

Wigle, D. T. (1977). Breast cancer and fertility trends in Canada. *Am. J. Epidemiol.*, 105, 428–38.

Wigle, D. T. (1978). Malignant melanoma of the skin and sunspot activity. *Lancet*, 2, 38.

Wilson, G. B. (1940). *Alcohol and the Nation. A Contribution to the Study of the Liquor Problem in the United Kingdom from 1800 to 1935.* Nicholson and Watson, London.

Wiseman, R. A. (1984). Absence of correlation between oral contraceptive usage and cardiovascular mortality. *Int. J. Fertil.*, **29**, 198–208.

World Health Organization (WHO) (1978). *Manual of the International Statistical Classification of Diseases, Injuries, and Causes of Death*. Ninth revision. WHO, Geneva.

Wrixon, A. D., Green, B. M. R., Lomas, P. R., Miles, J. C. H., Cliff, K. D., Francis, E. A., Driscoll, C. M. H., James, A. C., O'Riordan, M. C. (1988). *Natural Radiation Exposure in UK Dwellings*. (NRPB-R190). National Radiological Protection Board, Chilton.

Wynder, E. L. (1952). Some practical aspects of cancer prevention (concluded). *New Engl. J. Med.*, **246**, 573–82.

Wynder, E. L., Graham, E. A. (1950). Tobacco smoking as a possible etiologic factor in bronchiogenic carcinoma: a study of six hundred and eighty-four proved cases. *J. Am. Med. Assoc.*, **143**, 329–36.

Wynder, E. L., Fujita, Y., Harris, R. E., Hirayama, T., Hiyama, T. (1991). Comparative epidemiology of cancer between the United States and Japan. A second look. *Cancer*, **67**, 746–63.

Zahm, S. H., Tucker, M. A., Fraumeni, J. F. Jr. (1996). Soft tissue sarcomas. In: Schottenfeld, D., Fraumeni, J. F. Jr (eds.) *Cancer Epidemiology and Prevention*. Second edition. Oxford University Press, New York, 984–99.

Index

Page numbers in italic, e.g. *52*, signify references to figures. Page numbers in bold, e.g. **58**, denote references to tables.